NUTRITIONAL MANAGEMENT
The Johns Hopkins Handbook

MACKENZIE WALSER, M.D.

Physician, Johns Hopkins Hospital;
Professor of Pharmacology and Experimental Therapeutics;
Professor of Medicine,
The Johns Hopkins University School of Medicine, Baltimore

ANTHONY L. IMBEMBO, M.D.

Vice-Chairman and Professor of Surgery,
Case Western Reserve University School of Medicine, Cleveland;
Director, Department of Surgery,
Cleveland Metropolitan General Hospital, Cleveland

SIMEON MARGOLIS, M.D., Ph.D.

Physician, Johns Hopkins Hospital;
Professor of Medicine; Professor of Physiological Chemistry,
The Johns Hopkins University School of Medicine, Baltimore

GLORIA A. ELFERT, M.S., R.D.

Associate Director, Department of Nutrition,
The Johns Hopkins Hospital, Baltimore

1984
W. B. SAUNDERS COMPANY

Philadelphia, London, Toronto, Mexico City, Rio de Janeiro, Sydney, Tokyo

W. B. Saunders Company: West Washington Square
Philadelphia, PA 19105

1 St. Anne's Road
Eastbourne, East Sussex BN21, 3UN, England

1 Goldthorne Avenue
Toronto, Ontario M8Z 5T9, Canada

Apartado 26370 - Cedro 512
Mexico 4, D.F., Mexico

Rua Coronel Cabrita, 8
Sao Cristovao Caixa Postal 21176
Rio de Janeiro, Brazil

9 Waltham Street
Artarmon, N.S.W. 2064, Australia

Ichibancho, Central Bldg., 22-1 Ichibancho
Chiyoda-Ku, Tokyo 102, Japan

Library of Congress Cataloging in Publication Data
Main entry under title:

Nutritional management.

1. Diet therapy. I. Walser, Mackenzie. [DNLM:
1. Nutrition. 2. Diet therapy. WB 400 N9754]
RM 216.N863   1984   615.8'54   84-1221
ISBN 0-7216-1319-5

Last digit is the print number: 9 8 7 6 5 4 3 2 1

CONTRIBUTORS

ARNOLD E. ANDERSEN, M.D.

Assistant Professor of Psychiatry and Behavioral Sciences, Johns Hopkins School of Medicine; Physician and Director, Eating and Weight Disorders Clinic, Johns Hopkins Hospital.

Weight-Gaining Diets

ERNEST BARBOSA, M.D.

Chief Resident, Pediatric Neurology, Johns Hopkins Hospital.

Ketogenic Diets for Treatment of Childhood Epilepsy

MARK L. BATSHAW, M.D.

Associate Professor of Pediatrics, Johns Hopkins University School of Medicine; Developmental Pediatrician, John F. Kennedy Institute.

Congenital Hyperammonemia and Related Disorders

THEODORE M. BAYLESS, M.D.

Professor of Medicine, Johns Hopkins University School of Medicine; Physician, Department of Medicine, Johns Hopkins Hospital.

Fat-Restricted Diets in the Management of Gastrointestinal Disorders; Lactose Intolerance, Gluten Sensitivity, Gastrointestinal Reflux, Partial Obstruction, Peptic Ulcer Disease

BARBARA JEAN CAVAGNARO-WONG, R.D.

Formerly, Pediatric Nutritionist, Department of Nutrition, Johns Hopkins Hospital.

Phenylketonuria, Galactosemia, Maple Syrup Urine Disease, Homocystinuria from Cystathionine-β-Synthase Deficiency, Type I Glycogen Storage Disease

ELIZABETH C. CHANDLER, R.D.

Formerly Research Dietitian, Johns Hopkins Hospital.

Nutritional Aspects of Renal Failure; Phosphorus

GLORIA ELFERT, M.S., R.D.

Associate Director, Department of Nutrition, Johns Hopkins Hospital.

Normal Nutrition; Vegetarian Diets; Kosher Dietary Laws; Modifications in Consistency (Transitional Diets); Fat-Restricted Diets in the Management of Gastrointestinal Disorders; Dietary Modification of Plasma Lipid and Lipoprotein Levels; Sodium Restriction; Ketogenic Diets for Treatment of Childhood Epilepsy

JOHN M. FREEMAN, M.D.

Professor of Pediatrics and Neurology, Johns Hopkins University School of Medicine; Director, Birth Defects Treatment Center and Epilepsy Center, Johns Hopkins Hospital.

Ketogenic Diets for Treatment of Childhood Epilepsy

ANTHONY L. IMBEMBO, M.D.

Professor of Surgery and Vice-Chairman, Department of Surgery, Case Western Reserve University School of Medicine; Director, Department of Surgery, Cleveland Metropolitan General Hospital; Formerly Associate Professor of Surgery and Director, Department of Surgery, Johns Hopkins University School of Medicine; Physician, Johns Hopkins Hospital.

Nutritional Assessment; Modifications in Consistency (Transitional Diets); Enteral Alimentation; Parenteral Nutrition

MILLICENT T. KELLY, R.D.

Assistant Director, Department of Nutrition, Johns Hopkins Hospital.

Diabetes Mellitus

WILLIAM C. MACLEAN, JR., M.D., C.M.

Medical Director, Pediatric Nutrition, Ross Laboratories; Associate Clinical Professor of Pediatrics, Ohio State University College of Medicine; Staff Physician, Columbus Children's Hospital; Formerly Associate Professor of Pediatrics, Johns Hopkins University School of Medicine; Physician, Johns Hopkins Hospital.

Normal Pediatric Nutrition

SIMEON MARGOLIS, M.D., Ph.D.

Professor of Medicine and Physiological Chemistry, Johns Hopkins University School of Medicine; Physician, Johns Hopkins Hospital.

Food Allergies; Weight-Gaining Diets; Dietary Management of Obesity; Diabetes Mellitus; Symptomatic Postprandial Hypoglycemia; Dietary Modification of Plasma Lipid and Lipoprotein Levels; Modified Fiber Diets

SYLVIA V. McADOO, M.S., R.D.

Assistant Director, Department of Nutrition, Johns Hopkins Hospital.

Normal Pediatric Nutrition; Diet for Cystic Fibrosis

ALBERT I. MENDELOFF, M.D., M.P.H.

Professor of Medicine, Johns Hopkins University School of Medicine.

Modified Fiber Diets

FRANCIS D. MILLIGAN, M.D.

Associate Professor of Medicine, Johns Hopkins University School of Medicine; Physician, Johns Hopkins Hospital.

Dumping Syndrome

HELEN D. MULLAN, R.D.

Assistant Director, Department of Nutrition, Johns Hopkins Hospital.

Weight-Gaining Diets; Dietary Management of Obesity; Nutritional Aspects of Renal Failure; Partial Obstruction, Peptic Ulcer Disease

DAVID M. PAIGE, M.D., M.P.H.

Professor of Maternal and Child Health, Johns Hopkins University School of Hygiene and Public Health; Professor of Pediatrics, Johns Hopkins School of Medicine; Physician, Johns Hopkins Hospital.

Nutrition During Pregnancy and Lactation

BERYL J. ROSENSTEIN, M.D.

Associate Professor of Pediatrics, Johns Hopkins University School of Medicine; Physician and Director, Cystic Fibrosis Center, Johns Hopkins Hospital.

Diet for Cystic Fibrosis

K. M. MOHAMED SHAKIR, M.D., F.A.C.P, F.R.C.P., F.A.C.N.

Assistant Professor, Department of Medicine, USUHS; Staff Physician, Naval Hospital, Bethesda, Maryland; Formerly Instructor in Medicine, Johns Hopkins University School of Medicine.

Diabetes Mellitus

SYLVIA A. SMITH, M.S., R.D.

Pediatric Nutritionist, Department of Nutrition, Johns Hopkins Hospital.

Congenital Hyperammonemia and Related Disorders

DAVID L. VALLE, M.D.

Associate Professor of Pediatrics and Medicine, Johns Hopkins University School of Medicine, Physician, Johns Hopkins Hospital.

Dietary Management of Inborn Errors of Metabolism: Introduction, Phenylketonuria, Galactosemia, Maple Syrup Urine Disease, Homocystinuria from Cystathionine-β-Synthase Deficiency, Type I Glycogen Storage Disease

JEAN CLARK WAGNER, R.D.

Clinical Dietitian, Department of Nutrition, Johns Hopkins Hospital.

Lactose Intolerance, Gluten Sensitivity

JUDITH Z. WALKER, M.P.H., R.D.

Assistant Director, Department of Nutrition, Johns Hopkins Hospital.

Enteral Alimentation; Nutritional Aspects of Renal Failure

MACKENZIE WALSER, M.D.

Professor of Medicine and Pharmacology and Experimental Therapeutics, Johns Hopkins University School of Medicine; Physician, Johns Hopkins Hospital.

Normal Nutrition; Nutritional Assessment; Nutritional Aspects of Renal Failure; Protein Modifications in Other Disorders; Sodium Restriction, Potassium, Calcium, Phosphorus, Iron; Congenital Hyperammonemia and Related Disorders; Alcohol

LORA BROWN WILDER, M.S., R.D.

Clinical Nutritionist, Department of Nutrition, Johns Hopkins Hospital.

Modified Fiber Diets

PREFACE

Books on nutrition range from applied manuals—
which are primarily lists of diets with only brief references
to their usage or rationale—to multivolume discussions of
nutritional facts and principles, with little or no mention of
diets. Our aim was to produce a book that combined specific diet instructions with a description of major dietary
principles, the goals and rationale for each form of dietary
therapy, and criteria for patient selection.

The editors include two internists, a surgeon and a
chief of hospital nutrition. All chapter authors are (or
were) members of the faculty of the Johns Hopkins School
of Medicine or School of Hygiene and Public Health or
staff nutritionists from the Johns Hopkins Hospital. Thus
the book is very much a Johns Hopkins product. Nevertheless, points of view championed at other institutions have
been included. The editors are optimistic that the book will
be useful both in the United States and abroad to those
trained in or preparing for careers in medicine and nursing
as well as in nutrition. Although a basic knowledge of
medicine and medical terminology is assumed in the text,
many of the sections will be of interest also to the well-
read layman.

Most of the chapters concern specific disorders, such
as renal disease, and include recommendations for dietary
management. Each of these chapters is written by one or
more physicians and a dietitian. However, several sections
also address aspects of nutrition that do not involve specific diets; these include normal nutrition in adults, children,
pregnancy, and lactation; vegetarian and kosher diets and
food allergies; nutritional assessment; iron; and alcohol.

Our philosophy regarding the normal diet is similar to
that expressed in the following quotation from the preface

of the classic treatise Food, Nutrition and Health, by E. V. McCollum and J. E. Becker, from this institution (Lord Baltimore Press, 1947):

Unfortunately, the exaggerated claims of advertisers of ordinary food products and the faddists and graceless exploiters of nostrums, those seeking to exploit the common nutrients as medicines, and other self-appointed advisers on subjects relating to health, present to the public so much misinformation that a great deal of confusion exists about what is fact and what is fiction in matters relating to nutrition.

Likewise, in discussing nutritional therapy, we, like McCollum and Becker,

. . . have also attempted to point out some of the common fallacies about diets which have done and are still doing much harm to credulous and uninformed people.

We hope that the book will provide a useful summary of the current practice of nutrition, from the point of view of both medical science and practical dietetics. The union of these two disciplines into one integrated whole is perhaps the most unique aspect of this book and has been a highly educational experience for the editors.

This book was approved for use as the diet manual of Johns Hopkins Hospital by its Nutrition Advisory Committee on 22 September 1983.

We wish to thank all the contributors. We also acknowledge our gratitude to Tessie Ferkany, Rae Kopher, Joy Liken, Jean Stallings, and Milly Zublick for secretarial and bibliographic assistance.

THE EDITORS

Baltimore, Maryland
April 1984

CONTENTS

1
NORMAL NUTRITION

Normal Nutrition

Mackenzie Walser, M.D., and
Gloria Elfert, M.S., R.D.

INTRODUCTION

The role of nutrition in achieving optimal growth and development of children, in maintenance of optimal health in adults, and in prevention of disease has received increasing attention in recent years. Rigorous scientific study has now been applied to many aspects of these issues, which were formerly dealt with only in speculative terms, often with a commercial bias. However, major uncertainties still remain, and even those groups that have attempted to define goals for entire populations have been unable to reach a consensus on many major issues. Undocumented notions concerning the beneficial or harmful effects of one food or another are widespread. Such an atmosphere has fostered an enormous growth of the health food industry partly because of false or exaggerated claims for various products; most are harmless (and wasteful) but some are clearly detrimental to health.

NUTRITIONAL DEFICIENCIES

In healthy individuals, faulty nutrition may occur for several reasons. By far the most prevalent cause on a worldwide basis, and becoming more common even in the United States, is inadequate energy (caloric) intake or hunger. This is an enormous socioeconomic problem beyond the scope of this chapter.

Next in frequency are specific nutritional deficiencies occurring in diets adequate in energy intake. Some of these will be discussed in this chapter. In the United States, such deficiencies are far less common than might be assumed, judging from the plethora of books, newspaper columns, and advertisements that maintain that these deficiencies are of epidemic proportions.

1

Recommended Dietary Allowances

The nutritional needs of normal individuals are usually defined in terms of the Recommended Dietary Allowances, or RDAs. RDAs should not be confused with requirements; they are usually based on the upper limit of the requirement range of normal persons, to which is added a "safety factor" that permits sufficient increase of the nutrient in the body to delay the onset of a deficiency state should intake become inadequate. For example, the RDA of ascorbic acid, 60 mg per day, is far above the normal requirement of 5 to 10 mg per day. Diets providing at least two-thirds of RDAs are usually nutritionally adequate.

The RDAs set by the Food and Nutrition Board of the National Academy of Sciences are given in the Appendix. They include recommendations for the intake of energy, protein, and vitamins; the macroelements calcium, phosphorus, and magnesium; and certain microelements (iodine, iron, and zinc). In addition, "safe and adequate" ranges are given for the intake of the macroelements sodium, potassium, and chloride and for some microelements that are clearly essential in the human body (copper, manganese, molybdenum, selenium, and chromium). Other microelements that are probably essential—based on studies in animals—include tin, vanadium, silicon, nickel, and arsenic.

Macronutrients

Of the major nutrients (carbohydrate, fat, and protein), only protein is likely to be ingested in inadequate amounts by persons whose overall energy intake is adequate. By far the most common cause of protein deficiency (other than economic) is vegetarianism (see Vegetarian Diets).

The adult recommended dietary allowance (RDA) of protein of 0.8 g per kg per day is probably unnecessarily high, since a large segment of the world's population ingests significantly less than this amount and experiences no manifestations of protein deficiency except slower growth rates. On the other hand, if protein intake exceeds 5 g per kg per day or approximates half of the energy intake, symptoms (including nausea, headache, and lethargy) of "meat intoxication" may appear, probably signifying hyperammonemia.

The intake of fat is necessary only to meet the requirement for essential fats (linoleic, linolenic, and arachidonic acids). As little as 5 g per day of a fat with a relatively high proportion of unsaturated fats, such as corn oil, will meet these requirements.

Carbohydrate is not an essential requirement in the diet. However, even if a carbohydrate-free diet could be devised, using common foods, it would necessarily be high in protein or fat or both. Long-term high-fat diets can lead to premature coronary artery disease, and diets high in protein can result in the "meat intoxication" mentioned earlier. Diets in which carbohydrate is severely restricted may be vitamin-deficient.

It seems that widely varying proportions of these nutrients can be ingested without obvious ill effect. However, debate continues over whether high-protein or high-fat diets promote atherosclerosis and as to whether high-carbohydrate diets increase the probability of developing diabetes. (The latter view, in particular, has little to substantiate it; genetic factors or viral infection or both are considered to be the most likely causes of diabetes. There is little evidence that a high carbohydrate intake, in the absence of these other factors or obesity, causes diabetes.)

There is evidence that the incidence of certain types of cancer may correlate with dietary practices. For example, there is a relationship between fat intake and cancer of the colon, breast, and prostate. Ingestion of salt-cured, salt-pickled, and smoked foods is associated with increased incidence of cancer of the stomach and esophagus. It has not yet been confirmed whether reducing the intake of such foods will reduce the incidence of these forms of cancer.

The nutritional effects of alcohol are considered in Chapter 14.

Microelements

Two microelements deserve special comment: fluoride and iodide. Fluoride is present in all foods and water supplies, but the naturally occurring amounts are often too low to achieve the protection against tooth decay that this element affords. This effect is of particular importance in children, but fluoride may also reduce the incidence of other dental disorders in adults. Fluoridation of water supplies (to the extent of 1 mg per liter) is now widely practiced and is safe and effective. Persons consuming nonfluoridated water should receive supplemental fluoride in the RDA-specified amounts (see Appendix). Excess fluoride causes mottling of the teeth.

Iodine requirements (see Appendix) are generally met by the iodization of table salt, a process that furnishes 16 mcg iodine per gram of salt ingested. Individuals consuming uniodized salt (unless they live in coastal regions where iodine is more prevalent) could in theory become iodine-deficient. However, this appears to be quite rare in the United States.

The Importance of a Balanced Diet

When offered a "cafeteria-style" selection of foods, normal infants (as well as normal animals) will generally choose proportions of carbohydrate, fat, and protein close to the average normal United States proportions—about 40 per cent, 40 per cent, and 20 per cent, respectively, of the total energy intake. Thus, extreme deviations from these proportions usually represent idiosyncrasies or fads, rather than true dietary preferences.

It is, however, necessary to select from a variety of food groups in order to ensure adequate intake of all required nutrients. The major food groups and the daily servings from each group necessary to achieve adequate nutrition—both for persons who consume foods from all groups and for those with special dietary preferences—are shown in Table 1–1. These combinations of foods provide the RDAs for all nutrients except iron. The recommendations provide only 90 per cent of the RDA of iron for women, while providing 160 per cent of the RDA of iron for men. "Junk foods" and "fast foods" are compatible with adequate nutrition, as long as the requirements set forth in Table 1–1 are met.

TABLE 1–1.   FOOD GROUP COMBINATIONS THAT SATISFY RECOMMENDED DIETARY ALLOWANCES

Food Group	Type of Diet				
	All Foods	No Meat	No Milk	No Legumes	Low-Cost
	Servings per day*				
PROTEIN FOODS					
Animal	2	0	4	4	1
Legumes (peas, beans, nuts, and so on)	2	3	2	0	2
MILK AND/OR MILK PRODUCTS	2	4	0	1½	1½
FRUITS AND VEGETABLES					
Dark-green vegetables	1	1½	3	2	1½
Fruits/vegetables high in vitamin C	1	3	3	2½	0
Other fruits and vegetables	2	0	0	0	0
WHOLE-GRAIN CEREALS/CEREAL PRODUCTS	4	6	3	4	9
OILS AND FATS	1	0	0	0	1

*A serving equals 3 oz meat, poultry, or fish; 2 eggs; ¾ cup cooked legumes; 1 oz nuts; ¾ cup cooked or 1 cup raw leafy greens; 1 cup milk; 1 tbsp wheat germ; 1 oz dry cereal; ¼ cup cooked cereal or pasta; 1 slice bread; 1 tbsp vegetable oil.
Adapted from King, J.C., et al.: Evaluation and modification of the basic four food guide. J Nutr Educ 10:27–29, 1978.

Examination of this table shows that only the cereal food group, which includes breads, rice, pastas, and so forth, and the dark green vegetable group are indispensable. It should also be noted that consuming less than these recommended amounts will not necessarily result in nutritional deficiency, but it is clear that ingesting these amounts will prevent such a deficiency.

Vitamin Requirements

Among the specific nutritional deficiencies that may occur in normal persons who ingest adequate calories, vitamin deficiencies are alleged to be the most prevalent.

Vitamin supplements are ingested by a substantial fraction (about one-third) of the United States population hoping to improve health, vigor, or resistance to disease. Whenever this question has been scientifically examined, the same conclusion has been reached: vitamin supplements are of no value to healthy, nonpregnant adults ingesting adequate calories, unless they go out of their way to avoid whole groups of foods, such as fresh fruits and vegetables or milk and milk products. Persons who ingest a large portion of their calories in the form of alcohol develop characteristic vitamin deficiencies (see Chapter 14). The vitamin requirements of children and of women during pregnancy are discussed in succeeding sections on pediatric nutrition and nutrition during pregnancy and lactation. These groups are at risk of developing vitamin deficiencies and should receive supplements. But there is no evidence that increasing vitamin intake beyond requirements confers any benefit. Vitamin C, in particular, has not been shown to reduce the incidence of respiratory infections, although it may attenuate the symptoms. The possibly harmful effects of excessive vitamin intake are considered subsequently.

Mineral Requirements

The most common mineral deficiencies found in normal persons are those of calcium and of iron. The causes and prevention of dietary iron deficiency in normal persons are discussed in the section on iron in Chapter 9.

Osteoporosis is very common in older persons, particularly women, and its cause is not well understood. However, there is evidence suggesting that its incidence can be reduced by augmenting calcium intake. This goal is most readily accomplished by a daily supplement of calcium, such as calcium carbonate, 0.5 g/day. To what extent osteoporosis can be prevented by such long-term calcium supplementation is uncertain, but some benefit is highly probable and there is no known associated risk.

There is some evidence that diets of otherwise healthy Americans may commonly be deficient in zinc. However, the evidence for this conclusion is not sufficient to recommend zinc supplementation.

Fiber

As noted in Chapter 10, the relatively low fiber content of the average American diet (as compared with that in the developing countries) may cause Americans to be more susceptible to the premature development of atherosclerosis and to a greater incidence of diabetes, colonic polyps, and colonic cancer. Although most of these associations are incompletely proven, increased fiber intake is harmless except in the presence of acute colonic disease. Hence, it may be prudent to consume at least 25 g of fiber per day. This requires the daily consumption of some foods high in fiber, such as peas, beans, broccoli, prunes, peaches, berries, grapes, apricots, bran, almonds, or whole wheat bread.

NUTRITIONAL EXCESSES

Calories, Ethanol, and Saturated Fat

In developed countries, nutritional excesses can take the form of excess calories (see Chapter 5, section on obesity), excess alcohol (Chapter 14), and excess saturated fat (see Chapter 7). As noted in Chapter 5, obesity is the most common medical problem in the United States and contributes significantly to morbidity from hypertension, atherosclerosis, and diabetes. Caloric restriction is recommended for anyone more than 30 per cent overweight.

Alcohol comprises about 5 per cent of total calories ingested in the United

States, and is, therefore, a significant component of the American diet. The fraction of the population that consumes sufficient alcohol to affect their health adversely is uncertain, but probably at least 12 per cent of males and 6 per cent of females consume over 50 g of alcohol per day.

The effects on health of high intake of fat—especially of saturated fats— are discussed in Chapter 7. As noted therein, saturated fats in particular contribute significantly to the development of atherosclerosis and coronary heart disease. It may be advisable to restrict total fat to 30 per cent of an individual's caloric intake and to replace saturated fats with polyunsaturated fats.

Salt

Among the remaining specific dietary excesses in the United States (sodium, sugar, and vitamins) the most important is salt (see also Chapter 9). The average salt intake (about 4 g per day) exceeds the "safe and adequate" intake of 1.1 to 3.3 g per day recommended by the Food and Nutrition Board. Compelling evidence links high salt intake to the development of hypertension. Among different cultures outside the United States (and even between tribes within a single geographic area), the correlation between average salt intake and the incidence of hypertension is very strong. This close correlation has not been proved within the United States. Nevertheless, reduction of salt intake clearly ameliorates hypertension, which currently affects about one-fifth of the population (one-half of those over age 65). The incidence is twice as high in blacks as in whites.

The high value placed on sodium historically, dating back to the earliest civilizations, began with the shift of the primary foodstuff from meat to salt-poor cereals and with the discovery of the utility of salt as a food preservative. In the sixth century, salt was even traded, ounce for ounce, for gold in Africa. The excessive intake of salt in the United States (and in many other countries) is clearly an acquired habit. In many undeveloped and relatively isolated regions, salt intake is very low. Furthermore, infants show little interest in salt (although they clearly like sugar).

It is also clear that this habit can be broken. Many individuals who studiously avoid salt report that they soon become accustomed to low-salt foods and lose interest in salty foods. Low-salt cookbooks, courses in avoiding salty foods, and restaurants that will provide low-sodium meals are now common.

Salt substitutes, consisting chiefly of potassium chloride (often with glutamic acid), are also widely available. Since it is the sodium content of salt that contributes to the development of hypertension in susceptible individuals, and since there is preliminary evidence that the ratio of sodium to potassium intake may be as important as the sodium intake itself, such substitutes are a rational alternative for those who find their taste acceptable and who cannot become accustomed to a salt-free diet. However, potassium chloride is dangerous in patients with renal failure and in some with heart failure, because fatal hyperkalemia may result.

Common sources of sodium other than sodium chloride include baking

TABLE 1–2.   APPROXIMATE SODIUM CONTENT OF SOME NATURAL AND PREPARED FOODS

1 apple	1 cup applesauce	⅛ apple pie, frozen
2 mg	6 mg	208 mg
½ breast of chicken	1 chicken pie, frozen	1 chicken dinner, fast-food
69 mg	907 mg	2243 mg
1 potato	10 potato chips	1 cup instant mashed potatoes
5 mg	200 mg	485 mg
3 oz steak	1 jumbo hamburger, fast-food	1 meatloaf frozen dinner
55 mg	900 mg	1304 mg
3 oz tuna	3 oz canned tuna	1 tuna potpie, frozen
50 mg	384 mg	715 mg
1 tomato	1 cup tomato soup	1 cup tomato sauce
14 mg	932 mg	1498 mg

soda, baking powder, and absorbable antacids. To reduce sodium intake effectively, it is necessary to avoid these substances as well as salt itself.

A major obstacle in reducing salt intake is the absence of labels indicating the sodium content of most prepared foods. The Food and Drug Administration is at present attempting to convince the food industry of the need to label foods regarding their sodium content, to reduce the amount of sodium in processed foods, and to offer more low-sodium or salt-free products. Many processed foods contain far more sodium than do the natural foods from which they are prepared. A few examples are given in Table 1–2.

Table 9–2, in the section on sodium in Chapter 9, lists common food groups in order of their sodium content.

Sugar

Simple sugars such as sucrose promote the development of dental caries. Hence, the intake of these substances, particularly in children, should be limited. It is not true that sugar causes diabetes or heart disease, but it may contribute to obesity.

Vitamins

Owing to aggressive marketing, vitamin excesses are probably more common than vitamin deficiencies in the United States. The forms of vitamin toxicity seen most commonly are those caused by excessive vitamin A and vitamin D; those caused by other vitamins are uncommon. Excessive vitamin A causes retarded growth, brain damage, liver and spleen enlargement, hair and skin abnormalities, blindness, and aplastic anemia. Vitamin D overdosage is characterized by hypercalcemia, anorexia, nausea, vomiting, soft-tissue calcification, and renal failure. Excessive niacin causes severe flushing, liver damage, skin disorders, and gout. Megadoses of vitamin E can cause headaches, nausea, fatigue, gastrointestinal disorders, hypoglycemia, and bleeding tendencies (owing to the vitamin K deficiency it causes). There is no evidence that excess vitamin E improves sexual function; in rats, large doses even cause testicular atrophy. Vitamin C, the vitamin most commonly ingested in megadoses, may have some ameliorative effect against the symptoms of the common cold but can clearly also cause kidney stones, bone damage, and diarrhea.

"HEALTH FOODS"

One of the most prevalent nutritional myths in the United States today is the belief that "health foods" improve health and prevent disease. The term "health food" is used to include so-called organic foods, which are plant products grown in soil enriched in humus and compost, on which no pesticides, herbicides, or inorganic fertilizers have been used. The term "organic" obscures the fact that plants cannot utilize organic nutrients but only inorganic substances for growth. Numerous studies have shown no difference in pesticide levels between organic and inorganic foods. Thus, the ill effects of inorganic fertilizers are purely fanciful.

"Organic" meats are derived from animals grown without the aid of hormones or antibiotics. Other "natural" foods are those containing no artificial ingredients or food additives.

An individual's possible sensitization from exposure to traces of antibiotics in meats is the only adverse effect that may be avoided by consuming "organic" foods. On the other hand, many of the plant products sold in health food stores may be harmful. Examples are teas made from juniper berries, shave grass, horsetail, buckthorn, senna, dock, aloe, burdock root, jimson weed, chamomile, or ginseng.

FOOD ADDITIVES

The idea, championed by Feingold, that food-additive dyes may contribute to behavioral disturbances has recently been examined in controlled trials. Among children purported to be adversely affected by artificial food colors, abnormal behavioral responses were confirmed in only a few (unless unusually large doses were given). Only after extensive study of large doses in animals have the food additives in common use been approved for widespread consumption. Many food additives are essential to the proper preservation of foods.

Nutritional Assessment

Anthony L. Imbembo, M.D., and
Mackenzie Walser, M.D.

INTRODUCTION

Malnutrition can cause increased morbidity and mortality in patients who already suffer from a variety of underlying disorders. For example, poor nutrition impairs wound healing and delays the formation of bony callus following fracture. Indeed, wound and anastomotic dehiscences are common complications in malnourished subjects both in experimental and in clinical situations. Severe malnutrition increases the risk of sepsis by decreasing the replication rate of bone marrow and by impairing both antibody formation and delayed hypersensitivity.

The increase in gastrointestinal transit time resulting from malnutrition may cause spontaneous adynamic ileus and may thereby actually impede attempts at nutritional correction. In the same way, malnutrition may contribute significantly to inordinate prolongation of adynamic ileus after abdominal or retroperitoneal surgical procedures.

Some malnourished individuals have significant muscle wasting, which, in turn, contributes to a decrease in ventilatory and ambulatory capacities. These problems may lead to significant pulmonary complications, such as atelectasis and pneumonia, and to an increased incidence of deep venous thrombosis. When malnutrition impairs protein synthesis, the serum albumin level may fall sufficiently to cause generalized edema.

Malnutrition is a particular problem in the patient undergoing radiation treatment or chemotherapy for cancer. The malnourished patient may tolerate these forms of therapy poorly because of the body's reduced ability to repair associated sublethal injury to normal tissues.

Finally, in the pediatric and adolescent populations, significant impairment of growth and maturation may be added to all of the aforementioned potential risks.

Generally, the recognition of severe malnutrition is relatively easy. Usually, significant weight loss is confirmed by the patient's appearance. The clothing is loose and fits poorly; bony prominences are generally exaggerated, particularly in the face, with temporal wasting and prominence of the orbital ridges. Muscle wasting is apparent, there may be edema secondary to low serum albumin levels, hair may be thinned, and the patient may demonstrate both physical and mental lethargy.

However, borderline nutritional depletion may be more difficult to identify. Moderate degrees of weight loss may be overlooked or dismissed as inconsequential. Changes in body habitus may evolve so slowly that they escape notice. Subtle physical findings may elude the physician who is seeing the patient for the first time.

In view of the multiple adverse effects of malnutrition, it is important to recognize patients with a suboptimal nutritional status. In addition, since nutritional problems may develop during various forms of medical and surgical treatment, these changes must be recognized so that corrective measures can be undertaken before they become particularly significant.

Nutritional assessment is important. However, no single measurement or even group of determinations accurately assesses nutritional status under all circumstances. A variety of methods have proved useful under varying conditions. For example, Copeland et al. have suggested that changes in body weight, serum albumin level, and skin immunoreactivity be measured and followed in order to assess the efficacy of nutritional therapy. Blackburn et al. have proposed a more elaborate approach that includes various anthropometric measurements, determination of serum levels of albumin and transferrin, measurement of creatinine-height index and urinary excretion of nitrogen, and tests of skin immunoreactivity to various antigens. Neither method is clearly superior to the other, and a number of criticisms can be leveled at each component of the assessment procedure. These and other protocols are being followed and evaluated in a number of centers at the present time.

In this section, the possible components of a nutritional assessment protocol will be presented; their predictive value as well as their limitations will be discussed. Various protocols that may be of value will also be suggested.

COMPONENTS OF THE ASSESSMENT

History

A careful history may yield information suggesting the need for detailed nutritional assessment. As a history of weight loss may be important evidence of significant nutritional compromise, the patient should be questioned carefully about changes in weight or in the fit of clothing. Patients must also be asked about the use of medications, such as diuretics and corticosteroids, which may significantly affect their weight and may therefore detract from the reliability of the weight history for nutritional assessment.

A dietary history is taken as part of the nutritional assessment to identify those patients with inadequate intake. Poor dietary intake can develop for a variety of reasons including anorexia, nausea and vomiting, food aversion, changes in taste and smell, socioeconomic problems, lack of information about proper nutrition, and adherence to fad diets. Patients are asked to describe their usual diet and to specify their intake of food during the previous day. An effort is made to identify specific problems that may interfere with the intake or assimilation of foods. Specific assessment should be made of possible problems with chewing or swallowing or the presence of symptoms such as dysphagia, abdominal pain, early satiety, postprandial fullness, vomiting, diarrhea, or crampy abdominal pain following meals.

Anthropometric Determinations

Anthropometric measurements are of value in both initial nutritional assessment and in the follow-up of patients undergoing various forms of medical or surgical treatment. However, except for weight-height determinations, they are subject to considerable variation in measurement despite attempts to standardize each technique.

Height-Weight

Height and weight measurements are important indicators of somatic status, and abnormalities therein may suggest the need for further testing or patient evaluation. As a measure of nutritional status, weight can be expressed as absolute weight, weight for height, or, most commonly, as relative body weight (observed body weight/ideal body weight for the patient's height and build as provided in standard tables) (see Appendix). Generally, if a patient has lost over 10 per cent of his body weight during the previous 6 months or weighs less than 90 per cent of his ideal weight, nutritional support of some type is indicated.

However, in some instances weight alone may not be an accurate guide to nutritional status. At times during malnutrition, significant depletion of one body compartment accompanies expansion of another; as a result, overall weight changes little. For example, in some patients with protein malnutrition (kwashiorkor), marked depletion in lean body mass is almost matched by an increase in total body water because edema or ascites develops secondary to low serum albumin levels. On the other hand, although absolute weight loss may be a relatively crude assessment tool, it correlates positively with a 19-fold increase in the death rate of patients undergoing elective surgical procedures, in one study.

Evaluation of body weight and height as indicators of growth and nutritional status is of utmost importance in children and adolescents. Weight and height measurements are used to assess growth by plotting the values for age on the National Center for Health Statistics (NCHS) Growth Grids and determining the percentile level for a given child. Similarly, weight for height is determined for prepubescent children from NCHS tables; the standard is the 50th percentile. Both percentiles and standard deviations can be used to indicate how far a measurement deviates from the mean of a set of determinations. For any particular set of measurements, percentiles can be converted into standard deviations and vice versa. Some have preferred to determine a Z score for interpreting anthropometric measurements, particularly for children (see Figures 1–1 to 1–5).

$$Z \text{ score} = \frac{\text{Actual percentile} - \text{Mean percentile}}{\text{Standard deviation}}$$

Head Circumference

Head circumference should be measured in infants and in preschool children. A flexible tape, one-quarter-inch wide, is applied firmly around the head above the supraorbital ridges or the most prominent part of the frontal bulge,

Text continued on page 17

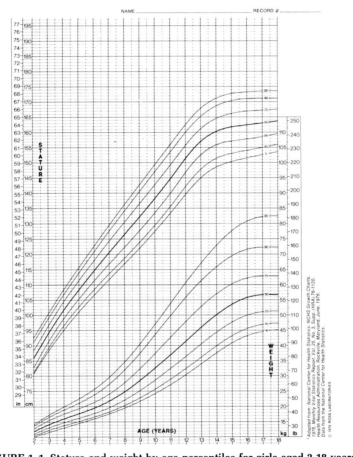

FIGURE 1–1. Stature and weight by age percentiles for girls aged 2-18 years.

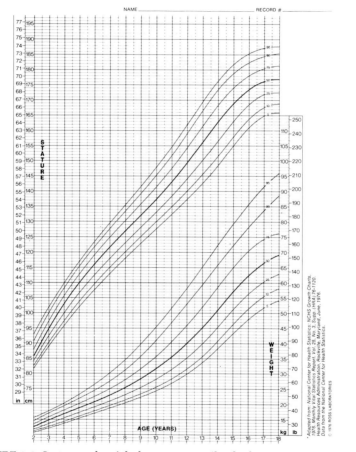

FIGURE 1–2. Stature and weight by age precentiles for boys ages 2 to 18 years.

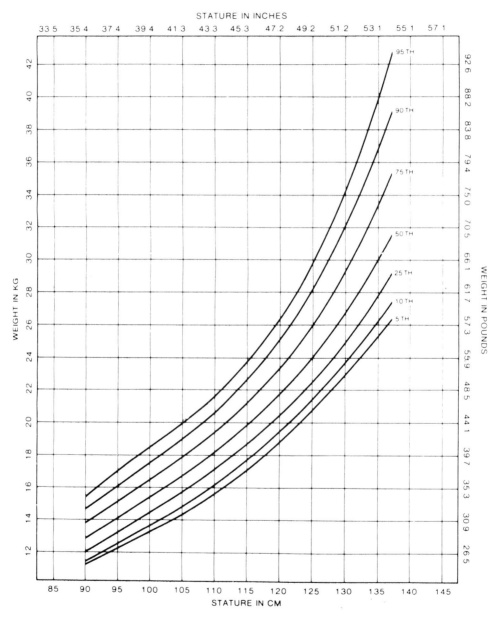

FIGURE 1–3. Weight by stature percentiles for prepubescent girls.

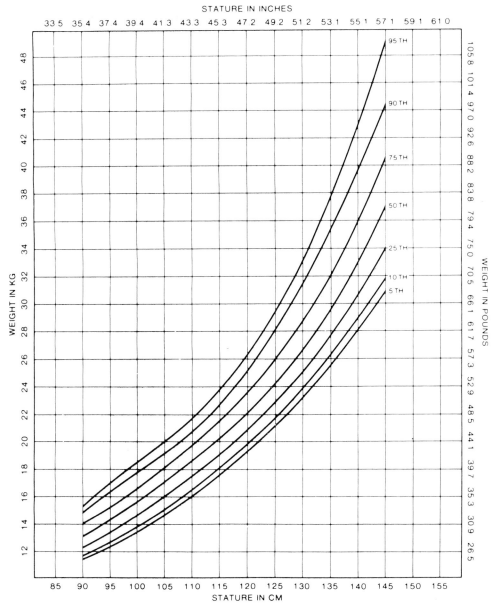

FIGURE 1–4. Weight by stature percentiles for prepubescent boys.

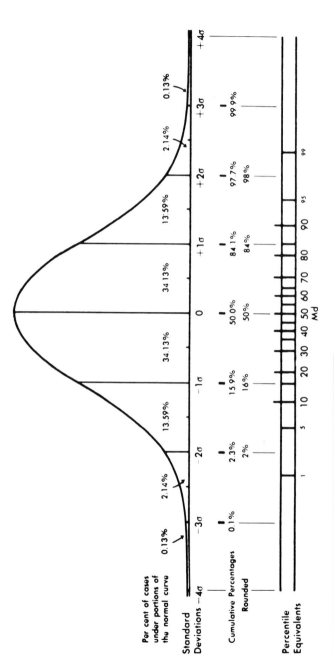

FIGURE 1-5. Normal curve showing relationship between standard deviations and percentiles. Both percentiles and standard deviations indicate how far a measurement deviates from the mean of a set of measurements. For any particular set of measurements, percentiles can be converted into standard deviations, and vice versa. (From Valadion, I., and Porter, D.: Physical Growth and Development, 1st Ed. Boston, Little, Brown and Co., 1977, p. 15.)

Z Score (S.D.)	Approximate (%)
+2	98
+1	84
−1	16
−2	2

anteriorly, and over the part of the occiput that gives maximum frontal-occipital circumference (measured to nearest 0.5 cm). The percentile is then determined from Figure 1–6 or 1–7.

Head circumference is significantly correlated with weight in the normal preschool population. A head circumference two standard deviations below the mean is positively related to nutritional problems (borderline biologic quality of protein in the diet, mechanical feeding problems and so forth).

Triceps Skinfold Thickness

Fat reserves may be estimated by measuring the triceps skinfold thickness. A fold of skin on the posterior aspect of the nondominant arm, midway between the shoulder and elbow, is grasped and gently pulled away from the underlying muscle. Calipers are applied to measure this skinfold. The measurement is then compared with a standard set of values to determine whether fat depletion or obesity is present (Table 1–3).

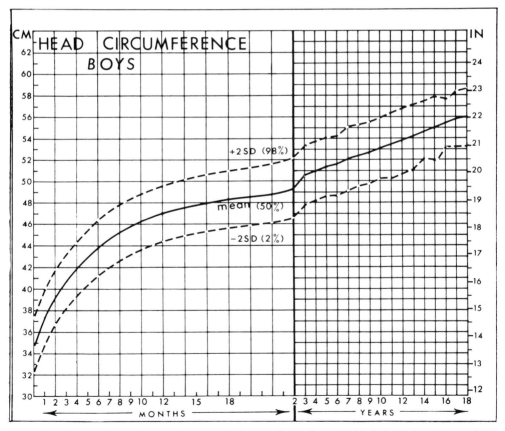

FIGURE 1–6. Composite graph of head circumference for males from birth through 18 years of age. (From Nellhaus, G.: Head circumference from birth to eighteen years. Pediatrics 41:106–114, 1968.)

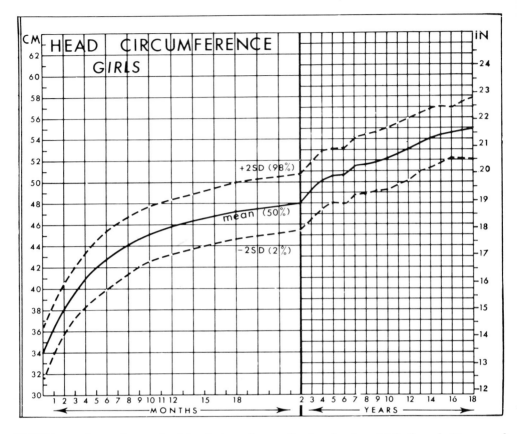

FIGURE 1–7. Composite graph of head circumference for females from birth through 18 years of age. (From Nellhaus, G.: Head circumference from birth to eighteen years. Pediatrics 41:106–114, 1968.)

Midarm Circumference

The midarm circumference is one measure of lean body mass or degree of somatic protein depletion. The midpoint of the upper arm is located halfway between the acromial process of the scapula and the olecranon process of the ulna. The mid–upper-arm circumference is measured and compared with standard values (Table 1–4).

Arm Muscle Circumference

The arm muscle circumference, which may correlate somewhat better with somatic protein deficits than does the midarm circumference, is calculated using the following formula:

$$\text{Arm muscle circumference (mm)} = \text{Midarm circumference (mm)} - (0.314 \times \text{triceps skinfold in mm}).$$

The value is then compared with the standards given in Table 1–4. Arm muscle

TABLE 1–3.   PERCENTILES FOR TRICEPS SKINFOLD FOR WHITES OF THE
UNITED STATES HEALTH AND NUTRITION EXAMINATION SURVEY I
OF 1971 TO 1974

Age Group	Triceps Skinfold (mm) Percentiles															
	n	5	10	25	50	75	90	95	n	5	10	25	50	75	90	95
	Males								Females							
1–1.9	228	6	7	8	10	12	14	16	204	6	7	8	10	12	14	16
2–2.9	223	6	7	8	10	12	14	15	208	6	8	9	10	12	15	16
3–3.9	220	6	7	8	10	11	14	15	208	7	8	9	11	12	14	15
4–4.9	230	6	6	8	9	11	12	14	208	7	8	8	10	12	14	16
5–5.9	214	6	6	8	9	11	14	15	219	6	7	8	10	12	15	18
6–6.9	117	5	6	7	8	10	13	16	118	6	6	8	10	12	14	16
7–7.9	122	5	6	7	9	12	15	17	126	6	7	9	11	13	16	18
8–8.9	117	5	6	7	8	10	13	16	118	6	8	9	12	15	18	24
9–9.9	121	6	6	7	10	13	17	18	125	8	8	10	13	16	20	22
10–10.9	146	6	6	8	10	14	18	21	152	7	8	10	12	17	23	27
11–11.9	122	6	6	8	11	16	20	24	117	7	8	10	13	18	24	28
12–12.9	153	6	6	8	11	14	22	28	129	8	9	11	14	18	23	27
13–13.9	134	5	5	7	10	14	22	26	151	8	8	12	15	21	26	30
14–14.9	131	4	5	7	9	14	21	24	141	9	10	13	16	21	26	28
15–15.9	128	4	5	6	8	11	18	24	117	8	10	12	17	21	25	32
16–16.9	131	4	5	6	8	12	16	22	142	10	12	15	18	22	26	31
17–17.9	133	5	5	6	8	12	16	19	114	10	12	13	19	24	30	37
18–18.9	91	4	5	6	9	13	20	24	109	10	12	15	18	22	26	30
19–24.9	531	4	5	7	10	15	20	22	1060	10	11	14	18	24	30	34
25–34.9	971	5	6	8	12	16	20	24	1987	10	12	16	21	27	34	37
35–44.9	806	5	6	8	12	16	20	23	1614	12	14	18	23	29	35	38
45–54.9	898	6	6	8	12	15	20	25	1047	12	16	20	25	30	36	40
55–64.9	734	5	6	8	11	14	19	22	809	12	16	20	25	31	36	38
65–74.9	1503	4	6	8	11	15	19	22	1670	12	14	18	24	29	34	36

From Frisancho, A.R.: New norms of upper limb fat and muscle areas for assessment of nutritional status. Am J
Clin Nutr 34:2540–2545, 1981.

circumference seems to be an excellent index of nutritional status and growth
in children.

Utility of Anthropometric Determinations

Although extremely valuable in the assessment of nutritional status and
growth changes in children and adolescents, anthropometric determinations are
not very sensitive to relatively slight deterioration of nutritional status in
adults. For example, despite the obligatory catabolism and negative nitrogen
balance that develops following all surgical procedures, it is most unusual for
anthropometric determinations to change by more than 10 per cent of the preoperative value. In comparison to other determinants of malnutrition, such as
plasma protein levels, anthropometry may be a less sensitive way to detect
mild nutritional depletion. Furthermore, the correlation between weight loss
and arm muscle circumference is weak. Anthropometric measurements may be
important indices, however, of severe malnutrition such as that seen in patients
who have postoperative complications following extensive procedures (sepsis,
enterocutaneous fistulae, and so on). Abnormal values for triceps skinfold

TABLE 1–4. PERCENTILES OF UPPER ARM CIRCUMFERENCE (mm) AND ESTIMATED UPPER ARM MUSCLE CIRCUMFERENCE (mm) FOR WHITES OF THE UNITED STATES HEALTH AND NUTRITION EXAMINATION SURVEY I OF 1971 TO 1974

Age Group	Arm Circumference (mm)							Arm Muscle Circumference (mm)						
	5	10	25	50	75	90	95	5	10	25	50	75	90	95
Males														
1–1.9	142	146	150	159	170	176	183	110	113	119	127	135	144	147
2–2.9	141	145	153	162	170	178	185	111	114	122	130	140	146	150
3–3.9	150	153	160	167	175	184	190	117	123	131	137	143	148	153
4–4.9	149	154	162	171	180	186	192	123	126	133	141	148	156	159
5–5.9	153	160	167	175	185	195	204	128	133	140	147	154	162	169
6–6.9	155	159	167	179	188	209	228	131	135	142	151	161	170	177
7–7.9	162	167	177	187	201	223	230	137	139	151	160	168	177	190
8–8.9	162	170	177	190	202	220	245	140	145	154	162	170	182	187
9–9.9	175	178	187	200	217	249	257	151	154	161	170	183	196	202
10–10.9	181	184	196	210	231	262	274	156	160	166	180	191	209	221
11–11.9	186	190	202	223	244	261	280	159	165	173	183	195	205	230
12–12.9	193	200	214	232	254	282	303	167	171	182	195	210	223	241
13–13.9	194	211	228	247	263	286	301	172	179	196	211	226	238	245
14–14.9	220	226	237	253	283	303	322	189	199	212	223	240	260	264
15–15.9	222	229	244	264	284	311	320	199	204	218	237	254	266	272
16–16.9	244	248	262	278	303	324	343	213	225	234	249	269	287	296
17–17.9	246	253	267	285	308	336	347	224	231	245	258	273	294	312
18–18.9	245	260	276	297	321	353	379	226	237	252	264	283	298	324
19–24.9	262	272	288	308	331	355	372	238	245	257	273	289	309	321
25–34.9	271	282	300	319	342	362	375	243	250	264	279	298	314	326
35–44.9	278	287	305	326	345	363	374	247	255	269	286	302	318	327
45–54.9	267	281	301	322	342	362	376	239	249	265	281	300	315	326
55–64.9	258	273	296	317	336	355	369	236	245	260	278	295	310	320
65–74.9	248	263	285	307	325	344	355	223	235	251	268	284	298	306
Females														
1–1.9	138	142	148	156	164	172	177	105	111	117	124	132	139	143
2–2.9	142	145	152	160	167	176	184	111	114	119	126	133	142	147
3–3.9	143	150	158	167	175	183	189	113	119	124	132	140	146	152
4–4.9	149	154	160	169	177	184	191	115	121	128	136	144	152	157
5–5.9	153	157	165	175	185	203	211	125	128	134	142	151	159	165
6–6.9	156	162	170	176	187	204	211	130	133	138	145	154	166	171
7–7.9	164	167	174	183	199	216	231	129	135	142	151	160	171	176
8–8.9	168	172	183	195	214	247	261	138	140	151	160	171	183	194
9–9.9	178	182	194	211	224	251	260	147	150	158	167	180	194	198
10–10.9	174	182	193	210	228	251	265	148	150	159	170	180	190	197
11–11.9	185	194	208	224	248	276	303	150	158	171	181	196	217	223
12–12.9	194	203	216	237	256	282	294	162	166	180	191	201	214	220
13–13.9	202	211	223	243	271	301	338	169	175	183	198	211	226	240
14–14.9	214	223	237	252	272	304	322	174	179	190	201	216	232	247
15–15.9	208	221	239	254	279	300	322	175	178	189	202	215	228	244
16–16.9	218	224	241	258	283	318	334	170	180	190	202	216	234	249
17–17.9	220	227	241	264	295	324	350	175	183	194	205	221	239	257
18–18.9	222	227	241	258	281	312	325	174	179	191	202	215	237	245
19–24.9	221	230	247	265	290	319	345	179	185	195	207	221	236	249
25–34.9	233	240	256	277	304	342	368	183	188	199	212	228	246	264
35–44.9	241	251	267	290	317	356	378	186	192	205	218	236	257	272
45–54.9	242	256	274	299	328	362	384	187	193	206	220	238	260	274
55–64.9	243	257	280	303	335	367	385	187	196	209	225	244	266	280
65–74.9	240	252	274	299	326	356	373	185	195	208	225	244	264	279

From Frisancho, A.R.: New norms of upper limb fat and muscle areas for assessment of nutritional status. Am J Clin Nutr 34:2540–2545, 1981.

thickness and arm muscle circumference occur in more than one-half of such patients.

Recently, the validity of weight-height, midarm circumference, and triceps skinfold thickness as measures of malnutrition was evaluated in a large number of adult patients whose body compositions were determined simultaneously. Weight-height correlated best with body cell mass. Triceps skinfold thickness correlated fairly well with body fat stores, but midarm circumference was a poor measure of muscle mass in adults ($r = 0.64$).

Others have found that anthropometry is reliable for the assessment of protein nutrition in epidemiologic surveys; however, most investigators agree that the great variability noted from patient to patient makes anthropometry a relatively less sensitive method for initial nutritional assessment and for following changes in body nitrogen in individual adult patients over short periods of time. Arm anthropometry seems to be most useful when evaluating individuals over long periods of time and in assessing populations.

Creatinine-Height Index

Creatinine is produced continuously in the body by the nonenzymatic dehydration of creatine. The rate of this reaction is a function of pH and temperature but under physiologic conditions is essentially constant. Approximately 1.7 per cent of body creatine is converted to creatinine daily. In normal subjects, creatinine is not metabolized and is, therefore, quantitatively excreted. The rate of creatinine excretion is a very accurate measure of the total body creatine pool, except in patients with chronic renal failure. Since creatine is located almost exclusively in muscle—the main constituent of lean body mass—creatinine excretion in normal subjects correlates well with lean body mass. It has been proposed that creatinine excretion might be a valid measure of lean body mass in diseased as well as in normal subjects. Although this is partially true, several other factors in addition to lean body mass can affect creatinine excretion.

The body creatine pool is affected by the intake of creatine, which is a component of meat. Subjects on a creatine-free diet exhibit a progressive fall in their body creatine pool and, therefore, in the rate of creatinine excretion. However, the magnitude of this decline has never been determined accurately. In addition, the cooking process itself may convert some meat creatine to creatinine; thus, a part of the total creatinine excreted is derived from preformed ingested creatinine. Consequently, when patients alter their diet to ingest less cooked meat, creatinine excretion decreases more rapidly than predicted by the reduced intake of preformed creatine.

In addition to these dietary factors, both age and sex can affect the amount of creatinine excreted per kilogram of lean body mass. Since the conversion of creatine to creatinine cannot be dependent upon age or sex, these data suggest that the muscle creatine pool per kilogram of muscle must be, to some degree, a function of both age and sex.

Information on creatinine excretion per kilogram of lean body mass as a

TABLE 1–5.   LINEAR REGRESSION OF CREATININE EXCRETION IN
MG/KG BODY WEIGHT (y) OR MG/KG IDEAL BODY WEIGHT (y′) ON
AGE IN YEARS (A) IN NORMAL ADULT SUBJECTS, ACCORDING TO
VARIOUS AUTHORS

Subjects	Authors	Equation
Men	Cockcroft and Gault	$y = 28.0 - 0.20\ A$ (n = 239)
Men	Norris et al.	$y' = 29.0 - 0.12\ A$ (n = 143)
Men	Ahlert et al.	$y = 26.7 - 0.17\ A$ (n = 97)
Men	Kampmann	$y = 29.2 - 0.20\ A$ (n = 149)
	Average regression	$y = 28.2 - 0.172\ A$
Women	Young et al.	$y' = 19.8 - 0.00\ A$ (n = 88)
Women	Kampmann	$y = 25.0 - 0.18\ A$ (n = 219)
Women	Ahlert et al.	$y = 18.7 - 0.11\ A$ (n = 155)
Women	Cockcroft and Gault	$y = 23.8 - 0.17\ A$ (n = 10)
	Average regression	$y = 21.9 - 0.115\ A$

function of age is almost nonexistent. However, several studies involving large numbers of normal individuals have clarified the relationship between creatinine excretion per kilogram of body weight and age, in both sexes. These studies were carried out in either healthy persons living in the community or hospitalized patients free of renal or hepatic disease. Since there are no consistent differences between these study types and since there is no obvious reason why the age-dependence of creatinine excretion should be affected by hospitalization, their results have been combined.

The average regression of creatinine excretion in mg per kg (y) with age (A) in men is $y = 28.2 - 0.172\ A$ and in women, $y = 21.9 - 0.115\ A$ (see Table 1–5). Thus, from age 20 to 80 creatinine excretion falls 42 per cent in men and 35 per cent in women. This is clearly greater than the decrease with age in muscle mass per kilogram of body weight; tissues other than muscle would have to more than double to account for such a change. Instead, it has been postulated, as noted earlier, that muscle creatine concentration declines with age, although this is purely speculative. Another factor, although probably of minor importance, may be lower consumption of meat by older persons. Whatever the explanation, it is clear that assessment of muscle mass on the basis of creatinine excretion must take both age and sex into account.

It has been proposed that creatinine excretion relative to height is a better measure of lean body mass than is creatinine excretion relative to weight. This proposal is based on the unproven concept that lean body mass varies linearly with height. In fact, there is little evidence for this, and anthropometric considerations would suggest that lean body mass should vary as a power of height. Nonetheless, the creatinine-height index is used as a measure of lean body mass and nutritional status. The creatinine-height index is calculated as follows:

$$\frac{\text{24-hr creatinine excretion of subject}}{\text{24-hr creatinine excretion of normal subject of same sex, height, and age}} \times 100$$

Table 1–6 gives creatinine excretion in relation to height of normal chil-

TABLE 1–6.   EXPECTED 24-HOUR CREATININE EXCRETION OF NORMAL CHILDREN

Height (cm)	24-Hr Urinary Creatinine (mg)	Height (cm)	24-Hr Urinary Creatinine (mg)
50.0	35.50	97.4	259.08
53.5	44.94	98.0	263.62
56.9	55.19	98.6	268.19
60.4	66.44	99.2	272.80
62.4	72.38	99.8	277.44
64.4	78.57	100.4	281.12
66.4	84.99	101.0	283.81
68.0	90.44	101.6	287.53
69.6	96.05	102.2	290.25
71.2	101.82	102.8	292.98
72.5	107.30	103.4	295.72
73.8	112.91	104.0	299.52
75.2	118.82	104.5	303.05
76.3	123.61	105.1	305.84
77.4	128.48	105.6	308.35
78.5	132.66	106.2	311.17
79.6	137.71	106.7	313.70
80.7	142.84	107.1	318.09
81.8	147.24	107.4	322.20
82.8	156.49	107.7	325.25
83.7	159.03	108.0	329.40
84.7	165.16	108.4	333.87
85.6	171.20	108.7	336.97
86.6	177.53	111.0	359.64
87.5	183.75	112.2	379.24
88.5	189.39	113.2	384.88
89.0	194.02	114.1	390.22
89.8	198.46	114.5	391.59
90.5	203.62	115.9	399.86
91.5	209.54	117.2	407.86
92.1	213.67	118.6	431.70
92.8	219.94	120.0	456.00
93.5	226.27	121.5	477.50
94.1	231.49	123.0	499.88
94.8	237.95	124.5	527.88
95.5	244.48	126.0	556.92
96.2	250.12	127.5	586.50
96.8	256.52	129.0	616.62

From Viteri, F.E., and Alvarado, J.: The creatinine height index: Its use in the estimation of the degree of protein depletion and repletion in protein calorie malnourished children. Pediatrics 46:696–706, 1970.

dren. Tables 1–7 and 1–8 give creatinine excretion in milligrams per day in relation to height and age for men and women of ideal weight. The values are derived from the ideal weights given in the Appendix and from the average regression equations given earlier. It should be noted that these values all refer to persons with normal diets. Vegetarians or persons with inadequate diets can be expected to excrete as much as 25 per cent less creatinine, depending upon the duration of these dietary habits.

TABLE 1-7. EXPECTED CREATININE EXCRETION, MG/DAY, IN MEN OF IDEAL WEIGHT

Height (cm)	Age (yrs)						
	20–29	30–39	40–49	50–59	60–69	70–79	80–89
146	1258	1169	1079	985	896	807	718
148	1284	1193	1102	1006	915	824	733
150	1308	1215	1123	1025	932	839	747
152	1334	1240	1145	1045	951	856	762
154	1358	1262	1166	1064	968	872	775
156	1390	1291	1193	1089	990	892	793
158	1423	1322	1222	1115	1014	913	812
160	1452	1349	1246	1137	1035	932	829
162	1481	1376	1271	1160	1055	950	845
164	1510	1403	1296	1183	1076	969	862
166	1536	1427	1318	1203	1094	986	877
168	1565	1454	1343	1226	1115	1004	893
170	1598	1485	1372	1252	1139	1026	912
172	1632	1516	1401	1278	1163	1047	932
174	1666	1548	1430	1305	1187	1069	951
176	1699	1579	1458	1331	1211	1090	970
178	1738	1615	1491	1361	1238	1115	992
180	1781	1655	1529	1395	1269	1143	1017
182	1819	1690	1561	1425	1296	1167	1038
184	1855	1724	1592	1453	1322	1190	1059
186	1894	1759	1625	1483	1349	1215	1081
188	1932	1795	1658	1513	1377	1240	1103
190	1968	1829	1689	1542	1402	1263	1123

For derivation of these data, see text.

TABLE 1-8. EXPECTED CREATININE EXCRETION, MG/DAY, IN WOMEN OF IDEAL WEIGHT

Height (cm)	Age (yrs)						
	20–29	30–39	40–49	50–59	60–69	70–79	80–89
140	858	804	754	700	651	597	548
142	877	822	771	716	666	610	560
144	898	841	790	733	682	625	573
146	917	859	806	749	696	638	586
148	940	881	827	768	713	654	600
150	964	903	848	787	732	671	615
152	984	922	865	803	747	685	628
154	1003	940	882	819	761	698	640
156	1026	961	902	838	779	714	655
158	1049	983	922	856	796	730	670
160	1073	1006	944	877	815	747	686
162	1100	1031	968	899	835	766	703
164	1125	1054	990	919	854	783	719
166	1148	1076	1010	938	871	799	733
168	1173	1099	1032	958	890	817	749
170	1199	1124	1055	980	911	835	766
172	1224	1147	1077	1000	929	853	782
174	1253	1174	1102	1023	951	872	800
176	1280	1199	1126	1045	972	891	817
178	1304	1223	1147	1065	990	908	833
180	1331	1248	1171	1087	1011	927	850

For derivation of these data see text.

The use of the creatinine-height index as a quantitative measure of protein depletion is supported by a highly significant negative correlation between nitrogen retention and creatinine-height index. In children, the creatinine-height index correlates well with intestinal absorption of protein, total circulating red blood cell and lean body mass, and recovery from malnutrition. Bistrian et al. have shown that the creatinine-height index is more sensitive than weight for height, nitrogen balance, or serum albumin levels in predicting the nutritional status of an adult population in epidemiologic studies. Others, however, have demonstrated a rather poor correlation between creatinine-height index and body cell mass as determined by multiple isotope dilution techniques.

Plasma Protein Determinations

There is some evidence that changes in the levels of certain plasma proteins correlate with visceral protein synthesis and malnutrition. Since the liver is the main site for most plasma proteins, low concentrations of prealbumin, transferrin, or albumin can reflect impaired hepatic function. However, in malnutrition decreased protein synthesis is usually due to limited availability of ingested amino acids. Plasma protein concentrations are dependent not only on synthetic rates but also on utilization, intravascular-extravascular transfer, catabolism, excretion, and state of hydration. The overall balance among these physiologic processes determines whether the plasma concentration of a specific protein accurately reflects the overall decrease in protein synthesis associated with both isolated protein and combined protein-calorie malnutrition.

Serum albumin is the primary protein responsible for the maintenance of intravascular oncotic pressure. If cardiac function is normal, a patient is prone to edema when the serum albumin level falls below 2 g/dl.

In patients with normal hepatic function, nutritional status is thought by some to correlate with the serum albumin level. Minimal nutritional impairment is considered to exist when the serum albumin level is between 3 and 3.5 g/dl, whereas severe impairment exists when the level is below 2.5 g/dl. One study has shown a significant relationship between arm muscle circumference, as a measure of muscle protein, and serum albumin levels. Since an abnormal serum albumin level also seems related to a striking increase in the rate of surgical complications and mortality, it has been suggested that the serum albumin level serves as a screening test for patients with potentially significant nutritional impairment.

However, other studies have shown a poor correlation between serum albumin and nutritional state. In nutritionally impaired individuals, the serum albumin level tends to be maintained somewhat by reduced catabolism; this compensatory change decreases the sensitivity of serum albumin as a determinant of malnutrition and, therefore, limits its usefulness. Albumin is a relatively insensitive index of early protein malnutrition and responds slowly to changes in nutritional status because of a large body pool and a long half-life.

Serum transferrin can be measured directly or estimated from the total iron binding capacity (TIBC) by utilizing this formula:

$$\text{Serum transferrin} = (0.8 \times \text{TIBC}) - 43$$

Mild nutritional impairment exists when serum transferrin levels are between 180 and 200 mg/dl, whereas severe impairment is associated with a level less than 160 mg/dl. The serum transferrin level is thought to be a more sensitive determinant of nutritional status than is serum albumin level because of the shorter biologic half-life of transferrin (about 8 days compared with the 17-day half-life of albumin). Serum transferrin levels are of limited value in the detection of protein-calorie malnutrition in the presence of severe iron-deficiency anemia, which itself causes an increase in serum transferrin level.

Assessment of Immune Competence

Total Lymphocyte Count

Because of the possible detrimental effect of malnutrition on certain immune functions, investigators have proposed evaluation of immune function as a component of nutritional assessment. The demonstration that nutritional restoration can improve immune function lends support to this idea. The total lymphocyte count has been proposed as a screening measure in the assessment of immune competence, using the following formula:

$$\text{Total lymphocyte count} = \frac{\% \text{ lymphocytes} \times \text{WBC}}{100}$$

A lymphocyte count between 1500 and 1800 constitutes mild impairment, whereas a count of less than 900 signifies severe derangement. In surgical patients, a low total lymphocyte count has been found to correspond with a statistically significant increase in operative mortality. A reduced total lymphocyte count is also associated with at least a twofold increase in the incidence of postoperative complications.

However, the reliability of the total lymphocyte count in nutritional assessment is difficult to determine for a number of reasons. Patients with marasmus (cachexia due to restricted intake) generally have no significant changes in total lymphocyte count. On the other hand, randomly selected postoperative surgical patients generally show significant decreases in their total lymphocyte counts despite a normal nutritional status. These reductions in total lymphocyte counts correlate with decreases in serum albumin. Marasmic children usually do not show lymphopenia, whereas those with kwashiorkor (protein malnutrition alone) show modest decreases. These data imply that injury-induced catabolism of protein may produce a protein depletion syndrome that affects immune function differently from the classic depletion syndromes secondary to various forms of restricted intake.

The interpretation of a decreased total lymphocyte count is complicated by a number of additional factors. A large wound may temporarily deplete the peripheral blood lymphocyte pool as a result of the migration of cells into the traumatized tissue. Massive blood loss also lowers the total peripheral lymphocyte pool.

It is unclear at what point a decrease in peripheral blood lymphocyte count starts to affect immune function. Many feel that moderate decreases in lymphocyte numbers may be irrelevant with respect to immune competence or nutritional status. It seems that dramatic decreases in amounts of either total lymphocyte or specific T or B cells do not usually occur as a result of malnutrition either in hospitalized patients or in children with kwashiorkor or marasmus. The observed changes in lymphocyte numbers correlate poorly with immune competence.

Skin Tests of Delayed Cutaneous Hypersensitivity (DCH)

These skin tests are widely used to assess immune function both prior to and following institution of nutritional support. However, much care must be exercised in interpreting the significance of anergy before concluding that nutritional depletion is responsible. The induration measured at the site of intradermal antigen injection is the end-result of a complex series of cell-cell interactions and mediator elaborations. For example, in the purified protein derivative (PPD) response, the manifestation of a maximally positive skin test requires functioning T cells, B cells, lymphokine production, effective monocyte chemotaxis, and macrophage activation. Obviously, a wide variety of metabolic derangements, in addition to nutritional depletion, can interfere with this complex process. Anergy occurs not only in immune deficiency states but also with conditions such as advanced age, uremia, bacterial or viral infection, liver disease, and immobilization. Finally, technical problems abound in the administration of skin tests, and the antigen preparation may vary widely in potency.

Clinical immunologists define anergy in the adult when only one response of at least 5 mm induration follows the injection of a panel of six skin test antigens (Candida, streptokinase-streptodornase, coccidioidin, mumps, PPD, dinitrochlorobenzene). A patient who fails to become sensitized after dinitrochlorobenzene (DNCB) administration (no second test reaction) is also defined as anergic, since only 20 per cent of normal controls are positive to this antigen on initial administration. When it is clinically undesirable to test patients with a panel of six antigens, the ability to become sensitized to DNCB is probably the most suitable single test.

Skin tests of delayed cutaneous hypersensitivity have been the method utilized most widely to assess the effects of nutritional depletion on cellular immunity. Protein-calorie malnutrition impairs delayed cutaneous hypersensitivity under certain circumstances.

Severe depression may occur in children with conditions resembling kwashiorkor and moderate depression in those with kwashiorkor-marasmus. No depression has been seen in patients with marasmus alone.

The data for adults are more difficult to interpret, because mixed patient groups have often been used and many of the study patients had coexisting conditions that in themselves could cause anergy. For example, in one study of cancer patients receiving total parenteral nutrition, 57 per cent converted from

DCH-negative to DCH-positive, but 28 per cent converted from DCH-positive to DCH-negative, presumably because of the effects of associated conditions. The variable results reported by others also suggest that skin testing is of borderline usefulness in assessing the effect of parenteral nutrition on restoration of optimal nutritional status.

In summary, the use of DCH as a means of assessing the effect of malnutrition on immune competence has the following drawbacks:

1. Anergy can be produced by a multitude of conditions, including uremia, liver disease and infection, which are often present simultaneously with nutritional deprivation.

2. The test itself assesses a very complex immune mechanism that often does not respond optimally even in healthy individuals.

3. When an actual immune dysfunction is detected, it is most likely in the accessory cell population. Accessory cells include macrophages and polymorphonuclear leukocytes that participate in the induction of immune mechanisms. Better techniques are available that specifically assess function of such accessory cells.

4. The techniques for accurate determination of anergy require either injection of multiple antigens or recall testing with DNCB. These procedures may not be feasible in many patients.

5. Impaired DCH testing may be due to low concentration of some trace element, such as zinc, at the skin site rather than to systemic depletion of protein.

6. The restoration of DCH response does not appear to be related to restoration of other metabolic parameters following nutritional therapy.

Finally, it seems that the basic immune mechanisms of blastogenesis, antibody production, and cell-mediated cytotoxicity have a high metabolic priority. Impairment occurs only with the most severe protein-calorie malnutrition syndromes. Significant reduction of serum albumin and transferrin is often present in the face of normal immunoglobulin levels, normal T- and B-cell levels, normal blastogenic response, and even normal DCH. Measurement of prime immunologic-lymphocyte function may be a poor way to determine whether nutritional support should be instituted.

NUTRITIONAL ASSESSMENT PROTOCOLS

A dietary history and physical examination can usually identify severe malnutrition. However, additional objective measurements of nutritional status are often necessary in order to diagnose moderate degrees of protein-calorie or isolated protein malnutrition. Although the objective measurements are epidemiologically useful and may correlate with morbidity and mortality, no single measurement is of consistent value in individual patients. Therefore, the nutritional assessment usually consists of a battery of tests, anthropometric measurements, and historic information.

TABLE 1-9. SAMPLE NUTRITIONAL ASSESSMENT PROFILE

I **Suggestive Physical Signs**

General Appearance: Thin ____ Well-Nourished ____ Obese _____

Edematous ____ Other _____

II **Anthropometircs**   Date _____   Date _____

MEASUREMENTS	Actual	Percentile	Actual	Percentile
Height for Age (cm)	____	____	____	____
Weight for Age (kg)	____	____	____	____
Weight for Height (kg)	____	____	____	____
Head Circumference (cm)	____	____	____	____
Midarm Circumference (mm)	____	____	____	____
Triceps Skinfold (mm)	____	____	____	____
CALCULATED VALUES				
Arm-Muscle Circumference (sq cm)	____	____	____	____

III **Laboratory Data**

	Actual	Percentile	Actual	Percentile
Serum Total Protein (g/dl)	____	____	____	____
Serum Albumin (g/dl)	____	____	____	____
Hemoglobin (g/dl)	____	____	____	____
Hematocrit (%)	____	____	____	____
TIBC (mcg/dl)	____	____	____	____
Serum Transferrin (mg/dl) (derived)	____	____	____	____
24 hr Urinary Creatinine (mg)	____	____	____	____
Total Lymphocyte Count	____	____	____	____

IV **Diet History** _____

_____

_____

V **Skin Tests** _____

_____

_____

VI **Assessment(s)** _____

_____

_____

_____

NUTRITIONIST _____

The following components are often included in the nutritional assessment profile (see Table 1-9).

A. History and Physical Examination
B. Evaluation of Height and Weight
    1. Height
    2. Weight
    3. Height for Age
    4. Weight for Age
    5. Weight for Height
    6. Relative Body Weight $= \dfrac{\text{Actual Weight}}{\text{Ideal Body Weight}} \times 100$

C. Estimation of Muscle Mass and Fat Stores (Anthropometric Measurements)
   1. Head Circumference (preschool children only)
   2. Midarm Circumference
   3. Triceps Skinfold Thickness
   4. Arm Muscle Circumference
D. Lean Body Mass—Creatinine-Height Index Corrected for Age
E. Visceral Protein Status
   1. Serum Albumin
   2. Serum Transferrin
F. Immune Function
   1. Total Lymphocyte Count
   2. Delayed Cutaneous Hypersensitivity Testing

On the basis of these variables, malnutrition has been classified into two general categories. Marasmus, a form of protein-calorie malnutrition, is characterized by depression of anthropometric measurements, decreased weight for height, and decreased creatinine-height index. These abnormalities reflect decreased lean body mass and fat stores. Visceral protein function, total lymphocyte counts, and delayed cutaneous hypersensitivity are within normal limits. A kwashiorkor-like syndrome is caused primarily by isolated protein deficiency. These patients may have depleted visceral protein synthesis and total lymphocyte count and impaired delayed cutaneous hypersensitivity. Lean body mass and fat stores may be relatively normal as is weight for height. Stress of any type results in increased morbidity and mortality in these patients. These two conditions commonly coexist in malnourished patients. In children, reasonable criteria for nutritional support have been suggested on the basis of these classifications (see Table 1–10).

TABLE 1–10.   INDICATIONS FOR NUTRITIONAL SUPPORT IN CHILDREN

Patients for Whom Nutritional Therapy Should Be a High Priority

Presence of any of the following:
1. Serum albumin <2.5 g/dl and transferrin <100 mg/dl (after 6 months of age)
2. Lymphocyte count <1000/mm³ (exclusive of patients on chemotherapy or radiation therapy)
3. Negative skin tests (beyond infancy, exclusive of patients on steroids)
4. Weight, height >2SD below median or <80% of standard (median)
5. Arm-muscle area <5th percentile
6. Creatinine-height index <60% standard

Patients Who Require at Least Maintenance Support and Continued Monitoring*

Presence of any of the following:
1. Weight, height >2SD below median or <80% of standard (median)
2. Arm-muscle area <5th percentile
3. Creatinine-height index <80% of standard
4. Serum albumin <3 g/dl or transferrin <150 mg/dl
5. Lymphocyte count <1500/mm³

*In the presence of sepsis or major injury, these patients should be placed in the high-priority group.
From Merritt, R. J.: Nutritional assessment and metabolic response to illness of the hospitalized child. *In* Suskind, R.M. (Ed.): Textbook of Pediatric Nutrition. New York, Raven Press, 1981.

CONCLUSION

This section not only has described the variety of methods and procedures presently used for nutritional assessment but also has detailed many of the difficulties encountered in their interpretation. No standard, validated procedures for the evaluation of nutritional status are applicable to all situations. Consequently, a number of measurements and laboratory tests are often added to the information obtained by history and physical examination. Although these data may be helpful in reaching practical clinical decisions, it is important to recognize that nutritional assessment presently remains inexact even when much information has been gathered.

Vegetarian Diets

Gloria Elfert, M.S., R.D.

INTRODUCTION

Traditional vegetarianism—followed either because of a limited supply of animal foods or adherence to religious or cultural principles—is practiced by only a small proportion of those who follow vegetarian diets in this country. Most vegetarians today are young adults who adhere to this dietary regimen for a variety of reasons, including health concerns, ethics, metaphysics, ecologic or political considerations, or simply preference. Although frequently differing in specific dietary practices and other attitudes, most vegetarians believe that purification of body and soul can occur through a lifestyle with vegetarianism as its essential element.

The most common vegetarian diets are

1. Vegan: Only foods of plant origin are allowed.
2. Lacto-vegetarian: Foods of plant origin as well as dairy products are permitted.
3. Lacto-ovo-vegetarian: Foods of plant origin and both eggs and dairy products are permitted.
4. New vegetarian: Avoidance of animal foods is required at least to some degree. Foods not considered "organic" or "natural" may be prohibited.

With each of these diets, the probability of meeting essential nutritional requirements increases as a wider variety of foods is ingested.

THE VEGAN DIET

ADEQUACY.   The vegan diet can be nutritionally adequate if it is planned with care. Some knowledge of nutrition and food composition is necessary to select plant foods that will supply all necessary nutrients in adequate amounts. Generally, inadequate diets are characterized by caloric deficiency, extreme limitation of variety, and excessive dependence on staples such as low-protein, starchy roots, tubers, and refined cereals.

CALORIES.   An adequate caloric intake is essential to prevent breakdown of body protein to meet energy requirements. Since most vegetarian diets are high in bulk, caloric needs may be difficult to meet, particularly in infants and children.

PROTEIN

Quantitative Considerations.   Vegans can easily ingest sufficient protein to satisfy the RDA for a normal adult of 0.8 g/kg of body weight.

Qualitative Considerations.   The essential amino acid content of a protein food determines its biologic value. Protein from animal sources is generally of high biologic value, containing the known essential amino acids in adequate proportions and in a utilizable form. Although many plant proteins are deficient in one or more of the essential amino acids, certain combinations of plant proteins can provide the essential amino acids necessary for growth and maintenance of life; such combinations are termed *complementary proteins.* For maximal utilization and benefit, complementary foods should be eaten together, at the same meal, since there are no reserves of amino acids that can be drawn upon (see Table 1-11).

The following example illustrates the way in which plant proteins can complement one another. Cereal proteins are high in methionine and relatively low in lysine, both essential amino acids. Legumes, such as dried beans and peas, contain ample amounts of lysine but are low in methionine. When cereal and legume proteins are eaten together, the methionine provided by the cereal grains and the lysine from the legumes improve the amino acid balance. The

TABLE 1–11.   COMPLEMENTARY AMINO ACID COMPOSITION OF SOME FOODS

Essential Amino Acids	Cheese Eggs Milk Meat	Corn	Cereal	Legumes	Whole Grains (with germ) Nuts	Seed Oils Soybeans	Sesame and Sunflower Seeds	Peanut Protein	Green Leafy Vegetable Protein	Gelatin	Yeast
Methionine	B	B	H	L	H	L	H	L	L	L	H
Isoleucine	H	B	B	B	B	B	B	B	B	B	B
Leucine	H	B	B	B	B	B	B	B	B	B	B
Lysine	H	L	L	H	H	H	L	L	B	L	B
Phenylalanine	B	B	B	B	B	B	B	B	B	B	L
Threonine	H	L	L	H	L	H	B	L	B	B	H
Tryptophan	B	L	B	L	B	B	H	B	B	L	B
Valine	H	B	B	B	B	B	B	B	B	B	B

H—Amino acid present in a high proportion in relation to other essential amino acids.
B—Amino acid present in a balanced proportion in relation to other essential amino acids.
L—Amino acid present in low proportion in relation to other essential amino acids.
Note: Be sure to complement a low–amino acid food with a food high in that amino acid at the same meal.
Adapted from Erhart, D.: Nutrition education for the now generation. J Nutr Educ 3:135–139, 1971.

combination of these two types of proteins results in protein of better quality than that provided by either food alone. Thus, through the judicious selection of plant protein combinations, their biologic nutritional value can be equivalent to that of high-quality animal protein foods.

FAT.   The vegan diet is low in cholesterol and saturated fats. The ratio of polyunsaturated fat to saturated fat in this diet tends to be higher than in diets containing animal protein.

MINERALS

Calcium.   The inclusion of 2 cups of fortified soybean milk per day will meet the adult daily calcium requirement. Although green leafy vegetables have essentially the same calcium content as milk, the absorption of calcium from plant sources may be inefficient. Other plant sources high in calcium include cabbage, broccoli, cauliflower, almonds, molasses, legumes (especially soybeans), and dried fruits.

Iron.   Heme iron is found only in animal foods. The bio-availability of nonheme iron in foods is generally less than that of heme iron and depends upon many factors, including the presence of ascorbic acid, which enhances absorption, in the meal (see Chapter 9, section on iron). Good sources of iron in foods permitted on a vegan diet include legumes, whole or enriched grain products, dark-green leafy vegetables, winter squash, and sweet potatoes. Iron-fortified soybean milk or an iron supplement may be used as well.

Iodine.   Deficiencies may occur in areas where the soil contains relatively little iodine. Iodized salt should be used.

Zinc and Copper.   Foods containing high concentrations of zinc and copper include legumes, soy products, whole grains and cereals, nuts, seeds, and sprouts. The bio-availability of these minerals may be adversely affected by the high fiber content of the diet. Soy protein products, such as tofu, are rich in zinc and copper and are low in fiber.

VITAMINS

With the possible exception of vitamin B_{12}, vegan diets utilizing a variety of foods provide the essential vitamins in adequate amounts. In order to prevent a possible deficiency of vitamin B_{12}, fortified meat substitutes or a vitamin supplement should be used.

VEGETARIANS AT SPECIAL RISK

PREGNANT AND LACTATING WOMEN.   Lacto-ovo-vegetarian diets usually provide adequate amounts of all the nutrients required by the pregnant or lactating woman; however, iron and folate supplementation is often necessary. On the other hand, the iron and folate intake of pregnant vegans is often considerably higher than that of pregnant omnivores owing to their high intake of legumes. Zinc intake may be below normal if foods low in zinc, such as fruits and vegetables, are used excessively. Increased consumption of zinc-rich foods such as legumes or soy protein products that are low in fiber, will help ensure adequate intake in a bio-available form.

INFANTS AND CHILDREN.   Vegan diets for the pediatric age group require careful planning to meet the energy, nitrogen, and essential amino acid requirements of a growing child. Lacto-ovo-vegetarian and lacto-vegetarian diets usually meet all growth requirements. However, iron deficiency is possible when milk products are used excessively because of the low iron content of milk compared with other foods. Vitamin D, vitamin B_{12}, and riboflavin may be inadequate in poorly planned vegan diets. Fortified soy milk supplements will help ensure an adequate intake of these vitamins and essential amino acids.

ADULT VEGETARIANS WITH SPECIAL HEALTH PROBLEMS

Lactose intolerance need not present a problem to the lacto-vegetarian. Lact-aid added to milk hydrolyzes lactose and prevents the untoward side effects of lactose ingestion. Lactose-free soy milks are available. Cheese is well tolerated by most lactose-intolerant persons.

Diabetes mellitus presents no additional problem, since it is relatively easy to plan both vegan and lacto-vegetarian diets that are nutritionally adequate.

Kosher Dietary Laws

Gloria Elfert, M.S., R.D.

INTRODUCTION

Familiarity with the basic principles of the kosher food laws is necessary in order to provide the best possible nutritional support to patients who follow these laws.

Observant Jews feel that the rules, which are known as kashruth and have been sacred since the time of Moses, are a means of self-purification and of service to God. The primary reason for adherence is the spiritual value of sanctification and self-discipline rather than the hygienic and ethical considerations often cited. The kosher dietary laws are based on Mosaic law and are specific with respect to the selection of types of meats and seafood and the modes of food preparation and service.

Orthodox Jews strictly adhere to the dietary laws listed here, which are based on biblical and rabbinical regulations. Conservative Jews follow the laws nominally but make a distinction between foods eaten at home and away from home. Reformed Jews place less emphasis on the ceremonial aspects and minimize the significance of the dietary laws.

Permitted Foods

1. Meats from quadrupeds that have cloven hooves and chew a cud (cows, sheep, goats, deer)
2. All poultry
(Note: All meats and poultry must be freshly slaughtered according to accepted ritual and soaked in salted water to remove all traces of blood.)
3. Fish with fins and scales

Prohibited Foods

1. All shellfish and eels
2. Pork in all forms, including lard and bacon

In planning meals for patients who follow the kosher dietary laws, these points must be considered:

1. Dairy and meat products are not eaten at the same meal. Milk or milk products may be taken just *before* a meal; however, there must be a 6-hour delay in taking dairy products *after* a meal that included meat.
2. "Pareve" foods are neutral foods, neither dairy nor meat products, which may be taken at any time and with any type of meal. These foods include fruits, vegetables, eggs, and fish.
3. Packaged, canned, and frozen products with the codes K and U are allowed. (K means the product is ritually fit for use according to liberal kosher law; U means that it has been approved by the Union of Orthodox Rabbis.)
4. Only unleavened products may be used during Passover. Utensils and dishes that have had contact with leavened products may not be used during this period.
5. Separate dishes and utensils are usually used for dairy and meat meals. For institutions without a kosher kitchen, single-service disposable dishes and utensils may be used. Prepackaged frozen kosher meals are also available.

Normal Pediatric Nutrition

Sylvia V. McAdoo, M.S., R.D. and
William C. MacLean, Jr., M.D.

INTRODUCTION

This section concentrates on guidelines for feeding normal infants and children but also includes information useful in specific therapeutic situations. The

TABLE 1–12.   SAMPLE HOSPITAL MEAL PATTERNS
FOR CHILDREN OF VARIOUS AGES

Foods	0.5–1 yr	1–3 yrs	4–6 yrs	7–10 yrs	11–14 yrs FEMALE	11–14 yrs MALE	15–18 yrs FEMALE	15–18 yrs MALE
Breakfast								
Fruit or juice	½ cup	½ cup	1 cup	1 cup	1 cup	1 cup	1 cup	1 cup
Cereal	½ cup	½ cup	½ cup	½ cup	½ cup	½ cup	½ cup	½ cup
Toast (slice)		1	1	2	2	2	1	2
Egg or exchange	½ oz	½ oz	1 oz	1 oz	1 oz	1 oz	1 oz	1 oz
Margarine	½ oz	1 oz	1 oz	2 oz	2 oz	2 oz	2 oz	2 oz
Milk		8 oz	8 oz	8 oz	8 oz	8 oz	8 oz	8 oz
Breast milk or formula	7 oz							
Noon meal								
Meat or exchange	½ oz	1 oz	1 oz	1½ oz	2 oz	2 oz	2 oz	2 oz
Vegetable		½ cup	½ cup	½ cup	½ cup	½ cup	½ cup	½ cup
Bread (slice) or exchange	1	1	2	3	3	4	3	4
Margarine		1 oz	1 oz	2 oz	2 oz	2 oz	2 oz	3 oz
Fruit or juice	½ cup	½ cup	½ cup	½ cup	½ cup	½ cup	½ cup	½ cup
Milk		8 oz	8 oz	8 oz	8 oz	8 oz	8 oz	8 oz
Breast milk or formula	7 oz							
Midafternoon								
Fruit juice	½ cup	½ cup	1 cup	1 cup	1 cup	1 cup	1 cup	1 cup
Evening meal								
Meat or exchange		1 oz	2 oz	2 oz	2 oz	4 oz	2 oz	3 oz
Potato or exchange	½ cup	½ cup	½ cup	½ cup	1 cup	1½ cups	½ cup	2 cups
Vegetable or salad	½ cup	½ cup	½ cup	1 cup	1 cup	1 cup	1 cup	1 cup
Bread (slice)		1	1	2	2	2	2	2
Margarine	½ oz	1 oz	2 oz	2 oz	2 oz	2 oz	2 oz	2 oz
Fruit or juice	½ cup	½ cup	½ cup	1 cup	1 cup	1 cup	1 cup	1 cup
Milk		8 oz	8 oz	8 oz	8 oz	8 oz	8 oz	8 oz
Breast milk or formula	7 oz							
Evening snack								
Meat or exchange							1 oz	2 oz
Bread (slice) or exchange			1	1	2	2	1	2
Fruit or juice		½ cup	½ cup	1 cup	1 cup	1 cup	1 cup	1 cup
Milk								1 cup
Breast milk or formula	7 oz							

underlying philosophy is that most normal children will consume sufficient food to meet their requirements if they are presented with a nutritionally balanced diet appropriate for their age. Consequently, dietary allowance tables for various age groups should be used as general guidelines only. Some children may wish to consume more; this should not be discouraged unless the child is becoming obese. Other normally growing children may consume substantially less than the amounts suggested. No attempt should be made to increase intake simply in order to conform to a set of dietary standards.

Although sample meal plans are presented for various age groups (Table 1–12), the nutritional requirements of most children can be met through a variety of foods. The dietitian or physician should attempt to meet a child's nutritional needs with foods that are in accord with taste preferences and eating habits. The least nutritious diet is the one that is returned uneaten.

Tables for standard basal calorie expenditure (Table 1–13) and for water and electrolyte losses (Table 1–14) are provided primarily to assist in calculat-

TABLE 1–13.   STANDARD BASAL CALORIE EXPENDITURES OF CHILDREN*

	Calories/24 Hrs	
Weight (kg)	MALE AND FEMALE	
3	140	
5	270	
7	400	
9	500	
11	600	
13	650	
15	710	
17	780	
19	830	
21	880	
	MALE	FEMALE
25	1020	960
29	1120	1040
33	1210	1120
37	1300	1190
41	1350	1260
45	1410	1320
49	1470	1380
53	1530	1440
57	1590	1500
61	1640	1560

Increments or Decrements
1. Add or subtract 12% of above for each degree Celsius (8% for each degree Fahrenheit) above or below rectal temperature of 37.8°C (100°F).
2. 0–30% increments for activity.

*This table and Table 1–14 are used primarily to calculate intravenous alimentation regimens. In some instances, such as renal failure, they may be useful for the calculation of oral regimens as well.

TABLE 1–14.   WATER AND ELECTROLYTE LOSSES PER 100 CALORIES
METABOLIZED

	Range			Usual		
	WATER (ML)	SODIUM (MEQ)	POTASSIUM (MEQ)	WATER (ML)	SODIUM (MEQ)	POTASSIUM (MEQ)
Evaporative*						
Lungs	10–60			15		
Skin	20–100	0.1–3.0	0.2–1.5	40	0.1	0.2
Total	30–160	0.1–3.0	0.2–1.5	55	0.1	0.2
Stool*	0–50	0.1–0.4	0.2–3.0	5	0.1	0.2
Urine*	0–400	0.2–30.0	0.4–30.0	65	3.0	2.0

*High values may also be considered to represent abnormal losses.

ing requirements for partial or complete parenteral alimentation. Under certain circumstances, such as chronic renal failure, the tables also may be useful for calculating oral intake.

INFANT NUTRITION

Breast Feeding

Human milk has supported newborns for centuries and is the optimal food for the normal full-term infant. The decision to breast feed an infant is, however, a personal one. Women should not be coerced to nurse their infants, since adequate nutrition can be provided through formula feeding. If possible, the question of whether to breast feed should be decided on prior to delivery. Table 1–15 shows various feeding alternatives in infancy.

Successful breast feeding, especially of a first child, is aided by a supportive atmosphere in the nursery setting. The new mother must have a comfortable, quiet place where she can spend uninterrupted time with her infant. Nursing may be started as soon as conditions of the mother and infant are stable. Feedings may be given either on demand or on a schedule of every 3 to 4 hours. Some studies suggest that mothers who nurse on demand initially tend to breast feed more successfully than those who try to schedule their feedings rigidly. In either case, most infants will evolve naturally into a schedule of feedings every 3 to 4 hours after they reach 3 to 4 weeks of age.

Supplementary feedings are usually indicated only if additional fluids or calories are required for conditions such as hypoglycemia or neonatal jaundice. A slower rate of weight gain, especially during the first 7 to 10 days of life, should be expected for breast-fed infants and is not an indication for supplementary feedings. In addition, breast-fed infants normally require a longer period of time to double their birth weight than do bottle-fed infants. It is not unusual for the breast-fed infant to gain weight at a slower rate during the first 4 to 6 months. If weight gain and linear growth are steady and the infant is satisfied, supplementary foods need not be offered.

Formula Feeding

Full-term infants who are healthy and growing normally vary considerably in their caloric and protein requirements. During the first several weeks of life, infants fed *ad libitum* consume 80 to 140 kcal/kg of body weight/day (120 to 210 cc of standard formula/kg/day). The range of normal intake narrows over the next 3 months. At 4 months of age, intake normally varies from 80 to 110 kcal/kg/day (120 to 155 cc of standard formula/kg/day). If allowed, most infants will regulate their intake to meet their needs. This process occurs naturally when the infant is breast fed but is more difficult to achieve with bottle feeding.

We suggest beginning with 90 to 120 cc (3 to 4 ounces) of formula per feeding, every 3 to 4 hours, depending on the child's apparent needs. Not all infants will consume the same amount at each feeding. Once the infant takes the amount offered at the majority of feedings, an additional 15 cc ($\frac{1}{2}$ ounce) can be added to each bottle. The infant should not be forced to finish this amount but should be allowed to take it spontaneously as desired. When this new intake is finished regularly at each feeding, the quantity offered may again be increased by 15 cc. In this way, the infant is allowed to regulate his own intake. The best test of the adequacy of intake is the rate of gain in weight and length of the growing child.

Initiation of Feedings

STERILE WATER.   Sterile water is generally given as the first feeding for all infants who are to be bottle fed. There is no uniformity of opinion concerning whether all breast-fed infants should have an initial feeding with sterile water.

The first feeding, usually by nursery personnel, is given within the first 4 hours after birth. Hungry infants may have sterile water whenever they awaken. An infant should always be offered some water during the first 24 hours; the physician is notified if this has not been possible.

If respiratory distress occurs during or following any feeding, withhold the next feeding and notify the physician.

Water feedings are given as follows:

1. Offer 30 cc sterile water.
2. If regurgitation or vomiting occurs during or following the first feeding —and there is no respiratory distress—give a second feeding of sterile water in 4 hours.
3. If regurgitation or vomiting occurs during or following the second feeding—and there is no respiratory distress—give a third feeding of sterile water in 4 hours.
4. Notify the physician if regurgitation or vomiting occurs during or after the third feeding of sterile water.

BREAST-FED INFANTS.   The infant to be breast fed may be brought to the mother when the conditions of both infant and mother are stable.

TABLE 1–15. ORAL FEEDING ALTERNATIVES IN INFANCY

Formula	Producer	Calories		Protein			Carbohydrate			Fat		
		per oz	per ml	GM/dl	Type	%CAL	GM/dl	Type	%CAL	GM/dl	Type	%CAL
Breast milk	—	22	0.71	1.1	Human	6	6.8	Lactose	38	3.8	Human	56
Goat milk	Meyenberg Brand	20	0.67	3.2	Goat	19	4.6	Lactose	27	4.0	Butter fat	53.6
Cow's milk	—	20	0.67	3.3	Bovine	19	5.0	Lactose	29	4.0	Butter	52
Advance	RL	16	0.54	2.0	Cow's milk with soy protein isolate	15	5.5	Corn syrup and lactose	40	2.7	Soy and corn oil	45
Similac with iron	RL	20	0.68	1.50	Cow's milk	9	7.2	Lactose	43	3.6	Soy and coconut oil	48
Enfamil with iron	MJ	20	0.68	1.5	Cow's milk/whey	9	6.9	Lactose	41	3.8	Coconut and soy oil	50
PM 60/40 "as fed"	RL	20	0.68	1.58	Whey/casein	9	6.9	Lactose	44	3.8	Coconut and corn oil	50
SMA 20	W	20	0.68	1.5	Cow's milk/whey	9	7.2	Lactose	43	3.6	Oleo and coconut, safflower, soy and bean oil	48
Isomil	RL	20	0.68	2.0	Soy protein isolate	12	6.8	Corn syrup and sucrose	41	3.6	Soy and coconut oil	48
Nursoy	W	20	0.68	2.1	Soy protein isolate	13	6.9	Sucrose	40	3.6	Oleo, coconut, safflower, and soy oil	48

Product	Source				Protein			Carbohydrate			Fat	
Prosobee	MJ	20	0.68	2.0	Soy protein isolate	12	6.9	Corn syrup solids	40	3.6	Soy and coconut oil	48
RCF	RL	*	*	2.0	Soy protein isolate	20	0*	*	0	3.6	Soy and coconut oil	80
Portagen	MJ	20	0.67	2.4	Sodium caseinate	14	7.8	Corn syrup solids, sucrose	44	3.2	MCT oil, 88%, corn oil, 12%	42
Pregestimil	MJ	20	0.68	1.9	Casein hydrolysate with added amino acids	11	9.1	Corn syrup solids, modified tapioca starch	54	2.7	Corn oil 60% MCT 40%	35
Nutramigen	MJ	20	0.68	2.2	Casein hydrolysate	13	8.8	Sucrose, modified tapioca starch	35	2.6	Corn oil	52
Enfamil Premature†	MJ	24	0.81	2.4	Demineralized whey and cow's milk	12	8.9	Corn syrup solids, lactose	44	4.1	MCT, corn and coconut oil	44
Similac LBW	RL	24	0.81	2.2	Cow's milk	11	8.5	Lactose	43	4.5	MCT, coconut, and soy oil	47
Similac Special Care†	RL	24	0.81	2.2	Demineralized whey and cow's milk	11	8.6	Lactose and glucose polymers	42	4.4	MCT, corn and coconut oil	47

RL = Ross Lab
MJ = Mead Johnson Products
W = Wyeth Lab
* = Varies depending on quantity of carbohydrate and water used.
†Also available at 20 cal/oz (0.68 cal/ml) dilution.
From Fomon, S.J.: Infant Nutrition, 2nd Ed. Philadelphia, W.B. Saunders Co., 1974, pp. 362–363.

Feedings are given "on demand" at routine clinical feeding times or by physician's order after the first water feeding (if one has been given) has been tolerated. The mother then may feed the infant on all occasions when it is clinically acceptable.

Although the infant may have supplementary feedings after each breast feeding, such feedings are not usually necessary.

FORMULA-FED INFANTS.   Formula feeding is started after the physician's order is written and after one sterile water feeding has been tolerated without regurgitation, vomiting, or respiratory distress.

Feedings are given "on demand," scheduled approximately every 4 hours, generally at 10 AM, 2 PM, 6 PM, 10 PM, 2 AM, and 6 AM. The infant may be brought to the mother for all feedings. However, the 2 AM and 6 AM feedings are often given in the nursery by nursing personnel if the infant is not staying in the mother's room.

Formula feedings are given as follows:

1. Give 90 cc of prescribed formula for the first feeding. No additional formula may be given with this feeding.
2. Subsequent feedings consist of 90 to 120 cc of prescribed formula. If the infant appears hungry, an additional 15 cc of formula may be given.

True formula intolerance is very rare at this age. Feeding problems usually reflect immaturity of the infant's intestinal tract rather than a reaction to an individual formula.

Formula Supplementation: Birth to One Year

Human milk or infant formula is nutritionally adequate for the growing infant for a period of at least 6 to 9 months. Although solid foods are frequently added to the infant's diet much earlier in life, there is a trend toward a later introduction of these foods because of the increasing concern about childhood and adult obesity.

The reflex protrusion of the infant's tongue during the first 3 to 4 months makes it difficult to feed solids at this time. By the age of 5 or 6 months, the child has good head control and is more capable of participation in the feeding of solids. There is no reason to recommend the introduction of solid foods earlier than 6 months in a healthy and growing infant who is consuming exclusively human milk or infant formula. Regardless of when solid foods are introduced, human milk or some sort of infant formula should be continued through 9 to 12 months of age.

An infant cereal such as rice or barley is most commonly the first solid food added to the diet. Many physicians and dietitians find that mothers make this addition spontaneously and without consultation. Strained fruits and vegetables are usually added then; meat is frequently the next food group given. This order of introduction of solids is based on custom rather than on nutritional principles. Perhaps the most important rules to follow are to add foods one at a time and not to add a new food until the child's tolerance to the prior item is verified for a period of several days.

The time for introduction of egg yolk is a matter of controversy. Some pediatricians suggest 3 months of age, while others advise waiting until the infant is closer to 1 year old. Egg white is often not fed before 1 year of age because of its alleged hyperallergenic tendency; this too is controversial.

When the infant tolerates a variety of solid foods during the second 6 months of life, the diet can be advanced from strained to junior foods and finally to table foods. This progression is best determined on an individual basis, depending on the presence or absence of teeth and the child's likes and dislikes.

The sodium content of commercially prepared baby foods was previously quite high. In the last few years, however, the major manufacturers have stopped using salt and sodium additives in the processing of these foods. Some studies have actually shown that the sodium content of homemade infant foods exceeds that of those currently on the market. Mothers who wish to prepare their own baby foods should be encouraged not to add salt during preparation.

Sugar was also frequently added to commercial baby foods. Depending on the manufacturer, added sugar has either been reduced considerably or omitted completely from baby foods.

Regular Infant Diet

This diet reflects nutritional requirements for children between approximately 6 and 12 months of age (see Table 1–16). Requirements are based on RDAs Appendix, but many infants will eat considerably less than these

Text continued on page 47

TABLE 1–16.   APPROXIMATE ALLOWANCES, 6–12 MONTHS OF AGE

Energy	80–135 kcal/kg
Protein[1]	8–15% of energy intake
Fat	35–50% of energy intake
Carbohydrate	35–50% of energy intake
Calcium[2]	350–500 mg
Phosphorus[2]	240–400 mg
Sodium[3]	46–69 mg (2–3 mEq) per kg
Potassium[3]	117–156 mg (3–4 mEq) per kg

[1]Protein requirements for infants and children are based on total energy intake. The requirement for protein is expressed as a percentage of total energy intake. The following formula is used to calculate the number of grams of protein required:

$$\text{Protein requirement (g)} = \frac{\text{Percentage of energy as protein} \times \text{Energy intake (kcal)}}{4 \text{ kcal/g}}$$

The distribution of fat and carbohydrate has been expressed as percentages of total energy intake. The grams of carbohydrate are calculated with the same formula as for protein, while 9 kcal/g is used as the denominator in calculating grams of fat.

[2]Calcium and phosphorus requirements are linked. The ratio of the two nutrients in the diet may be as important as the absolute amount.

[3]Requirements for sodium and potassium are generally met by any diet. When clinical situations dictate an alteration of sodium or potassium intake, a reduction of intake is usually necessary.

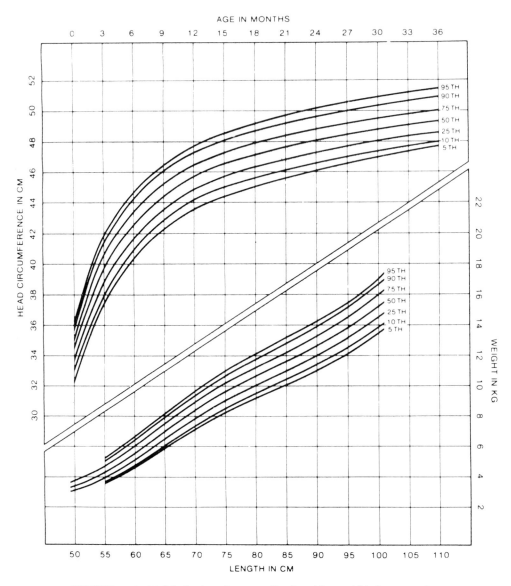

FIGURE 1–8A. Weight by length percentiles for girls aged birth-36 months.

FIGURE 1–8. continues on following page

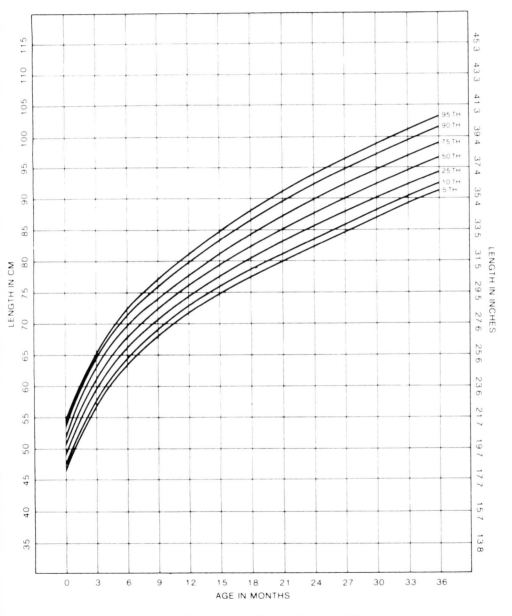

FIGURE 1–8B. Length by age percentiles for boys aged birth-36 months.

FIGURE 1–8. continues on following page

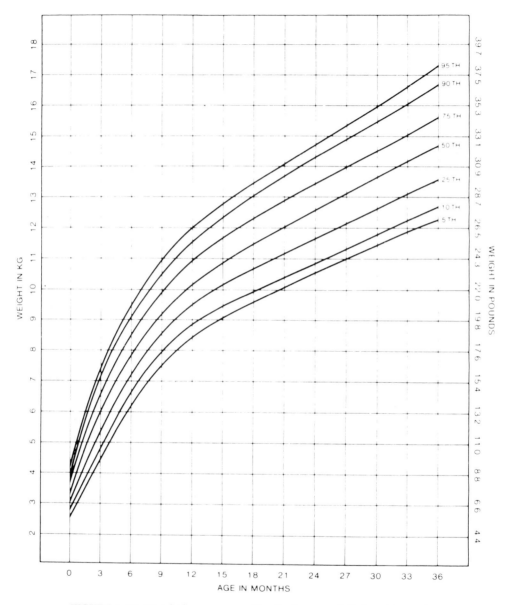

FIGURE 1–8C. Weight by age percentiles for boys aged birth to 36 months.

amounts. If growth is steady and adequate, their intake should be considered sufficient. Whenever possible, the diet should be adapted to the child's eating habits at home.

Formula Alterations

Increasing numbers of infants with malabsorption, short-gut syndrome, and so forth are being fed formulas altered by the addition of medium-chain triglycerides, glucose polymers, or other sources of nonprotein energy. These alterations are frequently made to increase the energy density of the formula without increasing the protein intake, or to provide a more readily absorbed diet as for infants with steatorrhea.

Such additions can present problems for physicians and dietitians unfamiliar with the calculation of infant diets. The desirable energy distributions for these formula alterations are protein, 9 to 16 per cent of energy; fat, 30 to 55 per cent; and the remainder from carbohydrate. The following guidelines are helpful in these calculations:

1. Most proprietary formulas supply between 9 and 16 per cent of energy as protein. When adding nonprotein calories (carbohydrate or fat), the proportion of calories supplied by protein should never be reduced to less than 6 per cent. Even this level is inadequate for some infants, especially premature ones.

2. When formulas provide a high percentage (85 per cent) of their fat as medium-chain triglycerides, at least 6 per cent of the total energy intake should consist of long-chain triglycerides. This will ensure that at least 3 per cent of total calorie intake is supplied by essential fatty acids.

3. The requirements for most vitamins are tied to the intake of proteins and calories. The consumption of "unaltered" proprietary formulas provides sufficient vitamins to meet RDAs. When large amounts of additional calories are included, the vitamin content of the formula may be insufficient to meet needs. In these cases, vitamin supplements should be added. Similarly, substantial alterations in the formula may require the addition of minerals to ensure the adequacy of their final concentrations.

4. Some elemental formulas may present an excessive osmotic load to the gastrointestinal tract and thus may serve as one of many factors associated with the development of necrotizing enterocolitis in the newborn. Formulas with higher osmotic loads may cause loose stools. For these reasons, we prefer formulas with an osmotic load of less than 450 mOsm/l.

5. *Renal solute load* is the collective term for solutes that must be excreted in the urine (nitrogenous substances and electrolytes). Dietary carbohydrates and fat do not contribute to renal solute. The amount of water obligated to excrete renal solutes becomes important when fluid intake is relatively low, extrarenal water losses are excessive, renal concentrating ability is decreased, or renal solute in the diet is excessive. Several of these conditions are often present concurrently in ill or low-birth-weight infants. Generally, water balance is adequate if urine specific gravity is less than 1.010 to 1.015. The renal solute loads (RSL) for many of the commonly used infant formulas are presented in Table 1–17.

TABLE 1-17. COMPOSITION OF HUMAN MILK AND INFANT FORMULAS

	Producer	Energy kcal/l	Protein g/l	CHO g/l	FAT g/l	Na mEq/l	K mEq/l	Ca mg/l	P mg/l	Iron mg/l	E:PUFA	RSL mOsm/l	Osmolality mOsm/kg
Human milk	—	710	11	68	38	7	13	333	133	1.5	0.7:1	75	300
Cow's milk	—	670	33	48	37	25	35	1200	946	1	0.1:2.1	220	270
Advance	RL	540	20	55	27	10	23	510	390	12	0.9:1	128	209
Similac PM 60/40–20	RL	680	16	69	38	7	15	400	200	1.5	1.3:1	96	260
Similac 20 w/iron	RL	680	15	72	36	10	21	510	390	12	1.0:1	105	290
Enfamil 20 w/iron	MJ	680	15	69	38	9	8	460	320	12	1.4:1	99	300
SMA 20	W	680	15	72	36	7	14	440	330	12	1.3:1	92	300
Isomil	RL	680	20	68	36	14	20	700	500	12	1.0:1	131	250
Nursoy	W	680	21	69	36	9	19	630	440	13	1.3:1	123	268
ProSobee	MJ	680	20	69	36	13	21	630	500	13	0.4:1	130	200
RCF*	RL	404	20	0	36	13	18	700	500	1.5	1.0:1	126	63
Pregestimil	MJ	680	19	91	27	14	18	630	420	13	1.6:1	122	348
Nutramigen	MJ	680	22	88	26	14	17	630	470	13	0.7:1	131	479
Portagen	MJ	680	24	78	32	14	22	630	470	13	9.8:1	146	158
Enfamil Premature Formula	MJ	680	20	74	34	12	19	790	400	1.1	1.1:1	128	244
Similac 24 LBW	RL	810	22	85	45	16	31	730	560	3	2.0:1	161	290
Similac Special/Care	RL	680	18	72	37	13	24	1200	600	3	2.5:1	128	250

RL = Ross Lab
MJ = Mead Johnson Products
W = Wyeth Lab
*This product should only be used with a carbohydrate source added.
From Fomon, S.J.: Infant Nutrition. 2nd Ed. Philadelphia, W.B. Saunders Co., 1974, pp. 362–363.

$$E:Pufa = \frac{\text{d-alpha tocopherol (mg)}}{\text{polyunsaturated fatty acids (g)}}$$

R.S.L. = estimated potential renal solute load = [Proteins (g) × 4] + [Na(mEq) + k(mEq) + Cl(mEq)]

Vitamin and Mineral Supplementation

Breast-fed infants are usually supplemented with vitamins A, C, and D, but only vitamin D supplementation is probably essential. Although infant skin can synthesize vitamin D in response to ultraviolet radiation, this source cannot be relied upon as adequate.

Human milk has a low iron content, but its high bio-availability fosters absorption of almost half of the iron ingested. For this reason, routine supplementation with iron is not recommended for exclusively breast-fed infants. Iron stores, plus the amount absorbed from human milk, are adequate until other foods are added to the diet in the second 6 months of life.

Fluoride consumed by nursing mothers is not present in any significant quantity in human milk. For this reason, all breast-fed infants should get routine supplements of fluoride. The supplemental fluoride dosage schedule is identical to that listed in Table 1–18 for a concentration of fluoride in drinking water less than 0.3 ppm.

Most formula-fed infants consume commercial, modified cow's milk formulas that contain adequate amounts of all vitamins and most minerals. Formulas supplemented with iron are generally in use and are recommended; if the formula intake satisfies the infant's requirements for energy and protein, iron needs will also be met. Fluoride supplementation may still be necessary, depending upon the fluoride concentration of the water used to prepare the formula (see Table 1–18).

Formulas based on evaporated milk are still used by some mothers; when prepared properly they provide good nutrition. Most milk sold in this country is fortified with vitamins A and D. Vitamin C supplementation is necessary when evaporated milk formulas are fed. Although the iron content of cow's milk is the same as that of human milk (about 0.5 mg/l), the low bio-availability of the iron in cow's milk makes it necessary to provide an additional source of iron for these infants. Again, the need for fluoride supplementation depends upon the fluoride content of the water used in formula preparation.

TABLE 1–18.   SUPPLEMENTAL FLUORIDE DOSAGE SCHEDULE (MG/DAY[1])

Age	Concentration of Fluoride in Drinking Water (ppm)		
	<0.3	0.3–0.7	>0.7
Under 2 wks	0	0	0
2 wks–2 yrs	0.25	0	0
2–3 yrs	0.50	0.25	0
3–16 yrs	1.00	0.50	0

[1]2.2 mg sodium fluoride contains 1 mg fluoride.
Note: The level of fluoride in water of large cities is adequate. Fluoride supplementation may be necessary with small town drinking water or if well water is used.
From: Pediatrics 63:150, 1979.

Nutrition During Pregnancy and Lactation

David M. Paige, M.D.

INTRODUCTION

Maternal nutrition may have a critical influence on the course and outcome of pregnancy. A well-balanced diet that includes ample increments in calories, protein, calcium, phosphorus, and other nutrients is recommended. The possible need for supplementary iron and folate should be considered in all pregnant women. Additional nutritional considerations may develop during pregnancy in teenagers and diabetics and in women with abnormal weight gain patterns, hypertensive disease, toxemia, aberrant dietary practices, and drug abuse.

GOAL AND RATIONALE OF THERAPY

The management goal is provision of a dietary intake that allows for optimal growth and development of the fetus, while preventing both nutritional deficiencies and excesses in the mother during the pregnancy and subsequent period of lactation.

DIETARY REQUIREMENTS

Energy

The energy requirements of a pregnant woman vary with age, level of activity, and nutritional status prior to pregnancy. Caloric intake must be sufficient to satisfy the energy required for the metabolism of fetal and maternal tissues, for the synthesis of new tissues, and for ambulation of the greater body mass. An additional 300 kcal per day is recommended by the National Research Council in order to ensure adequate weight gain and to meet the estimated total energy requirement of 80,000 kcal for an uncomplicated 9-month pregnancy.

Over the past decade it has become clear that an adequate weight gain reflecting appropriate caloric intake during pregnancy is associated with improved fetal growth, a decrease in the incidence of low birth weight, and other adverse outcomes of pregnancy. The National Academy of Sciences recommends an average weight gain of 12.5 kg during pregnancy and a weekly weight gain of 0.45 kg after the twentieth week of pregnancy. During the first trimester, a weight gain of 1 to 2 kg is adequate. It is considered inappropriate to recommend dietary restriction or initiate other efforts to limit weight gain during pregnancy.

While the mechanism is still unclear, the basis for an improved pregnancy outcome with increased weight gain appears to be a result of increased fat deposition reflecting a positive net energy balance. These maternal fat stores may represent almost 5 kg of the total 12.5 kg recommended weight gain during pregnancy and are rapidly deposited during the first two trimesters of pregnancy. These maternal fat stores represent an energy reserve of approximately 35,000 kcal, over 40 per cent of the total energy necessary for the entire pregnancy. Maternal fat reserves accumulated during the first two trimesters provide an important energy store for the last trimester when the fetus is undergoing maximal growth. Energy reserves unused in the latter phase of pregnancy can partially meet the energy requirements of lactation.

Energy requirements during lactation vary with milk production. The energy content of human milk approximates 70 kcal/100 ml. Since the utilization of energy for milk production is 80 per cent efficient, the cost to the mother is approximately 85 kcal/100 ml of milk produced. The National Academy of Sciences recommends that lactating women ingest an additional 500 kcal per day to meet this energy expenditure. Additional energy is also available to the lactating woman through the utilization of fat stores deposited during pregnancy.

Protein

The proper allowance during pregnancy remains somewhat unsettled. Nitrogen balance studies suggest that nitrogen absorption and retention may be lower than was formerly assumed. Epidemiologic studies suggesting that low protein intake frequently results in a poor outcome are confounded by the frequently coexistent low caloric intake in such diets. This association limits the conclusions that can be drawn regarding the level and quality of protein needed by a pregnant woman. Incomplete data account partially for the liberal protein intake currently recommended. The National Research Council recommends an additional 30 g of protein per day, beginning in the second month.

The amount of dietary protein required during lactation varies with the amount of milk produced. Conversion of maternal protein to milk protein is approximately 70 per cent efficient. The standard recommendation of an additional 20 g of protein per day during lactation is based on the average production of 1 liter per day of human milk containing approximately 1.2 g of protein per dl.

Minerals

The mineral intake of pregnant women requires particular attention. The recommended daily allowances for calcium, phosphorus and magnesium and the trace minerals iron, zinc, and iodine are increased during pregnancy. The higher turnover of both calcium and phosphorus during pregnancy requires increases of 400 mg per day while magnesium requires an increase of 150 mg per day over the RDA for a normal adult woman. Zinc and iodine levels are increased by 5 mg and 25 mg, respectively. Pregnant women can obtain their requirements for phosphorus and magnesium by eating a generally balanced diet, and iodine needs can be met by using iodized salt. Zinc intakes may generally be below recommended levels, but in the absence of evidence of depletion, these should not be supplemented. It may be difficult to meet the recommended intake for calcium unless milk products are regularly included in the diet.

The iron status of the pregnant woman must be considered and iron supplementation given when deficiencies are identified. The increased iron is required for deposition in the fetus and placenta, and blood losses at delivery. There is some controversy concerning the need for supplemental iron during pregnancy in women who have no evidence of iron deficiency. Since habitual American diets usually do not meet the increased requirement for iron during pregnancy and lactation, the National Research Council recommends the administration of 30 to 60 mg of supplemental iron daily. It is a common obstetric practice in this country to provide supplemental iron routinely during pregnancy and lactation, often in amounts considerably exceeding these recommendations. It is assumed that the increased requirement for iron during pregnancy cannot be met from usual dietary sources or from existing iron stores of many women.

Vitamins

Although all vitamin requirements increase during pregnancy, the caloric and protein supplementation recommended previously should also increase the intake of other nutrients and satisfy most vitamin needs of the pregnant woman in good nutritional state. However, folate deficiency, with resultant anemia, is particularly common during pregnancy. A daily supplement of 200 to 400 mg of folic acid is recommended in pregnant women with folate deficiency. It is a common obstetric practice in this country to supplement the diet during all pregnancies with a multivitamin preparation containing folate, although folate alone would probably be sufficient. Excessive intake of vitamins A, C, and D may have adverse effects on the fetus. This possibility should be weighed in women who are taking excessive vitamin supplementation. Women exclusively eating vegetarian diets that exclude all animal products require vitamin B_{12} supplements.

HIGH-RISK PREGNANCIES

The recommendations just described are for the normal, healthy pregnant woman. Many pregnant women, however, are high-risk patients because of nutritional or medical problems. Included in this group are:

1. Women with excessive weight gain during previous pregnancies
2. Women with inadequate weight gain during previous pregnancies
3. Women under 17 years of age
4. Women who abuse drugs, drink alcohol (see Chapter 14), or smoke cigarettes
5. Women with diabetes mellitus or an abnormal glucose tolerance

Excessive Weight Gain

Pregnant women who gain 3 kg or more per month are considered to have exessive weight gain. Such excessive weight gain may be due to accumulation of fluid or to deposition of fat.

The patient must be evaluated to check for the presence of edema, which may be a precursor to pre-eclampsia. Moderate to severe salt restriction, once standard treatment for edema and pre-eclampsia, has been abandoned as a result of recent studies that demonstrate no benefit. Instead, patients may be asked to reduce their salt intake to 5 to 6 g per day by avoiding excessive addition of salt to foods. The same treatment is usually recommended for most women with established hypertension prior to pregnancy.

Weight reduction during pregnancy is not recommended because any diet containing less than 1500 kcal increases the likelihood of having a low-birth-weight infant and causes maternal protein to be utilized as an energy source. Weight reduction diets also tend to cause ketosis, which may result in fetal neurologic damage. Weight loss should be delayed until after delivery or until breast feeding has been terminated.

Nonetheless, when edema is not responsible for excessive weight gain, the patient's dietary practices should be reviewed and suggestions made to restrict weight gain to less than 3 kg per month.

Inadequate Weight Gain

Women who have a problem gaining weight also present a nutritional risk. Women who are underweight before pregnancy or gain 1 kg or less per month after the first trimester have an increased risk of delivering a low-birth-weight infant. The expectant mother must be instructed to consume a diet sufficient in calories and nutrients to improve her own nutritional status and to allow for normal fetal growth. Increased calories should be provided by recommending a high-calorie diet apportioned into meals with snacks.

Adolescent Pregnancy

Pregnant adolescents may pose a major problem because they often follow nutritionally inadequate or fad diets. Teenagers are generally overly concerned about their weight and tend to restrict their caloric intake. Since they are still growing, teenagers must provide nutritional support for their own development as well as for that of their unborn child. The nutritional status of the adolescent must be assessed carefully and a diet planned accordingly. She must be made to understand that her eating habits can affect the health of her unborn baby.

Drug Abuse, Alcohol, and Smoking

Abuse of various drugs by pregnant women is another risk factor. Since most drugs depress appetite, their abuse can cause food intake to be reduced to an inadequate level.

Moderate to heavy intake of alcohol is associated with altered fetal growth and developmental retardation as part of the "fetal alcohol syndrome." A correlation between linear growth deficiency and retarded neurologic development has been noted in this syndrome. Little reported decreased birth weights of 91 g and 160 g associated with daily maternal consumption of 1 ounce of absolute alcohol during early and late pregnancy, respectively. These effects seem to be independent of those of cigarette smoking, which can also cause decreased birth weight.

Pregnant women should, therefore, be encouraged to avoid the use of non-prescribed drugs, minimize alcohol consumption, and eliminate cigarette smoking. Megadoses of vitamins should be avoided.

Glucose Intolerance and Diabetes

An abnormal maternal glucose tolerance curve is a major pregnancy risk factor. Glucose tolerance should be checked in women with a family history of diabetes, a previous stillborn, a previous high-birth-weight infant (over 4 kg), or recurrent glucosuria.

Some previously normal women develop abnormal glucose tolerance during pregnancy. The patient is classified as a gestational diabetic when blood glucose values exceed the following: 90 mg/dl when fasting, or 165 mg/dl, 145 mg/dl, or 125 mg/dl for specimens obtained 1, 2, or 3 hours, respectively, following glucose ingestion.

The pregnant diabetic must be carefully monitored during her entire pregnancy in order to minimize risk to both mother and baby. Early in pregnancy, when the mother normally tends to become hypoglycemic owing to transfer of glucose to the fetus, insulin dosage must be reduced. During the second half of pregnancy, increased serum levels of placental hormones may antagonize the effects of insulin, thereby increasing the mother's exogenous insulin requirement.

In order to maintain normal fetal weight and reduce perinatal mortality, every effort should be made to keep maternal glucose levels below 100 mg/dl at all times in both pregestational and gestational diabetics. This goal can often be accomplished by placing the patient on an 1800-calorie diet containing 100 g of protein, 200 g of carbohydrate, and 65 g of fat. Appropriate levels of energy intake for the pregnant diabetic are controversial. While many authorities advocate a normal pregnancy allowance of 36 kcal/kg for the pregnant diabetic, others suggest an intake of 30 kcal/kg of ideal body weight plus an added 300 kcal per day during gestation. The calories should be distributed as follows: approximately 20 per cent or 1.3 g/kg/day as protein, 200-250 g/day as carbohydrate, and the balance of energy as fat. Complex starches are recommended to reduce fluctuations in blood sugar since they are absorbed more slowly than simple sugars. Meals should be evenly distributed throughout the day. The skill and assistance of a qualified nutritionist in monitoring and adjusting the diet as pregnancy progresses is essential. If the patient develops hypoglycemia, develops ketonuria without glucosuria, or loses weight, the diet may be liberalized in increments of 200 kcal, not more than twice a week. Supplemental insulin treatment is required when hyperglycemia is not controllable by diet.

GENERAL CONSIDERATIONS

Nutritional counselling should be initiated at the first prenatal visit. Nutritional assessment should be carried out and additional studies ordered where appropriate. A personal food plan can then be adequately developed. Instruction should be provided when necessary in food purchase and preparation. Guidance may also be provided to pregnant women who are eligible for food stamps, other federal or local nutrition supplementation programs, and additional social service assistance.

Attention should be given to the dietary practices and food preferences of the patient. Preconceived dietary patterns, which may reflect the cultural bias of the nutritionist rather than the patient's preference, should be avoided. Instead, the patient's own dietary practices should be assessed and the nutrient content determined. This baseline information will permit modifications, when necessary, of the patient's regular dietary pattern rather than the imposition of an unfamiliar diet.

Food Allergies

Simeon Margolis, M.D., Ph.D.

INTRODUCTION

It has long been recognized that generally safe food substances can cause significant illness in susceptible individuals. In fact, in experiments by Prausnitz and Küstner, a substance in haddock was found to cause symptoms upon ingestion of the fish, and these studies were important landmarks in the history of clinical immunology.

Despite the voluminous literature on food allergy, estimates of its incidence vary widely because of differences in the criteria used for its diagnosis. One group of physicians limits the diagnosis of food allergy to those in whom the classic symptoms of anaphylaxis, asthma, hay fever, and hives occur repeatedly within a few hours of ingestion of a specific food. As discussed further on, others have attributed to allergy a group of nonspecific symptoms that may be associated with food intake but that often lack a consistent temporal relationship to its ingestion.

The former group has attempted to correlate a history of food sensitivity or an observed adverse response to foods with skin reactions to local injections of food allergens or with the presence of food-specific IgE antibodies in the serum. Individuals with other types of allergies have a higher frequency of skin reactions to a variety of food components. Despite a high incidence of false-positive reactions, there is a good correlation between the production of specific symptoms and a positive skin reaction to specific foods. Anaphylaxis, asthma, hives, irritation about the mouth, vomiting, diarrhea, and other gastrointestinal symptoms have been observed in response to a wide variety of specific foods in individuals with positive skin reactions to one certain food. These foods include egg white, fish (especially cod, pickerel, salmon, and halibut), shellfish (especially shrimp and lobster), peanuts, cow's milk, walnuts, brazil nuts, chocolate, tomatoes, spinach, asparagus, peas, oranges, bananas, corn, barley, strawberries, and garbanzo beans. In fact, more than 140 foods have been reported to cause typical allergic reactions.

Allergic reactions to fish can be considered as the prototype of food allergies mediated by IgE. The reactions are usually immediate and most commonly consist of hives or asthma or both. Other frequent symptoms include vomiting, colic, watery diarrhea, and conjunctival and nasal complaints. Fish myogens (sarcoplasmic proteins), which have compositions quite different from those of human proteins, may serve as potent allergens.

There is little doubt that a wide variety of food substances can cause predictable, IgE-mediated allergic reactions in sensitive individuals. In contrast, some physicians have attributed a different group of symptoms to food reactions that are not mediated by IgE. These symptoms commonly include aches, pallor, drowsiness, headache, enuresis, restlessness, and insomnia; however, almost any conceivable systemic symptom has been attributed to food intolerance.

The diagnosis of such food intolerances is complicated by both the diversity of symptoms and the fact that conventional skin tests are of little value. In addition, substances considered most likely to cause the symptoms are common foods or food additives that the patient eats regularly and has not necessarily associated with any ill effects. Approaches to the treatment of this form of food allergy have included elimination of foods and food additives from the diet and administration of so-called neutralizing doses of specific foods. The latter approach consists of intracutaneous injection of large volumes of food extracts and assessment of their ability to produce a local reaction or systemic symptoms. Subcutaneous injections of the extracts that provoked symptoms are then given in progressively increasing doses until the symptoms abate. Subsequently, injections of this neutralizing dose of food extract(s) are used to prevent symptoms. Many difficulties are encountered in evaluating the diagnosis and efficacy of treatment of this form of food intolerance. The pathophysiology is unclear, treatment is based on an empirical trial and error method, and assessment of clinical response is subject to both physician and patient bias. (Behavioral effects of food additives not based on allergy are discussed in the previous section on normal nutrition.)

PATIENT IDENTIFICATION

IgE-mediated food allergy should be considered as a possible cause or contributing factor in the development of classic allergic symptoms, anaphylaxis, asthma, hay fever, and hives or acute gastrointestinal complaints. Often the patient can identify the offending food, particularly if it is commonly served separately, as in the case of nuts or seafood. It is more difficult to recognize allergies to food substances, such as eggs or milk, which are often ingested mixed with other foods. A strongly positive skin reaction to a provocative test with food extracts may help to identify the offending agent. The ultimate diagnostic test is the disappearance of symptoms when the allergenic food is eliminated from the diet and their return upon its re-introduction into the diet.

Until the syndromes are better documented, attribution of symptoms to non–IgE-mediated food intolerance should be made with great care and circumspection. Treatment by administration of neutralizing doses of food extracts is still a highly questionable procedure.

DIETARY PRINCIPLES

1. Nutritional treatment of IgE-mediated food allergy involves elimination of the offending food from the diet.

2. Seafood, nuts, and other foods that are generally served by themselves are usually avoidable.

3. Great care must be exercised by patients allergic to foods that are often mixed with other foods.

4. Sensitivities to certain foods, especially milk, are manifested in infancy or early childhood but appear to diminish with age.

5. Treatment of the allergy by desensitization is rarely effective.

BIBLIOGRAPHY

Normal Nutrition

Anonymous: Toxic reactions to plant products sold in health food stores. Med Lett Drugs Ther 21:29–31, 1979.

Avioli, L.V.: Postmenopausal osteoporosis: Prevention versus cure. Fed Proc 40:2418–2422, 1981.

Committee on Diet, Nutrition, and Cancer; Assembly of Life Sciences, National Research Council: Diet, Nutrition, and Cancer. Washington, D.C., National Academy Press, 1982.

Denton, D.A.: The Hunger for Salt: An Anthropological, Physiological, and Medical Analysis. New York, Springer-Verlag, 1982.

Feingold, B.F.: Introduction to Clinical Allergy. Springfield, IL, Charles C Thomas Co., 1973.

Feingold, B.F.: Why Your Child Is Hyperactive. New York, Random House, 1975.

Gawthorne, J.M., Howell, J. McC., and White, C.L. (Eds.): Trace Element Metabolism in Man and Animals. Canberra, Australia, Australian Academy of Science, 1982.

Herbert, V., and Barrett, S.: Vitamins and "Health" Foods: The Great American Hustle. Philadelphia, George F. Stickley Co., 1982.

King, J.C., Cohenour, S.H., Corruccini, C.G., and Schneeman, P.: Evaluation and modification of the basic four food guide. J Nutr Educ 10:27–29, 1978.

Leverett, D.H.: Fluorides and the Changing Prevalence of Dental Caries. Science 217:26–30, 1982.

Shaw, J.H., and Roussos, G.G. (Eds.): Sweeteners and Dental Caries. Washington, D.C., Information Retrieval, Inc., 1978.

Simopoulos, A.P.: The scientific basis of the "goals": What can be done now? JADA 74:539–542, 1979.

Swanson, J.M., and Kinsbourne, M.: Food dyes impair performance of hyperactive children on a laboratory learning test. Science 207:1485–1487, 1980.

Walker, A.R.P., and Walker, B.F.: Recommended dietary allowances and third world populations. Am J Clin Nutr 34:2319–2321, 1981.

Weiss, B., Williams, J.H., Margen, S., Abrams, B., Caan, B., Citron, L.J., Cox, C., McKibben, J., Ogar, D., and Schultz, S: Behavioral responses to artificial food colors. Science 207:1487–1488, 1980.

Winter, S.L., and Boyer, J.L.: Hepatic toxicity from large doses of vitamin B_3 (nicotinamide). N Engl J Med 289:1180–1182, 1973.

World Health Organization: Elements in Human Nutrition. Geneva, 1973.

Nutritional Assessment

Ahlert, G., Brüschke, G., Dietze, F., Franke, H., and Haase, J.: Altersabhängige Veränderungen und normale Schwankungen der Kreatinin- und Kreatinausscheidung. Zschr Alternsforschung 20:113–118, 1967.

Bistrian, B.R., Blackburn, G.L., Sherman, M., and Scrimshaw, N.S.: Therapeutic index of nutritional depletion in hospitalized patients. Surg Gynecol Obstet 141:512–516, 1975.

Bistrian, B.R., Blackburn, G.L., Sherman, M., and Scrimshaw, W.S.: Therapeutic index of nutritional depletion in hospitalized patients. Surg Gynecol Obstet 141:512–516, 1975.

Bistrian, B.R., Blackburn, G.L., Vitale, J., Cochran, D., and Naylor, J.: Prevalence of malnutrition in general medical patients. JAMA 235:1567–1570, 1976.

Blackburn, G.L., Bistrian, B.R., Maini, B.S., et al.: Nutritional and metabolic assessment in the hospitalized patient. J Parent Ent Nutr 1:11–22, 1977.

Cockcroft, D.W., and Gault, M.H.: Prediction of creatinine clearance from serum creatinine. Nephron 16:31–41, 1976.

Collins, J.P., McCarthy, I.D., and Hill, G.L.: Assessment of protein nutrition in surgical patients—The value of anthropometrics. Am J Clin Nutr 32:1527–1530, 1979.

Copeland, E.M., Daly, J.M., and Dudrick, G.J.: Nutrition as an adjunct to cancer treatment in the adult. Cancer Res 37:2451–2456, 1977.

Faintuch, J., Faintuch, J.J., MacMado, M.C., and Raia, A.A.: Anthropometric assessment of nutritional depletion after surgical injury. J Parent Ent Nutr 3:369–371, 1979.

Forse, R.A., and Shizgal, H.M.: The assessment of malnutrition. Surgery 88:17–25, 1980.

Forse, R.A., and Shizgal, H.M.: Serum albumin and nutritional status. J Parent Ent Nutr 4:450–459, 1980.

Frisancho, A.R.: New norms of upper limb fat and muscle areas for assessment of nutritional status. Am J Clin Nutr 34:2540–2545, 1981.

Hill, G.L., Pickford, I., Young, G.A., Schorah, C.J., Blackett, R.L., Burkinshaw, L., Warren, J.V., and Morgan, D.B.: Malnutrition in surgical patients. Lancet 1:689–692, 1977.

Kampmann, J.P., Siersbaek-Nielsen, K., Kristensen, M., and Hansen, J.M.: Aldersbetingede variationer i urinkreatinin og endogen kreatininclearance. Ugeskrift Laeger 133:2369–2372, 1971.

Lykken, G.I., Jacob, R.A., Munoz, J.M., and Sandstead, H.H.: A mathematical model of creatine metabolism in normal males—comparison between theory and experiment. Am J Clin Nutr 33:2674–2685, 1980.

Miller, C.L.: Immunological assays as measurements of nutritional status: A review. J Parent Ent Nutr 2:554–566, 1978.

Nellhaus, G.: Head circumference from birth to eighteen years. Practical composite international and interracial graphs. Pediatrics 41:106–114, 1968.

Norris, A.H., Lundy, T., and Shock, N.W.: Trends in selected indices of body composition in men between the ages 30 and 80 years. Ann NY Acad Sci 110:623–639, 1963.

Ota, D.M., Copeland, E., Corriere, J.N., and Dudrick, S.J.: The effects of nutrition and treatment of cancer on host immunocompetence. Surg Gynecol Obstet 148:104–111, 1979.

Ringer, A.I., and Raiziss, G.W.: The excretion of creatinine by human individuals on a prolonged creatine-free diet. J Biol Chem 19:487–492, 1914.

Seltzer, M.H., Slocom, B.A., Cataldi-Betcher, E.L., Fileti, C., and Gerson, N.: Instant nutritional assessment: Absolute weight loss and surgical mortality. J Parent Ent Nutr 6:218–221, 1982.

Starker, P.M., Gump, F.E., Askanazi, J., Elwyn, D.H., and Kinney, J.M.: Serum albumin levels as an index of nutritional support. Surgery 91:194–199, 1982.

Viteri, F.E., and Alvarado, J.: The creatinine height index: Its use in the estimation of the degree of protein depletion and repletion in protein calorie malnourished children. Pediatrics 46:696–706, 1970.

Young, C.M., Blondin, J., Tensuan, R., and Fryer, J.H.: Body composition studies of "older" women, thirty to seventy years of age. Ann NY Acad Sci 110:589–607, 1963.

Young, G.A., and Hill, G.L.: Assessment of protein calorie malnutrition in surgical patients from plasma proteins and anthropometric measurements. Am J Clin Nutr 31:429–435, 1978.

Vegetarian Diets

American Dietetic Association: Position paper on the vegetarian approach to eating. JADA 77:61–69, 1980.

Anonymous: Nutrition and vegetarianism. Dairy Council Digest 50:1–6, 1979.

Bergan, J.G., and Brown, P.T.: Nutritional status of new vegetarians. JADA 76:151–155, 1980.

Dwyer, J.T., Andrew, E.M., Valadian, I., and Reed, R.B.: Size, obesity and leanness in vegetarian preschool children. JADA 77:434–439, 1980.

Ellis, F.R., and Montegriffo, V.M.E.: Veganism, clinical findings and investigations. Am J Clin Nutr 23:249–255, 1970.

Erhard, D.: Nutrition education for the now generation. J Nutr Educ 3:135–139, 1971.

Freeland-Graves, J.H., Bodzy, P.W., and Eppright, M.A.: Zinc status of vegetarians. JADA 77:655–661, 1980.

Freeland-Graves, J.H., Ebangit, M.L., and Bodzy, P.W.: Zinc and copper content of foods used in vegetarian diets. JADA 77:648–654, 1980.

Hardinge, M.G., and Crooks, H.: Non-Flesh Dietaries. JADA 45:537–541, 1964.

National Academy of Sciences: Vegetarian Diets: A Statement of the Food and Nutrition Board, Division of Biological Sciences, Assembly of Life Sciences, National Research Council. May, 1974.

Register, U.D., and Sonnenberg, L.M.: The vegetarian diet. JADA 62:253–261, 1973.

Vyhmeister, P.H., Register, U.D., and Sonnenberg, L.M.: Safe vegetarian diets for children. Pediatr Clin North Am 24:203–210, 1977.
Winick, M.: The vegetarian diet. Nutr Health 2:1–5, 1980.

Kosher Dietary Laws

Kashruth Handbook for Home and School. New York, Union of Orthodox Jewish Congregations of America, Rabbinical Council of America, 1972.
Robinson, C.H.: Basic Nutrition and Diet Therapy, 3rd Ed. New York, Macmillan Publishing Co., 1975.
Robinson, C.H.: Normal and Therapeutic Nutrition, 14th Ed. New York, Macmillan Publishing Co., 1972.
Siegel, R., Strassfield, M., and Strassfield, S.: The Jewish Catalogue. Philadelphia, The Jewish Publication Society of America, 1973.

Normal Pediatric Nutrition

American Academy of Pediatrics, Committee on Hospital Care: Care of Children in Hospitals, 2nd Ed., American Journal of Pediatrics, Evanston, IL, 1971.
Fomon, S.J.: Infant Nutrition, 2nd Ed. Philadelphia, W.B. Saunders Co., 1974.
Joint FAO/WHO Expert Group, Energy and Protein Requirements. World Health Organization, Technical Reports, Series No. 522; WHO, Geneva, 1973.
Food and Nutrition Board, National Research Council, Committee on Dietary Allowances: Recommended Dietary Allowances, 9th Ed. National Academy of Sciences, Washington, D.C., 1980.
Merritt, R.J.: Nutritional assessment and metabolic response to illness of the hospitalized child. *In* Suskind, R.M. (Ed): Textbook of Pediatric Nutrition. New York, Raven Press, 1981.
Owen, G.M., Kram, K., Garry, P.J., Lowe, J.E., and Lubin, A.H.: A study of nutritional status of preschool children in the United States, 1968–1970. Pediatrics 53:597–646, 1974.

Nutrition During Pregnancy and Lactation

Bailey, L.B., Maham, C.S., and Duniperio, D.: Folacin and iron status in low-income pregnant adolescents and mature women. Am J Clin Nutr 33:1997–2001, 1980.
Bergner, L., and Susser, M.W.: Low birthweight and prenatal nutrition: An interpretative review. Pediatrics 46:946–966, 1970.
Committee on Maternal Nutrition: Maternal Nutrition and the Course of Pregnancy. National Research Council/National Academy of Sciences, Washington, D.C., U.S. Government Printing Office, 1970.
Committee on Nutrition of the Mother and Preschool Child, National Research Council: Laboratory Indices of Nutritional Status in Pregnancy. Washington, D.C., 1978.
Coustan, D.: Recent advances in the management of diabetic pregnant women. Clin Perinatol 7:299–311, 1980.
Crosby, W.M., Metcoff, J., Costilloe, P., *et al.*: Fetal malnutrition: An appraisal of correlated factors. Am J Obstet Gynecol 128:22–31, 1977.
Eastman, N.J., and Jackson, E.: Weight relationships in pregnancy: The bearing of maternal weight gain and prepregnancy weight on birthweight in full term pregnancies. Obstet Gynecol Sur 23:1003–1065, 1968.
Food and Nutrition Board, National Research Council, Committee on Dietary Allowances: Recommended Dietary Allowances, 9th Ed. National Academy of Sciences, Washington, D.C., 1980.
Jacobson, H.N.: Current concepts in nutrition: Diet in pregnancy. N Engl J Med 297:1051–1053, 1977.
Jacobson, H.N.: Weight and weight gain in pregnancy. Clin Perinatol 2:233–242, 1975.
Pitkin, R.M.: Nutritional influences during pregnancy. Med Clin North Am 61:2–15, 1977.
Pitkin, R.M.: Vitamins and minerals in pregnancy. Clin Perinatol 2:221–232, 1975.
Thomson, A.M., Hytten, F.E., and Villewicz, W.Z.: The energy cost of human lactation. Br J Nutr 24:565–572, 1970.

Food Allergies

Bock, S.A., Buckley, J., Holst, A., and May, C.D.: Proper use of skin tests with food extracts in diagnosis of hypersensitivity to food in children. Clin Allergy 7:375–383, 1977.
Buckley, R.H., and Metcalfe, D.: Food allergy. JAMA 248:2627–2631, 1982.

Crook, W.G.: Food allergy—The great masquerader. Pediatr Clin North Am 22:227–238, 1975.

Editorial: Food allergy. Lancet 1:249–250, 1979.

Eriksson, N.E.: Food sensitivity reported by patients with asthma and hay fever. Allergy 33:189–196, 1978.

Haddad, Z.H., and Koratzer, J.L.: Immediate hypersensitivity reactions to food antigens. J Allergy Clin Immunol 49:210–218, 1972.

May, C.D., and Bock, S.A.: A modern clinical approach to food hypersensitivity. Allergy 33:166–188, 1978.

Prausnitz, D., and Küstner, H.: Studien über Überentfindlichkeit. Centralbl Bakteriol 86:160–169, 1921.

2
MODIFICATIONS IN CONSISTENCY (TRANSITIONAL DIETS)

Anthony L. Imbembo, M.D., and
Gloria Elfert, M.S., R.D.

INTRODUCTION

The three diets included in this section constitute a transitional program for the patient who is unable initially to ingest anything orally prior to the institution of a regular diet. The clear liquid diet is often the one prescribed during the first days of resolution of a paralytic ileus, because of still-abnormal bowel motility. The full liquid diet consists of foods that are liquid at room temperature, and it provides increased amounts of protein and fat. As a transitional diet it is not nutritionally adequate; however, if it is tolerated well, the patient may be advanced to a soft diet, which meets nutritional and caloric needs while minimizing fiber intake.

CLEAR LIQUID DIET

The clear liquid diet (Table 2–1) is used in conjunction with mechanical and pharmacologic agents to cleanse the bowel prior to colonic surgery or certain radiologic studies (including barium enemas, upper gastrointestinal series, and intravenous pyelograms). In this way, all nonabsorbable materials are eliminated, while the patient is permitted to maintain an adequate fluid intake.

This diet may also be the initial one prescribed after certain surgical procedures, particularly those involving the gastrointestinal tract. During the initial days of resolution of paralytic ileus, the patient may tolerate only a clear liquid diet, as bowel motility may not as yet have returned entirely to normal. As postoperative paralytic ileus resolves, there is a gradual increase in bowel motility and consequent ability to maintain the normal progression of gastrointestinal secretions and ingested nutrients.

TABLE 2–1.   CLEAR LIQUID DIET

Foods Permitted	Foods Omitted
Soups Clear broth, consommé (jellied or hot)	Cream soups
Desserts Fruit ice; clear gelatin	Custard; ice cream or sherbet
Sweets Sugar	
Beverages Fruit juices; carbonated beverages; coffee or tea; powdered fruit beverages	Milk

Sample Meal Plan

Breakfast
Clear broth
Citrus fruit juice (240 cc)
Clear gelatin (120 cc)
Coffee or tea
Sugar (10 g)

Mid-morning nourishment
Fruit juice (240 cc)
Clear gelatin (120 cc)

Noon meal
Clear broth (180 cc)
Fruit juice (240 cc)
Clear gelatin or fruit ice (120 cc)
Coffee or tea
Sugar (10 g)

Mid-afternoon nourishment
Fruit juice or carbonated beverage (240 cc)
Clear gelatin (120 cc)

Evening meal
Clear broth (180 cc)
Fruit juice (240 cc)
Clear gelatin or fruit ice (120 cc)
Coffee or tea
Sugar (10 g)

Evening nourishment
Fruit juice or carbonated beverage (240 cc)
Clear gelatin (120 cc)

Approximate Composition of This Sample Diet

Calories	1230	Iron	3–5 mg
Protein	12 g	Phosphorus	200 mg
Fat	0 g	Potassium	2000–3000 mg
Carbohydrate	300 g	Sodium	900
Calcium	100 mg		

TABLE 2–2. FULL LIQUID DIET

Foods Permitted (Select from this list.)

Soups
Broth, strained soup

Cereals
Strained cereals

Fats
Cream, butter, or margarine

Desserts
Any of the following without fruit, coconut, or nuts: clear gelatin, custard, pudding, junket, ice
   cream, fruit ice, sherbet, and plain yogurt

Sweets
Sugar, plain hard candies

Beverages
Milk, buttermilk, chocolate milk, milk shake, eggnog, cocoa, carbonated beverages, fruit and vegetable juices, coffee or tea

Sample Meal Plan

Breakfast
Citrus fruit juice (240 cc)
Strained cereal (180 cc)
Milk (240 cc)
Coffee or tea
Sugar (10 g)

Mid-morning nourishment
Fruit juice (240 cc)

Noon meal
Strained soup or broth (180 cc)
Custard, clear gelatin, ice cream, pudding, or
   sherbet (120 cc)
Fruit juice (240 cc)
Milk or eggnog (240 cc)
Coffee or tea
Sugar (10 g)

Mid-afternoon nourishment
Milk, eggnog, or protein supplement (240 cc)

Evening meal
Strained soup or broth (180 cc)
Milk or eggnog (240 cc)
Dessert (as at noon meal)
Fruit juice (240 cc)
Coffee or tea
Sugar (10 g)

Evening nourishment
Milk, eggnog, or protein supplement (240 cc)

Approximate Composition of This Sample Diet

Calories*	1730–2150	Iron	8 mg
Protein	55–65 g	Phosphorus	1500 mg
Fat	60–90 g	Potassium	4000 mg
Carbohydrate	240–250 g	Sodium	1000–1500 mg
Calcium	1500 mg		

*A variety of high-calorie beverages is available to increase the calories whenever necessary. (See also Tables 5–1 and 5–2.)

The clear liquid diet is inadequate in total calories and in all essential nutrients. The diet does provide adequate volume as long as sufficient liquid is ingested to meet insensible and urinary losses. It should not be used for long-term patient maintenance, however, unless adjuncts such as tube feedings, elemental diets, or parenteral nutrition are provided to obviate the nutritional and caloric deficits inherent in the clear liquid diet.

FULL LIQUID DIET

The full liquid diet (Table 2–2) is properly used in patients whose gastrointestinal function is sufficient to digest and absorb protein and fat loads but whose bowel residue must be restricted (e.g., in bowel preparation prior to surgery, in the transitional period after gastrointestinal surgery with anastomosis, or in treatment of inflammatory bowel diseases). It is commonly used as a transitional diet between diets of clear liquids and of solids in patients recovering from paralytic ileus of any etiology and particularly following gastrointestinal surgery.

The full liquid diet meets the patient's caloric needs to a greater extent than does the clear liquid program, by providing increased amounts of protein and fat. The fiber content remains minimal, and all foods are liquid at body temperature. The diet may still be inadequate in calories, depending upon patient intake, and it is inadequate in iron and niacin as well. Therefore, the full liquid diet is used only for short periods of time.

SOFT DIET

The soft diet (Table 2–3) is designed for patients recovering from surgery, trauma, or paralytic ileus of any etiology. It is most often the transitional diet just prior to the ingestion of foods of normal consistency. The patient is encouraged to select a nutritionally adequate diet from the foods offered. The diet is moderately low in indigestible carbohydrates and fiber. According to the recommended allowances, the diet is low in iron as well.

TABLE 2–3.   SOFT DIET

Foods Permitted	Foods Omitted
	All highly seasoned foods
MEATS	
Pureed, ground or tender beef, ham, veal, lamb, pork, poultry; tender steak and chops, fish, oysters, shrimp, lobster, clams, crabs, liver and organ meats (*Note*: Meats may be boiled, broiled, baked, but not fried)	

Table continues on following page

TABLE 2–3. SOFT DIET (Continued)

Foods Permitted	Foods Omitted
CHEESE	
American, cream, cottage, or any mild-flavored	
EGGS	
Soft- or hard-cooked, baked, scrambled, poached, creamed, fried, plain omelette or soufflé, low-cholesterol egg substitute	
MILK	
At least one pint (whole, skim, chocolate, buttermilk)	
FRUITS	
Fruit juices—All	Fresh fruits, other than those permitted
Canned fruits—Pears, peaches, Bing or Royal Anne cherries, apricots, applesauce, plums, pineapple, fruit cocktail, berries, rhubarb	
Fresh fruits—Ripe melon, ripe avocado, ripe banana, orange or grapefruit sections; ripe peeled peaches, apples, pineapple, pears, nectarines, seedless grapes	
Soft dried fruits—Prunes, apples, pears, or peaches	
Any pureed or blenderized fruits	
(*Note*: Foods containing seeds may be allowed, as tolerated)	
BREAD AND CEREAL PRODUCTS	
Whole-grain, made from finely milled flour, or enriched white bread; waffles, pancakes, French toast; any finely milled whole-grain or refined, cooked or ready-to-eat cereals; spaghetti, rice, macaroni, noodles; saltines, graham crackers, or plain crackers made with foods permitted	Any with whole grain, bran, cracked wheat
FATS	
Butter, margarine, salad oils, mayonnaise, boiled salad dressing, cream, crisp bacon, smooth peanut butter, and plain gravies	Crunchy peanut butter, nuts
SOUPS	
Strained or made with foods permitted, clear broth, bouillon, or consommé	
DESSERTS	
Any of the following without coconut or nuts: gelatin, puddings, custard, ice cream, cookies, cake, fruit on "permitted" list, any other smooth dessert (any flavor permitted), pie, and pastry	Any containing fruit not among those permitted, with coconut, or with nuts

Table continues on following page

TABLE 2–3.   SOFT DIET (Continued)

Foods Permitted	Foods Omitted
SWEETS	
Candy without coconut or nuts, jelly, jam, preserves without skins, syrup, sugar, honey, and molasses as desired	Any containing coconut or nuts

Sample Meal Plan

Breakfast
Citrus fruit or equivalent (120 cc)
Cereal (30 g dry or 180 g cooked)
1 egg or equivalent
1 slice toast with 5 g margarine
Milk (240 cc)
Coffee or tea
Sugar (10 g)

Noon meal
Soup as tolerated (180 cc)
Meat or equivalent (60 g)
Potato or equivalent (100 g)
Vegetable or salad (100 g, cooked)
1 slice bread with 5 g margarine
Dessert or fruit
Coffee or tea
Sugar (10 g)

Evening meal
Soup as tolerated (180 cc)
Meat or equivalent (60 g)
Potato or equivalent (100 g)
Vegetable or salad (100 g, cooked)
1 slice bread with 5 g margarine
Dessert or fruit
Milk (240 cc)
Coffee or tea
Sugar (10 g)

Evening nourishment
Fruit juice or milk (240 cc)

Approximate Composition of This Sample Diet

Calories	2000	Iron	12 mg
Protein	75 g	Phosphorus	1500
Fat	75 g	Potassium	3200
Carbohydrate	230 g	Sodium	4000–6000 mg
Calcium	800 g		

3

ENTERAL ALIMENTATION

Anthony L. Imbembo, M.D., and
Judith Z. Walter, R.D., M.P.M.

INTRODUCTION

The development of total parenteral nutrition has been a major break-through in nutritional technology. In many patients, however, adequate nutritional support can be given with specially formulated liquid diets administered by the enteral route. Enteral nutritional support avoids the potential technical, metabolic, and septic complications of parenteral nutrition. However, it is rather difficult to provide more than 3000 calories per day by this means. Therefore, parenteral nutrition remains necessary for patients with calorie and amino acid requirements of a significantly greater degree or in whom the gastrointestinal tract is not functional.

GOALS AND RATIONALE OF TREATMENT

The enteral route is both the preferred and most effective way of supplying nutrients when alimentary tract function is normal or only moderately impaired. When patients are unable to ingest or digest sufficient food to meet their needs, additional support may be given through the use of specially formulated liquid diets.

Oral administration of these diets is preferred; however, some patients with severe anorexia, nausea, malnutrition, or neurologic impairment may be unwilling or unable to ingest anything orally. Under such circumstances, supplemental nutrition may be administered by means of a tube or catheter placed in the gastrointestinal tract. Such feedings can be given through a small-bore nasoenteric tube or through a surgically placed gastrostomy or jejunostomy tube. The latter can be used to provide support when the disorder involves proximal gastrointestinal function, but the absorptive and motor capacities of the distal bowel are relatively normal.

Whether administered orally or by tube, specially formulated liquid diets

68

represent an intermediate step between high-calorie, high-protein total parenteral nutrition and oral ingestion and digestion of regular food. Formulated liquid diets are of greatest value in the nutritional support of patients who have at least a portion of the small intestine available for absorption.

Whenever feasible, enteral nutrition is preferred over parenteral nutrition, because it avoids many of the metabolic and all of the septic complications associated with the latter. In addition, enteral nutrition tends to maintain gastrointestinal structural integrity. Numerous animal studies have demonstrated atrophy of the small intestine and pancreas when nutrition is administered only parenterally. Enteral nutrition has been shown to be necessary to maintain the total mass, protein content, deoxyribonucleic acid content, and disaccharidase activity of the gastrointestinal tract. These effects seem to be mediated both directly by actual contact and indirectly by hormonal mechanisms.

PATIENT SELECTION

Patients who benefit from enteral alimentation via a feeding tube include those with normal gastrointestinal tract function who refuse oral alimentation (*e.g.,* geriatric patients, patients with senile dementia, and patients with anorexia nervosa). Patients with neurologic or muscular diseases who are unwilling or unable to swallow effectively will also benefit from this program—stroke patients; postoperative neurosurgical patients; and those with multiple sclerosis, myasthenia gravis, and dermatomyositis.

Enteral alimentation may be helpful in the treatment of patients with obstructing lesions of the proximal gastrointestinal tract—head and neck tumors, esophageal carcinoma, benign esophageal stricture, gastric carcinoma, and gastric outlet obstruction due to chronic duodenal ulcer disease. Such patients usually are fed liquid diets through an enterostomy tube placed distal to the obstructing lesion. In this way, significant malnutrition may be corrected prior to surgical treatment.

Postoperative patients with obstruction or dysfunction at proximal gastrointestinal suture lines may also require enteral alimentation. Prophylactic enterostomy tubes are often inserted when complicated esophagogastric, duodenal, pancreatic, or biliary surgery is performed or when the debility or mental or neurologic state of the patient suggests that postoperative feeding problems might ensue.

Patients with enterocutaneous fistulas and short-bowel syndrome can utilize elemental diets only, as do patients receiving immediate postoperative jejunal feedings.

DIETARY PRINCIPLES

Numerous enteral formulations are available. They differ in osmolarity, digestibility, caloric density, lactose content, viscosity, residue, fat content, taste, and expense. These special liquid diets can be classified as follows:

1. Blenderized regular food
2. Commercial, blenderized diets

3. Commercial, lactose-free diets
4. Defined formula diets
5. Elemental diets

BLENDERIZED REGULAR FOOD.   The simplest and most economical way to prepare tube feedings is to homogenize a regular diet or a diet with specific restrictions, *e.g.,* a renal diet. Blenderized tube feedings require normal alimentary tract function for utilization. They can be administered with appropriate amounts of additional free water, depending upon the patient's needs and level of oral intake. Blenderized tube feedings can be administered in divided portions of 200 to 400 cc every 4 to 6 hours or by continuous gravity drip infusion. The viscosity is high, necessitating administration through a large-bore tube, dilution with supplemental water, or both (see Table 3-1 for a sample formulation).

COMMERCIAL, BLENDERIZED DIETS.   These are commercially prepared homogenates of selected food items (see Table 3-2 for product information). Al-

TABLE 3-1.   SAMPLE TUBE FEEDING USING BLENDERIZED REGULAR FOODS, 2000 CALORIES

Ingredients	Grams	Household Measure
Applesauce	383	1½ cups
Egg*	57	1 large
Oil, corn	41	3 tbsp
Orange juice (unsweetened)	311	1¼ cups
Cereal (rice, infant [Gerber])	28	¾ cup
Instant potato flakes	56	1¼ cups
Skim milk powder†	91	1⅓ cups
Strained beef (Gerber)	300	3 jars

Water is added to above ingredients to make a total volume of 2000 cc or 8⅓ cups. This mixture may be blenderized, beaten, whipped, or stirred to mix the ingredients thoroughly. Mixture must be refrigerated until ready for use. Strain if necessary.

Approximate Composition of This Feeding

Calories	2000		Potassium	4.2	g
Protein	98	g	Sodium	1.1	g
Fat	65	g	Vitamin A	5228	IU
Carbohydrate	255	g	Thiamine	1.5	mg
Calcium	1.5	g	Riboflavin	20.3	mg
Phosphorus	1.8	g	Niacin	3.0	mg
Iron	24	mg	Ascorbic acid	203	mg
			Osmolarity	620	mOsm

Administration

When the patient is to be tube fed, the tube-feeding mixture must be shaken or thoroughly stirred. The prescribed amount should be carefully measured and allowed to stand at room temperature for 15–20 minutes. This feeding provides 1 kcal/cc.

* Egg may be fresh (cooked), frozen, or dried (amount equal to 1 egg).
† Check manufacturer's directions for weight or measure of skim milk powder to make 1 quart of liquid skim milk. Measures vary depending on density of product.

TABLE 3–2. COMMERCIAL BLENDERIZED DIETS. NUTRITIONAL SUPPORT SYSTEMS (COMPARISON/1000 CC STANDARD STRENGTH)

Product (Manufacturer)	Form	kcal	Osmolarity (mOs/kg)	CHO (g)	PRO (g)	FAT (g)	Na (mEq)	K (mEq)	Cl (mEq)	Fe (mg)	Ca (mg)	P (mg)
Compleat-B (Doyle)	L	1070	405	128 (48%)	42.7 (16%)	42.7 (36%)	56.1	36.8	24.5	12.0	667	1333
Compleat-Modified Formula (Doyle)	L	1070	Not available	141 (53%)	43.0 (16%)	37.0 (31%)	29.1	36.8	13.3	12.0	670	980
Formula 2 (Cutter)	L	1000	435–510	123 (49%)	37.5 (15%)	40.0 (36%)	26.0	46.0	53.6	12.6	720	560
Meritene Liquid (Doyle)	L	1000	560 (Vanilla)	115 (46%)	60.0 (24%)	33.3 (30%)	39.9	42.6	47.0	15.0	1250	1250
Meritene Powder (Doyle) [as prepared with whole milk]	P	1070	680 (Plain)	119 (45%)	69.2 (26%)	34.6 (29%)	41.8	75.8	61.8	17.3	2308	1923
Nutri 1000 (Cutter)	L	1060	500	101 (38%)	40.0 (15%)	56.0 (47%)	23.0	39.0	Not available	9.4	1198	Not available
Sustacal (Mead Johnson)	P	1010	625	136 (54%)	61.2 (24%)	24.8 (22%)	40.5	65.6	38.2	16.9	1636	1363
Vitaneed (Organon)	L	1000	375	125 (50%)	36.0 (14%)	40.0 (36%)	21.5	32.0	24.0	9.0	500	500

Table continues on following page

TABLE 3-2. COMMERCIAL BLENDERIZED DIETS, NUTRITIONAL SUPPORT SYSTEMS (COMPARISON/1000 CC STANDARD STRENGTH) (Continued)

Product (Manufacturer)	Carbohydrate	Protein	Fat	Flavors	Generic Description
Compleat-B (Doyle)	Hydrolyzed cereal solids, green peas, pea and peach purees, maltodextrin, orange juice	Beef purée, nonfat dry milk	Beef purée, corn oil	Unflavored	Meat-based blenderized tube feeding
Compleat-Modified Formula (Doyle)	Hydrolyzed cereal solids, green beans, pea and peach purees, orange juice	Beef purée, calcium caseinate	Beef purée, corn oil	Unflavored	Milk-based blenderized tube feeding
Formula 2 (Cutter)	Nonfat dry milk, sucrose, carrots, orange juice, green beans, wheat flour	Wheat, beef, egg, milk	Egg yolk, corn oil, beef fat	Orange	Oral or tube blenderized feeding
Meritene Liquid (Doyle)	Sweet skim milk, corn syrup solids, sucrose	Sweet skim milk, sodium caseinate	Corn oil	Vanilla, chocolate, eggnog	Supplemental or total diet
Meritene Powder (Doyle) (as prepared with whole milk)	Whole milk, nonfat dry milk, corn syrup solids	Whole milk, nonfat dry milk	Whole milk	Plain, vanilla, chocolate, eggnog	Supplemental or total diet
Nutri 1000 (Cutter)	Sucrose, lactose, corn syrup solids	Skim milk	Corn oil	Vanilla, chocolate	Oral or tube feeding
Sustacal (Mead Johnson)	Whole and nonfat dry milk, sucrose, corn syrup solids	Whole milk, nonfat dry milk	Whole milk	Vanilla, chocolate	Oral or tube feeding
Vitaneed (Organon)	Maltodextrin	Beef, sodium and calcium caseinates, vegetables	Soy oil	Unflavored	Blenderized tube feeding, low sodium, lactose-free

though the general composition of each diet is known, these are the least hydrolyzed or chemically defined of the enteral formulations. When administered in adequate amounts, these preparations can fully satisfy an individual's caloric and nutritional needs. The diets can also be used to supplement the intake of regular food. Administration may be oral, through a nasoenteric feeding tube, or through a surgically placed enterostomy tube or catheter. Since the lactose content of the milk-based preparations is high, they should not be used in patients with lactase deficiency.

The commercial, blenderized preparations contribute to fecal residue and are usually moderately hyperosmolar. When given through an indwelling tube, the feeding should be diluted to isotonicity and initially delivered at the relatively slow rate of 30 to 60 cc per hour (0.5 to 1 cc/kg body weight/hr). The concentration and volume can then be increased according to patient tolerance. Volume and concentration should not be increased simultaneously.

The major complications of this diet are diarrhea and crampy abdominal pain secondary to the high osmotic load or, occasionally, to an excessively rapid infusion rate. Diarrhea is best controlled by decreasing tonicity through the addition of free water. Other measures to control diarrhea include the administration of codeine, 15 to 30 mg every 4 to 6 hours, or the addition of tincture of opium, diphenoxylate (Lomotil), or loperamide HCl (Imodium) to the feeding. All of these substances may be useful in decreasing hyperperistalsis.

COMMERCIAL, LACTOSE-FREE DIETS.   These formulations contain protein, fat, and carbohydrate in high–molecular weight form and, therefore, require moderate digestive and absorptive capacity for utilization. They result in less residue than do the blenderized diets. Osmolarity is variable but some preparations are relatively isotonic and are, therefore, associated with a decreased incidence of diarrhea. The lactose-free preparations are indicated for patients with lactase deficiency (see Table 3–3).

Use of products with a caloric density of 1.5 or greater entails the risk of dehydration and prerenal azotemia because the solute load is high. Supplemental free water is necessary when using these preparations. Unless a patient has an indication for restriction, the usual fluid intake should approximate 1 ml/kcal/day. The osmolarity is also slightly higher than that of products with a standard caloric density.

DEFINED-FORMULA AND ELEMENTAL DIETS.   Defined-formula diets contain a more precisely defined protein, carbohydrate, lipid, vitamin, and mineral content than do the formulations previously described. Synthetic amino acids and hydrolyzed protein are used as amino acid sources. Calories are supplied as either oligo- or monosaccharides. Basal requirements for electrolytes, vitamins, and trace elements are included. When administered orally, various flavoring materials can be added to disguise the rather strong organic taste and odor of amino acid mixtures. Nonetheless, these high-protein, chemically defined diets are fairly unpalatable.

Elemental diets have several potential advantages over the other liquid diets. They are completely bulk-free, and some are almost fat-free (Table 3–4). Since minimal digestion is needed prior to absorption, most pancreatic, biliary,

Text continued on page 80

TABLE 3-3. COMMERCIAL, LACTOSE-FREE DIETS, NUTRITIONAL SUPPORT SYSTEMS (COMPARISON/1000 CC STANDARD STRENGTH)

Product (Manufacturer)	Form	kcal	Osmolarity (mOs/kg)	CHO (g)	PRO (g)	FAT (g)	Na (mEq)	K (mEq)	Cl (mEq)	Fe (mg)	Ca (mg)	P (mg)
Citrotein (Doyle)	P	660	496	129	43.0	22.0	31.0	19.0	Not available	37.5	1042	Not available
Ensure (Ross)	L, P	1060	460	146 (54.5%)	37.2 (14%)	37.2 (31.5%)	32.5	32.5	29.9	9.5	530	530
Ensure Plus (Ross)	L	1500	600	200 (53%)	56.0 (15%)	53.3 (32%)	46.1	48.6	44.8	14.3	630	630
Isocal (Mead Johnson)	L	1060	300	130 (50%)	34.2 (13%)	44.0 (37%)	23.0	33.8	29.6	9.5	630	530
Isocal HCN (Mead Johnson)	L	2000	740	225 (44%)	75.0 (15%)	91.0 (41%)	36.0	36.0	34.0	12.0	670	670
Magnacal (Organon)	L	2000	520	250 (50%)	70.0 (14%)	80.0 (36%)	43.5	32.0	31.3	18.0	1000	586
Nutri 1000 Lactose-Free (Cutter)	L	1060	380	101 (38%)	40.0 (15%)	55.0 (47%)	23.0	39.0	Not available	9.4	521	521
Nutri-Aid (American-McGaw)	L	1060	290	142 (53.7%)	39.2 (14.8%)	37.1 (31.5%)	33.0	32.4	29.8	9.5	548	548
Osmolite (Ross)	L	1060	300	145 (55%)	37.0 (14%)	39.0 (31%)	24.0	27.0	22.6	9.5	530	530
Osmolite HN (Ross)	L	1060	310	141 (53.3%)	44.3 (16.7%)	36.7 (30%)	40.4	39.9	44.1	13.9	760	760

Portagen (Mead Johnson)	P	983	357	115 (45%)	35.0 (14%)	47.6 (41%) (86% MCT)	20.0	31.0	Not available	19.0	936	Not available
Precision High Nitrogen (Doyle)	P	1050	557	216 (82%)	43.9 (17%)	1.3 (1%)	42.7	23.3	33.7	6.3	351	351
Precision Isotonic (Doyle)	P	960	300	144 (60%)	28.8 (12%)	30.1 (28%)	33.4	24.6	28.9	11.5	641	641
Precision Isotein HN (Doyle)	P	1190	300	156 (54%)	68.0 (24%)	34.0 (12%)	29.6	21.7	25.4	10.2	560	560
Precision Low Residue (Doyle)	P	1110	560	248 (89%)	26.3 (9.5%)	1.6 (1.5%)	30.5	22.4	31.3	10.5	585	585
Renu (Organon)	L	1000	330	130 (51%)	33.0 (13%)	40.0 (36%)	21.7	32.0	18.3	10.0	500	500
Traumacal (Mead Johnson)	L	1500	550	142 (38%)	82.3 (22%)	68.3 (40%)	51.4	35.6	45.3	8.9	747	747
Sustacal (Mead Johnson)	L	1000	625 (Vanilla)	138 (55%)	60.0 (24%)	23.0 (21%)	40.0	52.7	44.0	17.0	1000	920
Sustacal HC (Mead Johnson)	L	1500	650	190 (50%)	61.0 (16%)	58.0 (34%)	36.0	30.0	36.0	15.0	840	840
Travasorb (Travenol Labs)	L	1060	Not available	145 (54.5%)	37.2 (14%)	37.2 (31.5%)	32.3	32.5	29.9	9.5	530	530
Travasorb MCT (Travenol Labs)	P	1000	Not available	123 (50%)	49.2 (20%)	33.0 (30%)	15.2	44.5	34.3	9.0	500	500

Table continues on following page

TABLE 3–3. COMMERCIAL, LACTOSE-FREE DIETS, NUTRITIONAL SUPPORTS SYSTEMS (COMPARISON/1000 CC STANDARD STRENGTH) (Continued)

Product (Manufacturer)	Carbohydrate	Protein	Fat	Flavors	Generic Description
Citrotein (Doyle)	Maltodextrin, sucrose	Egg albumin	Partially hydrogenated soybean oil	Orange, grape	Supplemental: lactose, gluten, cholesterol-free
Ensure (Ross)	Corn syrup solids, sucrose	Sodium and calcium caseinates, soy protein isolate	Corn oil	Chocolate, vanilla, strawberry, coffee, black walnut	Supplemental diet; lactose-free tube feeding
Ensure Plus (Ross)	Corn syrup solids, sucrose	Sodium and calcium caseinates, soy protein isolate	Corn oil	Chocolate, vanilla, strawberry, coffee, eggnog	High-calorie, lactose-free; supplement or tube feeding
Isocal (Mead Johnson)	Glucose oligosaccharides	Calcium and sodium caseinates, soy protein isolate	Soy oil, medium-chain triglycerides	Unflavored	Isotonic, complete tube feeding
Isocal HCN (Mead Johnson)	Corn syrup	Calcium and sodium caseinates	Soy oil, MCT oil	Unflavored	High-calorie, high-nitrogen, concentrated tube feeding
Magnacal (Organon)	Maltodextrin, corn syrup solids, sucrose	Calcium and sodium caseinates	Soy oil	Vanilla	High-calorie, high-protein, complete liquid diet
Nutri 1000 Lactose-Free (Cutter)	Sucrose, corn syrup	Calcium and sodium caseinates, soy protein isolate	Corn oil	Chocolate, vanilla	Oral supplement or tube feeding; low-sodium and lactose
Nutri-Aid (American-McGaw)	Corn syrup solids, sucrose	Sodium and potassium caseinates	Corn oil	Vanilla, chocolate, strawberry	Isotonic oral supplement or tube feeding
Osmolite (Ross)	Corn syrup solids	Calcium and sodium caseinates, soy protein isolate	MCT oil, corn oil, soy oil	Unflavored	Isotonic liquid feeding
Osmolite HN (Ross)	Hydrolyzed corn starch	Sodium and calcium caseinates	Corn oil, soy oil, MCT oil	Unflavored	High-nitrogen, isotonic, oral supplement or tube feeding

TABLE 3-3. COMMERCIAL, LACTOSE-FREE DIETS, NUTRITIONAL SUPPORTS SYSTEMS (COMPARISON/1000 CC STANDARD STRENGTH) (Continued)

Product (Manufacturer)	Carbohydrate	Protein	Fat	Flavors	Generic Description
Portagen (Mead Johnson)	Maltodextrin	Sodium caseinate	MCT oil, corn oil	Unflavored	Supplement with high proportion MCT oil
Precision High Nitrogen (Doyle)	Maltodextrin, sucrose	Egg-white solids	MCT oil, soy oil	Citrus fruit, vanilla	Oral supplement or tube feeding; high-nitrogen, lactose-free, low-residue
Precision Isotonic (Doyle)	Glucose oligosaccharides, sucrose	Egg-white solids, sodium caseinates	Soy oil	Vanilla, orange	Oral supplement or tube feeding; isotonic
Precision Isotein HN (Doyle)	Maltodextrin, fructose	Lactalbumin	Soy oil, MCT oil	Vanilla	High-protein, isotonic oral supplement or tube feeding
Precision Low Residue (Doyle)	Maltodextrin, sucrose	Egg-white solids	MCT oil, soy oil	Cherry, lemon, lime, orange, vanilla	Oral supplement or tube feeding; low-residue
Renu (Organon)	Maltodextrin, corn syrup solids, corn and malt syrups	Sodium and calcium caseinates, soy protein isolate	Soy oil	Vanilla	Oral supplement or tube feeding
Traumacal (Mead Johnson)	Corn syrup	Sodium and potassium caseinates	MCT oil, soybean oil	Vanilla	Oral supplement or tube feeding; high-protein, high-calorie, rich source of branched-chain amino acids
Sustacal (Mead Johnson)	Sucrose, corn syrup	Calcium and sodium caseinates, soy protein isolate	Soy oil	Vanilla, eggnog, chocolate	High-protein supplement or tube feeding
Sustacal HC (Mead Johnson)	Corn syrup solids	Calcium and sodium caseinates	Soy oil	Vanilla, eggnog	High-calorie oral supplement; low-residue
Travasorb (Travenol Labs)	Sucrose, corn syrup solids	Sodium and calcium caseinates, soy protein isolate	Corn oil, soy oil	Vanilla, black walnut, eggnog	Whole protein liquid nutrition
Travasorb MCT (Travenol Labs)	Corn syrup solids	Lactalbumin, potassium caseinate	MCT oil, sunflower oil	Unflavored	Digestible protein MCT diet

77

TABLE 3–4. ELEMENTAL OR CHEMICALLY DEFINED DIETS, NUTRITIONAL SUPPORT SYSTEMS (COMPARISON/1000 CC STANDARD STRENGTH)

Product (Manufacturer)	Form	kcal	Osmolarity (mOs/kg)	CHO (g)	PRO (g)	FAT (g)	Na (mEq)	K (mEq)	Cl (mEq)	Fe (mg)	Ca (mg)	P (mg)
Criticare HN (Mead Johnson)	L	1060	650	222 (83%)	38.0 (14%)	3.0 (3%)	27.0	34.0	30.0	9.5	530	530
Traum-Aid HN (American-McGaw)	P	1000	800	180 (72%)	43.4 (17%)	12.4 (11%)	23.0	21.0	52.0	6.0	533	400
Travasorb STD (Travenol Labs)	P	1000	Not available	190 (76%)	30.0 (12%)	13.4 (12%)	40.0	29.9	42.3	9.0	500	500
Travasorb HN (Travenol Labs)	P	1000	Not available	175 (70%)	45.0 (18%)	13.4 (12%)	40.0	29.9	38.5	9.0	500	500
Vital High Nitrogen (Ross)	P	1000	460	188.3 (74%)	41.7 (16.7%)	10.8 (9.3%)	20.3	34.1	22.9	12.0	667	667
Vivonex (Norwich-Eaton)	P	1000	550 (Unflavored) 595–610 (Flavored)	230 (90.5%)	20.6 (8.2%)	1.5 (1.3%)	37.4	29.9	51.8	10.0	560	560
Vivonex High Nitrogen (Norwich-Eaton)	P	1016	810 (Unflavored) 860–865 (Flavored)	211 (81.5%)	43.3 (17.7%)	0.9 (0.8%)	33.5	17.9	52.4	6.0	333	333

TABLE 3–4. ELEMENTAL OR CHEMICALLY DEFINED DIETS, NUTRITIONAL SUPPORT SYSTEMS (COMPARISON/1000 CC STANDARD STRENGTH) (Continued)

Product (Manufacturer)	Carbohydrate	Protein	Fat	Flavors	Generic Description
Criticare HN (Mead Johnson)	Maltodextrin, modified corn starch	Hydrolyzed protein (30% oligopeptides, 70% free amino acids)	Safflower oil	Unflavored	Nutritionally complete tube feeding, considerable elemental nitrogen
Traum-Aid HN (American-McGaw)	Maltodextrin, sucrose	Synthetic amino acids (36% branched chain)	Partially hydrogenated soy oil, MCT oil	Berry, creme, grape, lemon	Chemically defined, high-nitrogen, high-branched-chain amino acid diet, oral or tube feeding
Travasorb STD (Travenol Labs)	Glucose oligosaccharides	Hydrolyzed lactalbumin, L-methionine	MCT oil, sunflower oil	Unflavored, beef broth, orange	Defined peptide diet
Travasorb HN (Travenol Labs)	Glucose oligosaccharides	Hydrolyzed lactalbumin, L-methionine	MCT oil, sunflower oil	Unflavored	High-nitrogen defined peptide diet
Vital High Nitrogen (Ross)	Hydrolyzed corn starch	Hydrolyzed whey, meat, soy; free amino acids	Safflower oil, MCT oil	Vanilla	Nutritionally complete, partially hydrolyzed diet; high nitrogen oral or tube feeding
Vivonex (Norwich-Eaton)	Glucose oligosaccharides	Crystalline amino acids	Safflower oil	Unflavored (flavor packs available)	Elemental diet
Vivonex High Nitrogen (Norwich-Eaton)	Glucose oligosaccharides	Synthetic amino acids	Safflower oil	Unflavored (flavor packs available)	Oral or tube feeding

and small intestinal secretions are not required for assimilation. In addition, absorption can occur even though minimal intestinal surface area is available. Elemental diets use only synthetic amino acids in their formulations.

The major complications of elemental diet administration—namely nausea, vomiting, and diarrhea—are most often related to nutrient concentration and rate of administration. (Although stool volume is reduced because of lack of bulk, diarrhea sometimes occurs when the concentration or rate of administration is too high.) Hypertonic dehydration and hyperosmolar nonketotic coma may develop when the diet is too concentrated and inadequate free water is provided. Hyperglycemia and glucosuria may occur in patients with diabetes, sepsis, or severe stress. Because of the high osmolarity of an elemental diet, it should be diluted to isotonicity when therapy is initiated. The concentration or volume administered can then be increased according to patient tolerance.

The indications for administration of an elemental diet are based upon its specific characteristics, *i.e.,* that it is bulk-free and is absorbed directly by the small intestine without the need for prior digestion by pancreatic or intestinal enzymes. It is estimated, however, that 100 cm of functional jejunum or 150 cm of functional ileum, preferably in association with an intact ileocecal valve, is necessary for absorption of an elemental diet in adequate amounts. Absorption of the diet is most efficient in the jejunum.

One of the most frequent specific indications for use of an elemental diet is the presence of an enterocutaneous fistula. Adequate nutritional support is one of many factors needed for successful treatment of such fistulas. Other factors necessary for fistula closure include (1) absence of distal intestinal obstruction, (2) control of intestinal secretions, (3) control of adjacent infection, and (4) a fistula diameter less than half the intestinal circumference. Total parenteral nutrition increases the spontaneous closure rate of intestinal fistulas and enhances the success of operative closure, and elemental diets can be used as an alternative mode of nutritional support once intestinal peristalsis has returned. The fistula output must be monitored carefully following institution of elemental alimentation; the technique must be abandoned if fistula output increases significantly, since this will only tend to keep the fistula open. Reported rates of spontaneous closure vary from 65 to 75 per cent in patients receiving elemental nutrition.

The short-bowel syndrome is a state of intestinal malabsorption resulting from (1) massive small-bowel resection following superior mesenteric artery occlusion, necrotizing enterocolitis, or midgut volvulus; (2) multiple small-bowel resections for conditions such as regional enteritis or recurrent small-bowel obstruction; or (3) the late changes of radiation enteritis.

Initial management following extensive small-bowel resection usually consists of total parenteral nutrition for 6 to 8 weeks while the remaining intestine undergoes compensatory hypertrophy. Once this period has passed, enteral feeding of an elemental diet may be instituted.

In order to minimize problems with diarrhea, the tonicity should be less than isotonic initially, and the solution should be infused at a slow, steady rate of 25 to 50 cc per hour. Absorption of the diet is variable and often slow; therefore, the rate of administration and concentration must be individualized.

In neonates, the short-bowel syndrome has been successfully treated with enterostomy feedings of defined-formula diets alone. A possibly important advantage of enteral nutritional therapy in these patients is maintenance of gastrointestinal structural and functional integrity. In animals, it has been demonstrated that intraluminal nutrition is mandatory for hyperplasia of the remaining intestine after a massive small-bowel resection. Others, however, have demonstrated mucosal atrophy in animals maintained on a defined-formula diet.

Administration of elemental diets in the immediate postoperative period has recently been advocated. Such diets are usually given through a standard jejunostomy tube or through a needle-catheter jejunostomy. Elemental diets can be started immediately after abdominal operations in many patients. In uncomplicated situations, postoperative ileus may affect the stomach for about 2 days and the colon for up to 5 days; the small bowel will not be affected unless there is also generalized peritonitis, small-bowel obstruction, extensive small-bowel adhesions, intrinsic small-bowel disease, or extensive retroperitoneal dissection. In the absence of these conditions, elemental diets may be administered directly into the small intestine immediately after surgery in an effort to achieve positive nitrogen balance. With this technique, positive nitrogen balance and preservation of both body weight and total protein levels have been demonstrated in patients undergoing extensive upper abdominal procedures or sustaining blunt abdominal trauma.

Recently, products enriched in branched-chain amino acids have been introduced. However, the use of such products is not supported to date by a plausible rationale, animal experiments, or clinical data.

ADMINISTRATION OF ENTERAL FEEDINGS

When a patient is unwilling or unable to ingest adequate nutrition orally, a feeding tube may be used to provide enteral nutritional support. Proper selection of enteral feeding equipment is essential to maximize patient tolerance, decrease nursing time, and optimize delivery of nutrient solutions. A nasoenteric feeding tube is generally chosen, particularly when enteral feeding is planned for a relatively short duration and there is no mechanical obstruction between the nasopharynx and stomach. A nasoenteric feeding tube is occasionally indicated when nocturnal feedings are required in patients with certain metabolic conditions (e.g., glycogen storage diseases), even though these patients can ingest feedings orally.

Use of the smallest tube that will allow for passage of the formula is essential to maximize patient comfort and tolerance. Nasoenteric feeding tubes are now generally made of silicone, silicone-rubber, polyurethane, or combinations of all three. Such tubes do not crack or stiffen after prolonged exposure to gastric secretions, a problem that was common with polyvinylchloride tubes. The most popular nasoenteric feeding tubes are weighted with elemental mercury or tungsten. The weight facilitates passage of a small-bore tube into the stomach; furthermore, a weighted tube can be passed through the pyloric sphincter to permit nasoduodenal or nasojejunal feedings in patients with malfunctions of the proximal gastrointestinal tract, such as disordered gastric motility.

When proximal gastrointestinal tract function or continuity is impaired, enterostomy tubes can be surgically placed directly into the stomach or jejunum. Such tubes are preferred to nasoenteric tubes in patients with long-term enteral feeding requirements because they are better tolerated by the patient, are generally easier to care for, and are socially more acceptable in the home environment. Gastrostomy tubes should be used with caution in patients with severe gastroesophageal reflux and are of limited value when gastric emptying is impaired. When proximal gastrointestinal continuity or function is impaired, jejunostomy tubes are generally required for nutritional support. Such tubes should be placed as proximal as possible, so that maximal digestion and absorption will minimize the risk of diarrhea.

Enteral feedings may be administered by constant drip or by intermittent gavaged bolus. Bolus feeding is certainly more convenient for chronic enteral nutrition in the home setting; however, constant drip feeding is generally preferable in the hospital setting, because it decreases the likelihood of diarrhea and permits more careful assessment of patient tolerance of the enteral formula.

When constant infusion is chosen, an enteral feeding pump should be used in order to maintain an accurate infusion rate and to facilitate delivery of the viscous solution through a small-bore tube by application of continuous positive pressure. The most frequently used pumps are of either the volumetric or the peristaltic-rotary type. Volumetric pumps are more accurate but also more costly, since they require the use of infusion cassettes. Peristaltic pumps, along with complete feeding sets, are less expensive and provide an acceptable degree of accuracy.

When enteral feedings are administered orally or through a nasogastric feeding or gastrostomy tube, aspiration of vomitus is a risk, particularly in elderly, weakened, or unconscious patients. Aspiration is usually preventable by elevating the head of the bed, avoiding night feedings, placement of the distal end of the tube beyond the pylorus, and careful evaluation for possible gastric retention. Tube feedings should not be administered when residual volume from a previous feeding is greater than 75 to 100 ml.

BIBLIOGRAPHY

Andrassy, R.S., and Woolley, M.M.: Progress in the use of elemental diets in infants and children. Surg Gynecol Obstet 147:701–704, 1978.

Christie, D.L., and Ament, M.D.: Dilute elemental diet and continuous infusion technique for management of short bowel syndrome. J Pediatr 87:705–708, 1975.

Chrysomilides, S.A., and Kaminski, M.V.: Home enteral and parenteral nutritional support: A comparison. Am J Clin Nutr 34:2271–2275, 1981.

Delany, H.M., Carnevale, N., Garvey, J.W., and Moss, C.M.: Postoperative nutritional support using needle catheter feeding jejunostomy. Ann Surg 186:165–170, 1977.

Dunn, E.L., Moore, E.E., and Bohus, R.W.: Immediate postoperative feeding following massive abdominal trauma — the catheter jejunostomy. J Parent Ent Nutr 4:393–396, 1980.

Freeman, J.B., Egan, M.C., and Ellis, B.J.: The elemental diet. Surg Gynecol Obstet 142:925–932, 1976.

Hoover, H.C., Ryan, J.A., Anderson, E.J., and Fischer, J.E.: Nutritional benefits of immediate postoperative jejunal feeding of an elemental diet. Am J Surg 139:153–158, 1980.

Kaminski, M.V.: Enteral hyperalimentation. Surg Gynecol Obstet 143:12–16, 1976.

Levine, G.M., Deren, J.J., and Yezdimir, E.: Small bowel resection; oral intake is the stimulus for hyperplasia. Am J Dig Dis 21:542–546, 1976.

McArdle, A.H., Echave, W., Brown, R.A., and Thompson, A.G.: Effect of elemental diet on pancreatic secretion. Am J Surg 128:690–692, 1974.

McArdle, A.H., Palmason, C., Morency, I., and Brown, R.S.: A rationale for enteral feeding as the preferable route for hyperalimentation. Surgery 90:616–622, 1981.

Nealon, T.F., Jr., Grossi, C.E., and Steier, M.: Use of elemental diets to correct catabolic states prior to surgery. Ann Surg 180:9–13, 1974.

Rocchio, M.A., Chung-Ja, M.C., et al.: Use of chemically defined diets in the management of patients with high output gastrointestinal cutaneous fistulas. Am J Surg 127:148–156, 1974.

Torosian, M.H., and Rombeau, J.: Feeding by tube enterostomy. Surg Gynecol Obstet 150:918–927, 1980.

Young, E.A., Cioletti, L.A., Winborn, W.B., Traylor, J.B., and Weser, E.: Comparative study of nutritional adaptation. A defined formula for diet in rats. Am J Clin Nutr 33:2106–2118, 1980.

4
PARENTERAL NUTRITION

Anthony L. Imbembo, M.D.

INTRODUCTION

The term *parenteral nutrition* is used here to denote infusion of a source of calories plus an amino acid solution. Provision of carbohydrate or fat without amino acids is used only in special situations, such as acute hyperammonemia. *Total parenteral nutrition* is a term meaning provision of all nutritional requirements by the parenteral route. Total parenteral nutrition can be administered by peripheral venous access but is more commonly given via a central venous catheter.

Since its introduction by Dudrick and associates in 1968, this technique has become an invaluable tool in the management of certain complicated nutritional problems. Available parenteral nutrition methodologies differ in their prime source of calories; either hypertonic dextrose or a lipid emulsion can be used to meet energy needs for both maintenance and protein synthesis.

PATIENT SELECTION

Parenteral nutrition is used in the preoperative preparation of certain malnourished patients when the oral or enteral route is not deemed appropriate— *e.g.,* patients with stricture or carcinoma of the esophagus, severe peptic ulcer disease with gastric outlet obstruction, or Crohn's disease with partial intestinal obstruction or chronic malabsorption. It is used as well in postoperative or post-trauma patients, and in those with enterocutaneous fistulas, short-bowel syndrome, transmural type of inflammatory bowel disease, acute renal failure with increased catabolic or metabolic needs, and burns. Cancer patients receiving chemotherapy also benefit from this technique. Enteral nutrition is preferred for patients refusing to ingest food orally in adequate amounts, as long as the gastrointestinal tract is functional, however.

GOALS AND RATIONALE OF TREATMENT

PREOPERATIVE PREPARATION OF THE MALNOURISHED PATIENT. Malnutrition may have many adverse effects on the postoperative course of a patient, including prolongation of postoperative adynamic ileus, relative obstruction at anastomoses due to edema, impairment of wound healing, increased susceptibility to infection secondary to reduced antibody formation and bone marrow replication, decreased ventilatory reserve with a higher incidence of atelectasis and pneumonitis, and decreased ambulatory capacity with a possible increase in the incidence of deep venous thrombosis. It is likely that preoperative correction of existing nutritional deficits can decrease the incidence of these complications. Nutritional support is best accomplished via either the oral or enteral route. However, parenteral correction may be necessary for patients who are unable to take nutrition orally or for those in whom the enteral route is unavailable.

In deciding whether to institute total parenteral nutrition in these patients, the state of the patient's disease and overall nutritional status, as well as the degree and duration of catabolism expected, must be considered. For example, a well-nourished patient for whom the predicted duration of limited oral intake is short and in whom only moderate catabolism is expected should not be given preoperative parenteral nutritional support. On the other hand, mortality and morbidity rates for surgery and trauma increase with age, while tolerance of starvation and catabolism decreases. Therefore, an older patient, even in a borderline-adequate nutritional state, might be a candidate for nutritional support when major surgical trauma and the consequent need for postoperative total parenteral nutrition are anticipated.

SUPPORT OF THE COMPLICATED POSTOPERATIVE OR POST-TRAUMA PATIENT. The nutritional requirements of postoperative or post-trauma patients differ strikingly from those of fasting individuals. A fasting 70-kg adult utilizes approximately 1800 kcal/day under basal conditions. This requirement normally is met by the metabolism of adipose tissue triglycerides and of protein, predominantly derived from skeletal muscle. Under basal conditions, about 85 per cent of energy requirements in prolonged fasting are met by the complete oxidation of fatty acids to carbon dioxide or by partial oxidation in the liver to acetoacetic acid or beta-hydroxybutyric acid (the ketone bodies). Remaining energy needs are met by oxidation of amino acids derived from proteolysis and by glucose synthesized from certain amino acids by the gluconeogenic pathways of the liver. This endogenously synthesized glucose is used primarily by the central nervous system, leukocytes, erythrocytes, bone marrow, and peripheral nerves.

The postsurgical or post-trauma patient deviates from this pattern, however. While the rate of fat oxidation is not significantly different from the normal starvation state, inordinate breakdown of tissue protein occurs consistently following operations, trauma, burns, and fractures and during sepsis. This protein loss, termed the *catabolic response,* can approach 30 g of nitrogen per day (or approximately 1 kg of muscle per day) during periods of severe stress. The cause of the catabolic response remains unclear. The degree of negative balance clearly is related to the severity of the illness or injury, ranging from 3 to 4 g of nitrogen per day following inguinal herniorrhapy to 30 g of nitrogen per day in complicated situations. Moreover, decreased muscle uptake of the branched-chain amino acids (valine, leucine, and isoleucine) suggests that protein synthesis by muscle also may be impaired.

Protein and calorie requirements of post-trauma patients can be still greater under certain circumstances. Significant direct loss of protein can result from external hemorrhage, leakage of protein from enterocutaneous fistulas or open wound surfaces, colloid losses into the peritoneal cavity secondary to peritonitis, and plasma protein losses into soft tissues following crush injuries. The total caloric expenditure of complicated postoperative and post-trauma patients is frequently increased strikingly by the presence of hypermetabolic states, such as fever or sepsis; by the direct loss of heat from open wounds or burns; or secondary to hyperventilation. Calories are also necessary for tissue synthesis and protein replenishment. Since 100 to 150 kcal/g of nitrogen are required for tissue synthesis, a patient who is markedly catabolic or who has excessive protein losses requires a considerable number of calories to support synthesis. By satisfying these increased caloric needs, total parenteral nutrition can often ameliorate the degree of negative nitrogen balance.

ENTEROCUTANEOUS FISTULAS.   Prior to the availability of total parenteral nutrition, the mortality rate from enterocutaneous fistulas was about 50 per cent, particularly with those arising from the duodenum or jejunum. The spontaneous closure rate of such fistulas may increase to 50 to 70 per cent when positive nitrogen balance is achieved through the use of intravenous nutritional support. Even if the fistula fails to close after a course of total parenteral nutrition, operative intervention is more apt to be successful because of the patient's improved nutritional status.

In one large study of small-bowel fistulas, the spontaneous closure rate was over 50 per cent in those receiving total parenteral nutrition as opposed to 27 per cent in patients receiving conventional fluid replacement. Others, however, have noted that surgical closure is still necessary in 70 per cent of enterocutaneous fistulas even after a course of total parenteral nutritional support. However, the mortality rate in such patients after operative fistula closure has been lowered considerably, now ranging from 8 to 21 per cent.

Total parenteral nutrition benefits the management of intestinal fistulas both by improving wound healing and, possibly, by decreasing the volume of gastric, pancreatic, and biliary secretions, thereby secondarily promoting spontaneous closure.

SHORT-BOWEL SYNDROME.   This syndrome is a state of severe intestinal malabsorption that may arise in a number of ways. Most often, the syndrome occurs following massive small bowel resection for mesenteric ischemia or in the setting of multiple resective procedures for regional enteritis. Initial management following extensive small bowel resection usually consists of total parenteral nutrition for a period of 6 to 8 weeks while hypertrophy of the remaining intestine occurs. Even in patients with minimal lengths of small intestine remaining (15 to 30 cm of jejunum), the bowel will usually hypertrophy to such an extent that intravenous nutritional support can eventually be discontinued.

INFLAMMATORY BOWEL DISEASE OF THE TRANSMURAL TYPE.   This form of inflammatory bowel disease may be benefited by total parenteral nutrition. Crohn's disease frequently is associated with partial intestinal obstruction, intestinal fistulas, intra-abdominal abscess, and chronic malabsorption. These patients often are markedly malnourished, depleted of protein and electrolytes, and severely catabolic.

In this setting, total parenteral nutrition may be a valuable tool. The nutritional status of the patient can be improved at the same time as the bowel is placed at rest. The correction of malnutrition, coupled with bowel rest and intensified medical therapy, may result in a higher remission rate. Remission may avert the ultimate development of a short-bowel syndrome that is seen occasionally after multiple small-bowel resections for extensive disease. Such remission may be of particular importance in those patients who have had previous resections for inflammatory bowel disease. Even if the complications of inflammatory bowel disease persist after several weeks of total parenteral nutrition, the patient has become an improved operative candidate following at least partial correction of nutritional deficits.

ACUTE RENAL FAILURE (SEE ALSO CHAPTER 8, SECTION ON RENAL FAILURE). The improved management of acute renal failure during the past several years, which includes hemodialysis, has not reduced the overall mortality rate from this condition. Acute renal failure is of particular significance in postoperative or post-trauma patients whose catabolic rates are frequently greater than those of anuric patients with otherwise normal metabolism.

The management of acute renal failure in the patient with an increased catabolic rate and caloric requirement may be facilitated by the intravenous infusion of a 5 per cent essential amino acid preparation along with 70 per cent dextrose. The administration of such a solution in patients with acute renal failure may result in improved wound healing, shorter duration of renal dysfunction, and the need for fewer dialysis treatments for control of azotemia and hyperkalemia.

It remains to be established whether survival is improved by such therapy. Some feel that the main advantage of this regimen is its high ratio of calories to nitrogen. It is not clear whether the infusion of only essential amino acids is of greater efficacy than infusion of a balanced amino acid preparation.

When acute renal failure is not complicated by abnormally high metabolic or catabolic demands, peripheral intravenous alimentation utilizing dextrose (5 or 10 per cent), or a lipid emulsion (10 or 20 per cent), or both, along with an essential amino acid preparation may provide adequate nutritional support.

BURNS. High catabolic rates and severe negative nitrogen balance are observed consistently in burn patients. Adequate nutrition is often difficult to achieve, at least partly because of frequent and prolonged postburn ileus. Total parenteral nutrition in burn patients has been achieved with either hypertonic dextrose or lipid as the prime calorie source.

CHEMOTHERAPY OF MALIGNANT DISEASE. Although increasingly effective chemotherapeutic agents offer hope in the treatment of some disseminated malignant diseases, poor nutritional status and possible gastrointestinal side effects of chemotherapy may preclude this form of treatment. Total parenteral nutrition has become a useful adjunct to management under these circumstances. These patients can have their nutritional needs met safely by the parenteral route despite their high potential risk of sepsis. Furthermore, increased nutrient intake may not cause a significant increase in tumor protein synthesis; instead protein synthesis by many other host tissues is improved. A further benefit that may be of particular importance in these patients is improved cell-mediated immune competence secondary to correction of nutritional deficits.

ACUTE HEPATIC FAILURE AND ENCEPHALOPATHY (SEE ALSO CHAPTER 8, SECTION ON PROTEIN MODIFICATIONS). Abnormal plasma amino acid patterns have been noted in many patients with various degrees of hepatic failure and acute hepatic encephalopathy. In patients with cirrhosis of the liver and moderate impairment in hepatic function, the concentrations of the branched-chain amino acids (leucine, isoleucine, and valine) decrease, while the aromatic amino acids, especially phenylalanine, tend to accumulate in the plasma. As hepatic encephalopathy develops, tryptophan concentrations also seem to rise, but to a variable degree, and plasma levels of methionine are often strikingly increased. Corresponding changes in amino acid levels are noted in the cerebrospinal fluid and central nervous system.

The etiology and significance of these abnormalities have not been definitively established. It is known that some amino acids or their derivatives may have adverse effects on central nervous system function. For example, methionine sulfoxide and methanethiol (arising from metabolism of methionine by gut flora) are cerebrotoxic. Excess plasma methionine may also be toxic to the central nervous system owing to either depletion of adenosine triphosphate secondary to excessive synthesis of S-adenosylmethionine or to accumulation of methylated amino compounds that are known to be extremely toxic. The possible inability of the body of the encephalopathic patient to hydroxylate phenylalanine to form tyrosine impairs the synthesis of norepinephrine and dopamine, which are both believed to be important for brain neurotransmission. Increased concentrations of phenylalanine and tyrosine also promote synthesis of centrally active p-hydroxyphenolic acids and of false neurotransmitters, such as octopamine and phenylethanolamine. It has been postulated that such false neurotransmitters compete with the usual neurotransmitters dopamine and epinephrine for receptor sites in the central nervous system.

Excessive plasma phenylalanine levels may further contribute to deficient central nervous system neurotransmitter levels by competitive impairment of tyrosine uptake. A rise in the free tryptophan component in plasma stimulates the cerebral synthesis of serotonin, a product that may account for some of the neurologic abnormalities observed.

Finally, branched-chain amino acids compete with phenylalanine, tyrosine, and tryptophan for active transport across the blood-brain barrier. A decrease in branched-chain amino acid levels possibly increases transport of aromatic amino acids into the brain, thereby contributing to the encephalopathic picture.

A recent approach advocated by some for the treatment of acute hepatic encephalopathy is the normalization of plasma amino acid levels by techniques of parenteral nutrition. It has been suggested that the administration of a solution rich in branched-chain amino acids might improve hepatic encephalopathy by competing with aromatic amino acids for transport across the blood-brain barrier. Similarly, phenylalanine, tryptophan, and methionine should be restricted in patients with hepatic encephalopathy.

PRINCIPLES OF TOTAL PARENTERAL NUTRITION

Hypertonic Dextrose–Synthetic Amino Acids

In order to satisfy caloric requirements without exceeding a patient's daily fluid tolerance, dextrose must be administered as at least a 20 or 25 per cent solution. Therefore, solutions containing 200 to 250 g of dextrose per liter and supplying 680 to 850 kcal/l are markedly hyperosmolar (1000 to 1350 mOsm/l). Administration of 3 to 5 l of such a solution per day generally satisfies a patient's caloric needs.

Even though sufficient hypertonic dextrose can be administered to provide adequate calories, positive nitrogen balance cannot be achieved unless amino acids are administered along with a calorie source. Protein is generally supplied as a solution of synthetic amino acids. These preparations are biologically efficacious, since all of the nitrogen is in a utilizable form, owing to the absence of oligopeptides. The commercial preparations have amino acid compositions similar to those occurring in natural proteins of high biologic value, such as egg albumin. The free ammonia level is low, yet encephalopathy is still an occasional complication following infusion. Hypersensitivity reactions are virtually nonexistent. Generally, most hospitalized patients require between 200 and 250 mg of nitrogen per kilogram of body weight per day (Tables 4–1 to 4–5).

Recently, amino acid preparations containing branched-chain amino acids in slightly higher concentrations have been introduced (FreAmine III and Aminosyn). It has been shown that the branched-chain amino acids play an important role in the regulation of nitrogen balance in muscle by decreasing protein degradation and increasing protein synthesis in a dose-dependent fashion. Although branched-chain amino acids are minimally utilized by the liver, kidney, and gut, they do lead to *de novo* synthesis in muscle of alanine and glutamine, which, in turn, can be metabolized by these organs as a source of energy. The branched-chain enriched solutions are designed to improve nitrogen sparing in the postoperative period. However, there is still no convincing evidence that branched-chain enriched products achieve any greater nitrogen sparing than do the conventionally balanced amino acid solutions.

With the exception of potassium and phosphorus, mineral and electrolyte requirements are probably about the same for patients on total parenteral nutrition as they are for those receiving oral or enteral nutrition. Glucose utilization is accompanied by an intracellular shift of potassium, and, consequently, maintenance potassium requirements may be increased for patients on total parenteral nutrition with hypertonic dextrose. In addition, supplemental phosphate is usually necessary; almost all patients receiving phosphate-free solutions will develop low serum phosphate levels over a 7- to 10-day period. There are data

Text continues on page 95

TABLE 4–1. TRAVASOL AMINO ACID SOLUTIONS (TRAVENOL)

	3.5% with Electrolytes	5.5%	5.5% with Electrolytes	8.5%	8.5% with Electrolytes	10%
Total nitrogen (g/100 ml)	0.59	0.92	0.92	1.42	1.42	1.68
Approximate pH	6.0	6.0	6.0	6.0	6.0	6.0
Osmolarity (mOsm/l)	450.0	520.0	850.0	860.0	1160.0	1060.0
ESSENTIAL AMINO ACIDS (MG/100 ML)						
Isoleucine	168	263	263	406	406	600
Leucine	217	340	340	526	526	730
Lysine	203	318	318	492	492	580
Methionine	203	318	318	492	492	400
Phenylalanine	217	340	340	526	526	560
Threonine	147	230	230	356	356	420
Tryptophan	63	99	99	152	152	180
Valine	161	252	252	390	390	580
NONESSENTIAL AMINO ACIDS (MG/100 ML)						
Alanine	728	1140	1140	1760	1760	2070
Arginine	364	570	570	880	880	1150
Glycine	728	1140	1140	1760	1760	1030
Histidine	154	241	241	372	372	480
Proline	147	230	230	356	356	680
Tyrosine	14	22	22	34	34	40
Serine	—	—	—	—	—	500
ELECTROLYTES (MEQ/L)						
Acetate	54	35	100	35	135	44
Chloride	25	22	70	22	70	20
Magnesium	5	—	10	—	10	—
Phosphate (as HPO_4^-)	15	—	60 (30 mM)	—	60 (30 mM)	—
Potassium	15	—	60	—	60	—
Sodium	25	—	70	—	70	—

TABLE 4–2.   FREAMINE AMINO ACID SOLUTIONS (AMERICAN-MCGAW)

	FreAmine III 3%	FreAmine III 8.5%	FreAmine III 10%
Total nitrogen (g/100 ml)	0.46	1.3	1.53
Osmolarity (mOsm/l)	405	810	950
ESSENTIAL AMINO ACIDS(MG/100 ML)			
Isoleucine	210	590	690
Leucine	270	770	910
Lysine	219	620	1020
Methionine	160	450	530
Phenylalanine	170	480	560
Threonine	120	340	400
Tryptophan	46	130	150
Valine	200	560	660
NONESSENTIAL AMINO ACIDS (MG/100 ML)			
Alanine	210	600	710
Arginine	290	810	950
Histidine	85	240	280
Proline	340	950	1120
Serine	180	500	590
Glycine	420	1190	1400
Cysteine	—	< 20	< 24
ELECTROLYTES (MEQ/L)			
Acetate	44	74	86
Chloride	40	< 2	< 2
Magnesium	5	—	—
Phosphate (as HPO_4^-)	3.5	10	20
Potassium	24.5	—	—
Sodium	35	10	10

TABLE 4–3.   VEINAMINE 8% AMINO ACID
SOLUTION (CUTTER)

Amino acids	8%
Total nitrogen (g/100 ml)	1.33
Approximate pH	6.2–6.6
Osmolarity (mOsm/l)	950

ESSENTIAL AMINO ACIDS (MG/100 ML)

Isoleucine	493
Leucine	347
Lysine	667
Methionine	427
Phenylalanine	400
Threonine	160
Tryptophan	80
Valine	253

NONESSENTIAL AMINO ACIDS (MG/100 ML)

Alanine	—
Arginine	749
Aspartic acid	400
Cysteine	—
Glutamic acid	426
Glycine	3387
Histidine	237
Proline	107
Serine	—
Tyrosine	—

ELECTROLYTES (MEQ/L)

Acetate	50
Chloride	50
Magnesium	6
Phosphate	—
Potassium	30
Sodium	40

TABLE 4–4.   NOVAMINE AMINO ACID SOLUTIONS (CUTTER)

	8.5%	11.4%
Total nitrogen (g/100 ml)	1.35	1.8
Acetate (mEq/l)	88	114
Osmolarity (mOsm/l)	785	1049

ESSENTIAL AMINO ACIDS (MG/100 ML)

	8.5%	11.4%
Isoleucine	420	570
Leucine	590	790
Lysine (acetate)	673	900
Methionine	420	570
Phenylalanine	590	790
Threonine	420	570
Tryptophan	140	190
Valine	550	730

NONESSENTIAL AMINO ACIDS (MG/100 ML)

	8.5%	11.4%
Alanine	1200	1590
Arginine	840	1120
Aspartic Acid	250	330
Cysteine	40	60
Glutamic Acid	420	570
Glycine	590	790
Histidine	500	680
Proline	500	680
Serine	340	450
Tyrosine	20	30

TABLE 4–5.   AMINOSYN AMINO ACID SOLUTIONS (ABBOTT)

	3.5%	5%	7%	7% with Electro-lytes	8.5%	8.5% with Electro-lytes	10%
Total Nitrogen (g/100 ml)	0.55	0.78	1.1	1.1	1.34	1.34	1.57
Approximate pH	5.3	5.3	5.3	5.3	5.3	5.3	5.3
Osmolarity (mOsm/l)	460	500	700	1013	850	1160	1000
ESSENTIAL AMINO ACIDS (MG/100 ML)							
Isoleucine	252	360	510	510	620	620	720
Leucine	329	470	660	660	810	810	940
Lysine (acetate)	252	360	510	510	624	624	720
Methionine	140	200	280	280	340	340	400
Phenylalanine	154	220	310	310	380	380	440
Threonine	182	260	370	370	460	360	520
Tryptophan	56	80	120	120	150	150	160
Valine	280	400	560	560	680	680	800
NONESSENTIAL AMINO ACIDS (MG/100 ML)							
Alanine	448	640	900	900	1100	1100	1280
Arginine	343	490	690	690	850	850	980
Histidine	105	150	210	210	260	260	300
Proline	300	430	610	610	750	750	860
Serine	147	210	300	300	370	370	420
Tyrosine	31	44	44	44	44	44	44
Glycine	448	640	900	900	1100	1100	1280
ELECTROLYTES (MEQ/L)							
Sodium	47	—	—	70	—	70	—
Potassium	13	5.4	5.4	66	5.4	66	5.4
Magnesium	3	—	—	10	—	30	—
Phosphorus (mM)	—	—	—	30	—	30	—
Chloride	40	—	—	96	35	98	—
Acetate	68	86	105	124	90	142	148

suggesting that repletion of protoplasm and extracellular fluid of wasted adults by total parenteral nutrition is retarded or abolished if nitrogen, phosphorus, sodium, or potassium is deficient in the infusate. Repletion of bone does not occur in the absence of sodium or phosphorus.

In order to prescribe additives properly, the mineral and electrolyte content of the amino acid solution must be known, as it varies considerably from preparation to preparation. In general, a liter of solution for total parenteral nutrition should contain at least 30 mEq sodium, 20 mEq potassium, 5 mEq calcium, 10 mEq phosphate, and 5 mEq magnesium (Table 4–6).

Various multivitamin preparations for intravenous administration are available for use in long-term total parenteral nutrition therapy. At the present time, the vitamins recognized as essential for humans are

1. Fat soluble—retinol (vitamin A), cholecalciferol and ergocalciferol (vitamin D), alpha-tocopherol (vitamin E), and phytonadione (vitamin K_1)

2. Water soluble—ascorbic acid (vitamin C), thiamine (vitamin B_1), riboflavin (vitamin B_2), niacin, pyridoxine (vitamin B_6), pantothenic acid, folacin, cyanocobalamin (vitamin B_{12}), and biotin

The recommended multivitamin dosage for parenteral use is detailed in Table 4–7. Sample preparations for intravenous use in total parenteral nutrition are given in Table 4–8.

The RDAs reflect the needs of healthy people and do not necessarily reflect possible special requirements that arise secondary to infection, metabolic disorders, or chronic disease. Minimal vitamin requirements in most disease states have not been defined. Most water-soluble vitamins are provided in amounts that are approximately twice the highest RDA. For adults, the amounts of parenteral vitamin A given are less than the oral allowance, since the RDAs are based, in part, on the variable absorption and conversion of ingested carotenes. Care must be taken to avoid vitamin A or D excess, since problems can result from overdosage with these slowly excreted vitamins.

TABLE 4–6. SAMPLE TOTAL HYPERALIMENTATION SOLUTION—JOHNS HOPKINS HOSPITAL

Stock:	500 ml FreAmine III 8.5%			
	500 ml dextrose 50% injection			
Yielding:	1000 ml dextrose 25%, amino acids 4.25%			
Provides:	Amino acids	42.5 g		
	Total nitrogen	6.5 g		
	Calories from dextrose	850		
	Nonprotein calories/g nitrogen	131:1		
Electrolytes (mEq/l):				
	Sodium	30	Chloride	30
	Potassium	20	Phosphate	10
	Magnesium	5	Acetate	67
	Calcium	5		
Trace Elements:				
	Copper	1–2 mg/day	Chromium	12 mcg/day
	Zinc	3 mg/day	Manganese	0.3 mcg/day

**TABLE 4–7.   RECOMMENDED DAILY MULTIVITAMIN DOSAGE FOR INTRAVE-
NOUS THERAPY (ADULTS AND CHILDREN AGED 11 YEARS AND ABOVE)**

Vitamin	Dose	
Vitamin A	3300	IU
Vitamin D	200	IU
Vitamin E	10	IU
Vitamin K	1	mcg/kg
Ascorbic acid	100	mg
Folacin	400	mcg
Niacin	40	mg
Riboflavin	3.6	mg
Thiamine	3	mg
Pyridoxine (vitamin B_6)	4	mg
Cyanocobalamin (vitamin B_{12})	5	mcg
Pantothenic acid	15	mg
Biotin	60	mcg

From American Medical Association Nutrition Advisory Group: Multi-vitamin preparation for parenteral use. J Parent Ent Nutr 3:258–262, 1979.

**TABLE 4–8.   PARENTERAL MULTIVITAMIN PREPARATIONS FOR USE IN TOTAL
PARENTERAL NUTRITION**

M.V.C. 9+3 (Lypho-Med Inc., Chicago, IL 60651)
M.V.I.-12 (USV Laboratories, Division USV Pharmaceutical Corp, Tuckahoe, NY)
Each product consists of two 5-vials, labeled Vial 1 and Vial 2, containing the following:

Vial 1			Vial 2	
Ascorbic acid	100	mg	Biotin	60 mcg
Vitamin A (retinol)	3300	IU	Folic acid	400 mcg
Vitamin D (ergocalciferol)	200	IU	Vitamin B_{12}	5 mcg
Thiamine (vitamin B_1)	3.0	mg		
Pantothenic acid	15.0	mg		
Riboflavin (vitamin B_2)	3.6	mg		
Niacinamide	40	mg		
Vitamin E (dl-alpha tocopheryl acetate)	10	IU		
Pyridoxine HCl (vitamin B_6)	4.0	mg		

MVC Plus (Ascot Pharmaceuticals, Inc.)

Contained in Lower Chamber:			Contained in Upper Chamber:	
Ascorbic acid	100	mg	Biotin	60 mcg
Vitamin A	3300	IU	Folic acid	400 mcg
Vitamin D (ergocalciferol)	200	IU	Vitamin B_{12}	5 mcg
Thiamine (vitamin B_1)	3.0	mg		
Pantothenic acid	15	mg		
Riboflavin	3.6	mg		
Niacinamide	40	mg		
Vitamin E	10	IU		
Pyridoxine	4.0	mg		

Solutions containing 20 to 25 per cent dextrose as a calorie source must always be administered through a central venous catheter. These solutions are markedly hypertonic and, consequently, must be infused through a large-diameter, high-flow vessel. In this way, the solution is diluted rapidly and the risk of venous thrombosis is minimized. The superior vena cava is the most suitable route and can be cannulated satisfactorily via the subclavian or internal jugular vein. It is essential to ensure proper catheter position by examining a chest x-ray before starting the hypertonic infusion.

Total parenteral nutrition is often instituted with 10 per cent dextrose in water, 1 liter over 24 hours. Glucose tolerance is assessed by following the patient's urinary and blood sugars. If there is no evidence of glucose intolerance, the patient is initially given 1 liter of total parenteral nutrition solution per day. This is then increased at the rate of an additional liter per day until the desired level is reached. Once established, the final infusion rate is kept constant, usually through the use of an infusion pump. The patient's weight is followed daily, and urine sugars, serum electrolytes, calcium, phosphorus, and magnesium are carefully monitored.

Lipid Emulsion, Dextrose, and Amino Acids

An alternate regimen for total parenteral nutrition utilizes lipid as the prime calorie source. Intralipid (Table 4–9), until recently the only intravenous lipid preparation available in this country, consists of either 10 or 20 per cent soybean oil emulsified with 1.2 per cent egg yolk phospholipids, and 2.25 per cent glycerin in water. Soybean oil is a mixture of triglycerides containing predominantly unsaturated fatty acids. The major component fatty acids are linoleic (50 to 54 per cent), oleic (26 per cent), palmitic (9 to 10 per cent), and linolenic (7 to 8 per cent). The solutions have an osmolarity of 280 to 330 mOsm/l and a caloric value of 1.1 to 2.0 kcal/ml. Thus, Intralipid is relatively isotonic and contains emulsified fat particles approximating the size of a chylomicron (0.5 micron). Travamulsion is a new 10 per cent soybean oil intravenous fat emulsion with similar characteristics (Table 4–10).

Recently, an alternative fat emulsion based on safflower oil has been introduced. Liposyn consists of 10 or 20 per cent safflower oil emulsified with 1.2 per cent egg phosphatides and 2.5 per cent glycerin in water (Table 4–11). Safflower oil is also a mixture of triglycerides containing predominantly unsaturated fatty acids. The fatty acids forming the major component of the emulsion are linoleic (77 per cent), oleic (13 per cent), palmitic (7 per cent), and stearic (2.5 per cent). The solutions have an osmolarity of 300 to 340 mOsm/l and a total caloric value of 1.1 to 2.0 kcal/ml.

The safflower oil emulsion provides more linoleic acid than is provided in an equal volume of soybean emulsion, thereby ensuring, to a greater degree, a source of essential fatty acids; it is unlikely that this represents any distinct advantage. The safflower oil emulsion, however, contains no linolenic acid; recently, a case has been reported of human linolenic acid deficiency in the pediatric age group, causing episodic numbness, paresthesias, weakness, inabil-

Text continues on page 99

TABLE 4–9.   INTRALIPID (CUTTER)

Intralipid 10%	Intralipid 20%
Soybean oil 10%	Soybean oil 20%
Egg yolk phospholipids 1.2%	Egg yolk phospholipids 1.2%
Glycerin 2.25%	Glycerin 2.25%
Osmolarity 280 mOsm/l	Osmolarity 330 mOsm/l
Total caloric value 1.1 kcal/ml	Total caloric value 2 kcal/ml

Total Fatty Acid Pattern—Intralipid 10%

		SOYBEAN OIL %	PHOSPHOLIPIDS %
Myristic acid	C_{14}	0.035	0.090
Palmitic acid	C_{16}	9.18	32.51
Palmitoleic acid	$C_{16:1}$	0.026	0.37
Stearic acid	C_{18}	2.87	15.69
Oleic acid	$C_{18:1}$	26.41	32.03
Linoleic acid	$C_{18:2}$	54.27	11.33
Linolenic acid	$C_{18:3}$	7.81	0.297
Arachidic acid	C_{20}	0.12	0.132
Arachidonic acid	$C_{20:4}$	—	0.15
Behenic acid	C_{22}	0.059	3.41
Unidentified acids		—	0.222

TABLE 4–10.   TRAVAMULSION (TRAVENOL)

Soybean oil	10%	
Egg phosphatides	1.2%	
Glycerin	2.25%	
Osmolarity	270	mOsm/l
Total caloric value	1.1	kcal/ml
Fatty Acid Pattern		
Linoleic acid	56%	
Oleic acid	23%	
Palmitic acid	11%	
Linolenic acid	6%	

TABLE 4–11.   LIPOSYN (ABBOTT)

Safflower oil	10%		20%	
Egg phosphatides	1.2%		1.2%	
Glycerin	2.5%		2.5%	
Osmolarity	300	mOsm/l	340	mOsm/l
Total caloric value	1.1	kcal/ml	2.0	kcal/ml
Fatty Acid Pattern				
Linoleic acid	77%		77%	
Oleic acid	13%		13%	
Palmitic acid	7%		7%	
Stearic acid	2.5%		2.5%	

ity to walk, and blurring of vision. The requirement for linolenic acid is now estimated to be 0.54 per cent of calories.

In general, a fat emulsion should comprise no more than 60 per cent of the patient's total caloric input. Remaining calories are supplied by a 20 per cent solution of dextrose, primarily to meet the glucose requirements of the central nervous system. Fat emulsions, which are all nearly isotonic, may be infused through a peripheral vein without the rapid development of venous thrombosis, but the catheter site should be changed every 1 or 2 days to minimize the risk. To achieve positive nitrogen balance, lipid emulsions must be administered along with a carbohydrate–amino acid solution (500 ml 7 to 8 per cent synthetic amino acids plus 500 ml 20 per cent dextrose).

Appropriate vitamin and electrolyte additives should be placed in the dextrose–amino acid bottle rather than added to the lipid emulsion. The solutions are infused simultaneously into the same vein through an external Y-connector immediately adjacent to the venipuncture device; adding either dextrose or amino acids directly to the emulsion would alter its stability. Travenol Laboratories has recently introduced containers suitable for admixtures of Travamulsion—Travasol amino acid injection and dextrose; this system eliminates the need for the Y-connector and for simultaneous dual administration.

The initial infusion rate of any lipid emulsion in adults should be 0.5 ml/minute for the first 15 to 30 minutes. If no immediate adverse reactions occur—namely, dyspnea, cyanosis, urticaria, nausea, or vomiting—the rate can be increased so that 500 ml of a 10 per cent solution will be infused over 8 hours. The dosage can then be increased again on the following day, but the daily adult dosage should not exceed 3 g/kg of body weight.

In pediatric patients, the initial infusion rate should be 0.05 ml/minute for the first 10 to 15 minutes. If no untoward reactions occur, the rate can be increased to permit infusion of 1 g/kg of body weight over 4 hours, but the daily dosage should not exceed 4 g/kg of body weight. Premature and small-for-gestational-age infants clear intravenous fat emulsions poorly, and free fatty acid plasma levels increase following infusion. Therefore, the infant's ability to eliminate the infused fat from the circulation must be monitored by following serum triglyceride levels and by making sure that lipemia clears between infusions.

Many reports have shown that intravenous fat emulsions are metabolized and biologically utilized. Positive nitrogen balance and weight gain with a fat emulsion as the prime calorie source have been attained in a variety of pathologic settings, including inflammatory bowel disease, enterocutaneous fistulas, burns, and premature births.

Although fat can be used as a calorie source, the optimal ratio of fat to carbohydrate calories has not been determined. Some suggest that carbohydrate calories should be given in amounts sufficient to approximate the metabolic rate, thereby minimizing protein catabolism. Fat can then be used as a source of essential fatty acids and of additional calories necessary to meet synthetic caloric requirements. However, the distribution of administered amino acids appears to be altered when calories are supplied as fat. When carbohydrate alone is used, most of the administered amino acids are utilized by skeletal muscle.

When both fat and carbohydrate are used as calorie sources, amino acids are distributed both to skeletal muscle and to viscera, especially the liver. Some evidence suggests that optimum hepatic protein levels may be maintained when 20 to 25 per cent of the administered calories are given as lipid.

Adverse effects of the long-term use of intravenous fat emulsions are uncommon. In animals, hemoglobin and red blood cell counts may decrease slightly. Some have reported a mild decrease in the platelet count, while others have observed only a reduction in platelet adhesiveness. Liver function is occasionally impaired. Isolated patients receiving fat emulsions have developed hyperbilirubinemia, elevated serum glutamic oxaloacetic transaminase levels, and a prolonged prothrombin time. Liver biopsies in patients receiving fat emulsions for extended periods often show pigment deposition but no other abnormalities; the significance of the pigment is not known.

In patients receiving long-term lipid infusions, significant reduction in pulmonary membrane diffusing capacity has been demonstrated, with no change in lung volumes, airway resistance, and steady-state diffusion capacity. However, others have shown that use of fat to decrease the respiratory quotient may be helpful in weaning patients from ventilatory support. A very high rate of glucose infusion over several weeks may result in excessive CO_2 production, which, in turn, increases the respiratory work and may not be cleared by patients with compromised pulmonary function. Burke *et al.* demonstrated, in a group of burn patients, that at the highest rates of glucose infusion only 40 per cent of the glucose was oxidized completely; the remainder was handled by other metabolic pathways, the most likely being incorporation into fat.

The exact role of fat emulsions in the management of complex nutritional problems remains unclear at this time. The use of a fat emulsion as the prime calorie source has the theoretic advantage of obviating the need for a central venous catheter, thereby minimizing the associated technical and septic complications. The risk of developing either the hyperosmolar syndrome or rebound hypoglycemia is markedly reduced, since the glucose administered is relatively isotonic. The inclusion of fat in the hyperalimentation regimen prevents essential fatty acid deficiency. However, it remains difficult to achieve a caloric intake of greater than 3000 kcal/day utilizing a fat emulsion as the major calorie source. Thus, adequate nutritional support often cannot be achieved for prolonged periods by using peripheral access alone.

COMPLICATIONS

Technical Complications of Central Venous Catheters

Although subclavian venous cannulation is frequently used for the administration of hyperosmolar total parenteral nutrition solutions, the technique is not without possible complications. These include pneumothorax, arterial puncture, hydrothorax, catheter embolization, and brachial plexus injury. Infusion of a hyperosmolar solution should never be started until chest x-ray confirms the correct positioning of the central venous catheter in the superior vena cava.

The overall complication rate of subclavian venous cannulation ranges between 3 and 10 per cent; experience is the major factor in minimizing complications. The internal jugular vein can be used as an alternate site for long-term central venous catheterization. Facility with this technique makes two additional sites available for use during a prolonged course of total parenteral nutrition. Many feel that fewer technical complications occur with internal jugular venous cannulation; however, it is more difficult to stabilize and secure the internal jugular vein catheter and, therefore, the risk of contamination may be higher than with subclavian venous lines.

Central Venous Thrombosis

Thrombosis secondary to long-term indwelling catheters has been reported occasionally. The etiology remains unclear. Endothelial damage at the time of catheter insertion may serve as a nidus for thrombus formation. Alternatively, progressive aggregation of fibrin and platelets to an indwelling catheter sheath could lead to the development of a large thrombus. Sepsis, with its associated hypercoagulability, may be an important factor, particularly in cases where obstructive venous signs are associated with fever. Venous thrombosis seems unrelated to the length of time the catheter is in place. Treatment consists of removal of the central venous catheter and anticoagulation, unless contraindicated by other patient problems. Anticoagulation is designed to minimize propagation of the thrombus and should probably be continued for a period of 6 to 12 weeks.

Infectious Complications

Sepsis is one of the most serious complications of nutritional support through a central venous catheter. Potentially, the solution is a rich culture medium, especially for fungal organisms. The possibility of solution contamination can be minimized by daily preparation in the pharmacy under laminar flow hoods with rigid aseptic technique. In addition, an in-line final filter is usually used as a safeguard against the infusion of contaminated solution. The final filter consists of a cellulose membrane with an average pore size of 0.22 micron; this membrane is an absolute bacterial and fungal filter and also acts as a sieve for particulate matter. The filter should be changed daily.

Catheter-related sepsis, defined as positive blood cultures along with microbial growth from the cultured catheter sheath, is a much more frequent problem than is solution contamination. Indwelling catheters can become contaminated in a variety of ways, including administration of infusions other than the parenteral nutrition solution, measurement of central venous pressure, incorporation of a stopcock into the system, and failure to change the final bacterial filter on a regular basis. Contamination occurs readily if rigid aseptic techniques are not observed during both catheter insertion and its subsequent maintenance. The incidence of catheter sepsis can be as low as 3 to 5 per cent, provided that the infusion line is used only for parenteral nutrition and dressings are changed regularly in conjunction with skin care of the catheter site by specially trained personnel.

Catheter sepsis is heralded by the sudden appearance of fever, along with positive blood cultures and, in many cases, positive catheter cultures. The appearance of fever during total parenteral nutrition therapy should be viewed as an urgent problem because of the possibility of catheter sepsis, but a thorough fever work-up should first be performed to determine possible causes other than from the catheter. If no explanation of the fever can be found, then the central venous catheter should be removed and cultured, since any delay in removing an infected catheter is associated with a significant risk of septic shock. Catheter-related sepsis usually resolves within 24 to 36 hours after removal of the catheter, and antibiotic therapy is generally not necessary.

Metabolic Complications

HYPOGLYCEMIA. On occasion, sudden cessation of a long-term hypertonic dextrose infusion can result in rebound hypoglycemia. This is particularly apt to occur in infants or in patients with marked negative nitrogen balance, because both groups characteristically have decreased glycogen stores. Rebound hypoglycemia can result in convulsions, coma, and permanent neurologic deficits. Hypoglycemia is caused by the high levels of endogenous insulin generated to metabolize the hyperosmolar glucose solution. Hypertonic glucose infusions should never be interrupted completely for the administration of glucose-free fluids. Postinfusion hypoglycemia can be avoided by gradually decreasing the infusion rate over a few hours or by infusing isotonic glucose for several hours after cessation of hypertonic glucose.

HYPEROSMOLAR NONKETOTIC HYPERGLYCEMIC COMA. The basic pathophysiologic event in hyperosmolar nonketotic hyperglycemic coma is hyperosmolarity secondary to hyperglycemia. Hyperosmolarity produces an osmotic diuresis, dehydration, a shift of fluid and sodium from the intracellular to the extracellular space, and resultant coma. The causes of this complication include excessive rate of glucose infusion, impaired glucose tolerance associated with sepsis, latent or frank diabetes mellitus, acute or chronic renal failure, and pancreatic disorders. Premature infants with immature islets also may demonstrate glucose intolerance.

The risk of developing the hyperosmolar state is minimized by initial administration of hypertonic glucose at a slow, constant rate, along with careful assessment of glucose tolerance. The infusion rate is increased only gradually; once the desired level is reached, infusion is maintained at a constant rate by the use of a mechanical infusion pump. In patients with glucose intolerance, supplemental insulin is usually necessary to ensure utilization of the hypertonic solution.

Hyperosmolar nonketotic coma is treated by cessation of the glucose infusion and vigorous rehydration with half-normal or normal saline. Insulin should be administered cautiously, probably at a rate of no more than 25 units crystalline zinc insulin per hour. Excess insulin administration results in rapid lowering of the blood glucose, which may be detrimental, since it creates a reverse osmotic gradient between the central nervous system and the vascular space. The resulting rapid shifts of water into the central nervous system may, in the setting of total body depletion of sodium, produce cerebral edema, convulsions, and death.

METABOLIC ACIDOSIS.   Infusion of synthetic amino acid preparations can cause metabolic acidosis. The acidosis results neither from excessive gastrointestinal or renal losses of base nor from the infusion of preformed hydrogen ion as judged by the low titratable acidity (approximately 10 mEq/l) of these preparations. The synthetic amino acid mixtures contain an excess of cationic amino acids in relation to anionic amino acids or other organic anions. Metabolism of basic amino acids (lysine, histidine, and arginine) when given as chloride salts produces a net excess of hydrogen ion and resultant metabolic acidosis. In patients with normal renal function, acidosis can be avoided by administering sodium and potassium requirements in the form of their acetate or lactate salts. Bicarbonate administration is rarely required. Many of the current total parenteral nutrition preparations already contain 30 to 75 mEq/l of acetate; this should prevent acidosis in most patients.

HYPERAMMONEMIA.   Hyperammonemia has been observed during amino acid infusion, particularly in neonates and in patients with hepatic disorders. The free ammonia in synthetic amino acid solutions is low and cannot be responsible for this problem. Hyperammonemia can result from an insufficient arginine content of the preparation; relative arginine deficiency decreases the efficiency of the urea cycle and interferes with the conversion of ammonia to urea. The problem can be corrected by the addition of arginine glutamate, 2 mmol/kg/day, or arginine hydrochloride, 3 mmol/kg/day, to the infusate.

ESSENTIAL FATTY ACID DEFICIENCY.   An essential fatty acid deficiency can develop during hyperalimentation with hypertonic dextrose–amino acids, since this regimen is fat-free. The typical biochemical findings consist of decreased plasma levels of linoleic and arachidonic acids, while the levels of oleic, palmitoleic, and 5,8,11 eicosatrienoic acids are increased.

In infants, the clinical signs and symptoms of essential fatty acid deficiency include impaired wound healing, thrombocytopenia, growth retardation, increased incidence of intercurrent illness, and a dry, scaly dermatitis. The dermatitis has also been observed in adults.

Essential fatty acid deficiency can be corrected by the infusion of 500 ml of 10 per cent lipid emulsion per day for at least 7 to 10 days. Essential fatty acid deficiency can also be eliminated by the daily cutaneous application of sunflower-seed oil (approximately 230 mg per day), since sunflower-seed oil is a rich source of linoleic acid. The deficiency can be prevented by using lipid as a calorie source or by the infusion of 500 ml of 10 per cent lipid emulsion twice weekly in conjunction with a hypertonic dextrose–amino acid regimen.

HYPOPHOSPHATEMIA.   Hypophosphatemia can develop when phosphate-free solutions are utilized for total parenteral nutrition. The probable mechanism is the cellular influx of phosphate ions during anabolic metabolism. Hypophosphatemia can cause paresthesias, weakness, lethargy, dysarthria, seizures, abnormal respiratory patterns, and respiratory failure. Other consequences include impaired platelet function and decreased phagocytic and bactericidal activity of granulocytes.

Addition of 10 to 15 mEq of phosphate (expressed as $HPO_4^=$) to each liter of the total parenteral nutrition solution will prevent hypophosphatemia. For most adult patients, a solution containing 5 mEq calcium, as calcium gluconate, is compatible with up to 30 mEq phosphate (as $HPO_4^=$) per liter. Care must be taken to avoid calcium phosphate crystallization, which results from excess phosphate or calcium additions to the total parenteral nutrition preparation. Additional calcium or phosphate, if needed, should therefore be administered as a separate solution. Too rapid infusion of supplemental phosphate can result in tetany.

TRACE METAL DEFICIENCY STATES. Until recently, trace metals were not ordinarily included in total parenteral nutrition solutions. However, zinc deficiency can develop during prolonged total parenteral nutrition therapy; this is particularly apt to occur in patients with large gastrointestinal fluid losses (*e.g.,* enterocutaneous fistulas, diarrhea, or excessive ileostomy output). Zinc deficiency can produce the syndrome of acrodermatitis enteropathica, characterized by dry, scaly dermatitis of the face and extremities, diarrhea, and alopecia. Zinc deficiency may also retard wound healing, diminish cellular replication, and decrease taste acuity.

Many now recommend that zinc be administered as a routine component of parenteral nutritional therapy, particularly in children, debilitated adults, or the patient with large gastrointestinal losses. While the daily intravenous requirements have not been definitively established, the recommended dosage schedule for intravenous zinc is given here. (Zinc is administered as a zinc sulfate solution.)

DAILY ZINC REQUIREMENTS IN TOTAL PARENTERAL NUTRITION

Pediatric Patients	Stable Adult	Adult in Acute Catabolic State	Stable Adult with Intestinal Losses
Premature infants 300 mcg/kg (up to 3 kg)	2.5–4.0 mg	Additional 2.0 mg	Add 12 mg/l small-bowel fluid lost Add 17 mg/kg of stool or ileostomy output
Full-term infants and children 100 mcg/kg			

The intravenous administration of zinc presents some risk for the development of toxic side effects, since by this method the normal regulatory absorptive mechanism of the intestinal mucosa is bypassed. Renal excretion normally minimizes the danger of a modest excess of zinc. However, when renal dysfunction is present, caution is necessary to protect against excess dosage. The routine monitoring of serum zinc levels is essential in patients receiving intravenous replenishment. The normal serum zinc level is 90 to 120 mcg/ml. The frequently propounded idea that periodic infusions of fresh plasma will maintain adequate levels of body zinc is unfounded.

Copper deficiency may also develop during prolonged nutritional support with solutions free of trace elements. Copper deficiency results in neutropenia, anemia, and neurologic deficits. The recommended daily intravenous intake of copper (as copper sulfate) is 20 mcg/kg of body weight for pediatric patients and 0.5 to 1.5 mg for adults. Since copper is excreted primarily via the biliary tract, it is essential to avoid copper overdose in patients with biliary obstruction. Serum copper levels should be monitored during parenteral nutritional therapy; the normal level is 100 to 120 mcg/dl.

The trace element chromium helps to maintain normal glucose metabolism and peripheral nerve function. Trivalent chromium is a constituent of the glucose tolerance factor, an essential activator of insulin-mediated reactions. The chromium deficiency state is characterized by impaired glucose tolerance, ataxia, peripheral neuropathy, and a confusional state similar to mild hepatic encephalopathy. Serum chromium is bound to transferrin in the betaglobulin fraction. The normal blood values range from 1 to 5 mcg/l; however, blood levels are not indicative of tissue stores. Excretion of chromium is primarily via the kidneys; biliary excretion occurs but is definitely a less significant excretory route.

The usual adult dose of chromium is 10 to 15 mcg/day, while for children the suggested additive dosage is 0.14 to 0.20 mcg/kg/day. Trivalent chromium administered intravenously to adult patients receiving total parenteral nutrition has been shown to be nontoxic when given at dosage levels of up to 250 mcg/day for 2 consecutive weeks; however, reported toxic reactions to chromium include nausea, vomiting, renal and hepatic injury, seizures, and coma.

Manganese is also an essential microelement; it serves as an activator for enzymes such as polysaccharide polymerase, hepatic arginase, cholinesterase, and pyruvate carboxylase. Manganese administration to patients on total parenteral nutrition helps to prevent development of deficiency symptoms, such as nausea, vomiting, weight loss, dermatitis, growth retardation, and changes in hair color. Manganese is widely distributed but concentrates in mitochondria-rich tissues, such as brain, kidney, pancreas, and liver. The normal whole-blood concentration of manganese is 6 to 12 mcg/l with most of the blood manganese being bound to a specific beta-1-globulin transport protein. Excretion of manganese is mainly biliary. In the event of biliary obstruction, ancillary excretory routes include pancreatic and intestinal secretions. Urinary excretion of manganese is negligible.

For the adult patient receiving total parenteral nutrition, the suggested additive dosage for manganese is 0.15 to 0.8 mcg/day. For pediatric patients, a dosage of 2 to 10 mcg/kg/day is recommended. Manganese supplementation should probably be omitted in patients with severe liver dysfunction or biliary tract obstruction.

Commercial products containing trace elements for parenteral administration are available.

TOTAL PARENTERAL NUTRITION IN ACUTE RENAL FAILURE

An advance in the management of acute, potentially reversible renal failure, in the setting of increased catabolic and metabolic rates, is the intravenous infusion of essential amino acids along with a concentrated calorie source. Nephramine (American-McGaw) is a 5.4 per cent solution of 8 essential amino acids, which should be infused with 70 per cent dextrose ($D_{70}W$) as a calorie source. Nephramine also contains histidine, an amino acid that may be essential in all individuals but that certainly is essential in those with renal failure. A 250-ml unit of Nephramine should be diluted with 500 ml of $D_{70}W$ to provide a total daily volume of 750 ml that is consistent with the usual insensible water losses and oliguric urine output seen in patients with acute renal failure. The patient receives 1190 nonprotein calories with a minimal electrolyte load of less than 2 mEq sodium (Table 4–12). The solution is markedly hyperosmolar and must, therefore, be administered via a central venous catheter using techniques described earlier. Alternately, lipid emulsion can be used as the major energy source, thereby permitting administration via a peripheral vein, if fluid limitations permit.

The infusion of the aforementioned solution in patients with potentially reversible acute renal failure may decrease the rate of rise of blood urea nitrogen, minimize or reverse hyperkalemia, and minimize elevations of serum phosphorus and magnesium. Serum potassium levels in patients with hypermetabolic renal failure are ordinarily elevated because of release of intracellular potassium secondary to tissue catabolism that occurs when protein intake is inadequate. Clinical studies of Nephramine–$D_{70}W$ therapy in patients with acute tubular necrosis have shown a significant decrease in serum potassium levels, since circulating potassium is apparently incorporated into newly synthesized tissue. There has been some suggestion that treatment with essential amino acids shortens the duration of renal dysfunction and decreases the morbidity associated with acute renal failure. Essential amino acid–dextrose therapy is not in-

**TABLE 4–12.   NEPHRAMINE
(AMERICAN-MCGAW)**

Essential Amino Acid Solution		
	G/100 ML	G/250 ML
Isoleucine	0.56	1.40
Leucine	0.88	2.20
Lysine	0.64	1.60
Histidine	0.25	0.62
Methionine	0.88	2.20
Phenylalanine	0.88	2.20
Threonine	0.40	1.00
Tryptophan	0.20	0.50
Valine	0.65	1.60
Osmolarity 420 mOsm/l		

TABLE 4–13.   AMINOSYN-RF, 5.2%
(ABBOTT)

Essential Amino Acid Solution — Renal
Formula

	G/100 ML
Isoleucine	0.46
Leucine	0.72
Lysine acetate	0.54
Methionine	0.73
Phenylalanine	0.73
Threonine	0.33
Tryptophan	0.17
Valine	0.53
Arginine	0.60
Histidine	0.43
Osmolarity 475 mOsm/l	

tended as a substitute for dialysis but may decrease the frequency of dialysis treatment necessary for control of azotemia or hyperkalemia.

Nephramine should be used with particular caution in pediatric patients, especially in low-birth-weight infants. Laboratory and clinical monitoring must be frequent. The initial total daily dose should be low and increased very slowly. Dosage should not exceed 1 g of essential amino acids per kilogram of body weight per day. Frequent monitoring of blood glucose is required in low-birth-weight or septic infants who have an increased risk of hyperglycemia. Finally, the absence of arginine in Nephramine may increase the risk of hyperammonemia in infants.

Aminosyn-RF (Abbott Laboratories) is another synthetic essential amino acid solution designed for the patient with potentially reversible acute renal failure who cannot ingest adequate calories orally (Table 4–13). For hypercatabolic individuals in acute renal failure, 300 ml of Aminosyn-RF (5.2 per cent) is mixed with 500 ml of 70 per cent dextrose. This mixture provides a calorie-to-nitrogen ratio of 502:1 and a total nitrogen content of 2.4 g. Aminosyn-RF does contain arginine (0.6 g/dl).

The availability of these essential amino acid preparations has generated renewed interest in the study of the nutritional support in patients with renal failure. A recent randomized study compared the efficacy of an essential amino acid solution with that of a balanced amino acid preparation, both in combination with a high-density caloric solution, in patients with impaired renal function. There were no significant differences in mortality, serum potassium and phosphate levels, serum urea nitrogen, and creatinine levels over the 10-day test period. These results raise some doubt regarding whether the essential amino acid solutions are a significant improvement in the management of reversible acute renal failure.

There is a new amino acid solution for use in the management of renal failure that contains both essential amino acids and certain nonessential ones.

TABLE 4–14.   RENAMIN AMINO ACID
SOLUTION—RENAL FORMULA
(TRAVENOL)

	G/100 ML
Amino acids	6.5
Total nitrogen	1.0
Essential amino acids	
Isoleucine	0.50
Leucine	0.60
Lysine (hydrochloride)	0.42
Methionine	0.50
Phenylalanine	0.49
Threonine	0.38
Tryptophan	0.15
Valine	0.82
Histidine	0.42
Nonessential amino acids	
Arginine	0.63
Alanine	0.56
Glycine	0.30
Proline	0.35
Serine	0.30
Tyrosine	0.04
Anions	
Acetate	60 mEq/l
Chloride	31 mEq/l
Osmolarity	600 mOsm/l

RenAmin (Travenol) includes some nonessential amino acids—arginine, ala-nine, glycine, proline, serine, and tyrosine—in an effort to enhance nitrogen uti-lization in uremic patients (Table 4–14). It has been suggested, for example, that low concentrations of an amino acid may be rate limiting for protein synthesis. In patients with uremia, low intracellular pools of valine, threonine, histidine, and tyrosine may have this undesirable effect. In addition, others maintain that inclusion of nonessential amino acids results in better nitrogen balance than does use of an essential amino acid solution. Controlled, randomized studies are needed to compare essential amino acid and mixed amino acid solutions in the management of acute renal failure.

TOTAL PARENTERAL NUTRITION IN HEPATIC FAILURE

In patients with acute hepatic encephalopathy, total parenteral nutritional support is not generally used unless indicated for other reasons. When such support is necessary, modification in the pattern of the amino acid infusate may be indicated.

Uncontrolled clinical studies have suggested that a parenteral amino acid solution rich in branched-chain amino acids and restricted in aromatic amino acids may be beneficial in the therapy and nutritional support of patients with hepatic encephalopathy. HepatAmine (American-McGaw) is a recently introduced 8 per cent amino acid solution that is high in branched-chain amino acid content (36 per cent) but low in both aromatic amino acids and methionine. It has been suggested that infusion of HepatAmine along with hypertonic dextrose (25 per cent) may be effective in the treatment of hepatic encephalopathy and in nutritional management of chronic liver disease patients. When compared with neomycin and isocaloric glucose in a prospective, randomized, double-blind trial, HepatAmine resulted in significantly greater improvement in hepatic encephalopathy, electroencephalogram pattern, nitrogen balance, and plasma amino acid patterns. The recommended dosage is 80 to 120 g of amino acids as HepatAmine per day. HepatAmine (500 ml) is usually combined with 50 per cent dextrose (500 ml) to yield a solution with a final concentration of 25 per cent dextrose, 4 per cent amino acids. For reasons that are unclear, this solution contains three amino acids—methionine, phenylalanine, and tryptophan—which are believed to contribute to hepatic encephalopathy; the amino acids are present in reduced quantities, however (Table 4–15).

The role of branched-chain amino acids or of branched-chain amino acid–enriched solutions in the management of hepatic encephalopathy has not been established. Other studies have suggested that when a similar solution is given as the sole protein source, unusual new amino acid profiles can be produced and that hepatic encephalopathy may not be consistently ameliorated.

TABLE 4–15. HEPATAMINE (AMERICAN-MCGAW)

8% Amino Acid Solution

ESSENTIAL AMINO ACIDS	MG/100 ML
Isoleucine	900
Leucine	1100
Lysine (as acetate)	610
Methionine	100
Phenylalanine	100
Theonine	450
Tryptophan	66
Valine	840

NONESSENTIAL AMINO ACIDS	MG/100 ML
Alanine	770
Arginine	600
Histidine	240
Proline	800
Serine	500
Glycine (amino acetic acid)	900
Cysteine hydrochloride	< 20

ELECTROLYTE CONTENT	MEQ/L
Sodium	10
Phosphate (HPO$_4$)	20
Acetate	62
Chloride	< 3

HYPOCALORIC PERIPHERAL PARENTERAL NUTRITION

It has been known for many years that the provision of 400 to 600 kcal of carbohydrate per day will achieve virtually the same degree of nitrogen-sparing as does provision of total energy needs. These observations have been made in normal subjects, not in hypercatabolic patients. It is widely believed, on the basis of clinical observations, that the provision of total energy needs in catabolic states is associated with reduced morbidity. However, controlled studies of this question are lacking.

In certain situations, administration of isotonic amino acid solutions (3 to 5 per cent) and 400 to 600 kcal of carbohydrate per day by a peripheral vein may indeed be indicated. Generally, this is done only in the fasting normal or minimally catabolic patient.

The major problem with this form of therapy is that it tends to be used indiscriminately, even in patients who have no need for infusions of amino acids. As noted earlier, the use of a peripheral line avoids the potential complications of central venous catheterization. However, the availability of lipid emulsions, which will permit the provision of *total* energy needs by a peripheral route in many cases, casts further doubt on the role of hypocaloric regimens in parenteral nutrition. Controlled studies comparing hypocaloric with isocaloric infusions are awaited.

Until recently, whenever hypocaloric peripheral parenteral nutrition was utilized, the traditional source of carbohydrate was dextrose. The dextrose solution must be stored separately from the amino acid solution and then mixed under sterile conditions prior to use. However, glycerol has been shown to be a nonprotein calorie source that can be autoclaved with amino acids and then stored with a reasonably long shelf life.

Glycerol is primarily metabolized by the liver (75 per cent) and kidneys (20 per cent). Glycerol kinase converts glycerol to glycerol-3-phosphate, which is then oxidized by glycerophosphate dehydrogenase to dihydroxyacetone phosphate. This compound can be metabolized to carbon dioxide by the glycolytic pathway and tricarboxylic acid cycle or serve as a substrate for gluconeogenesis.

It has recently been shown that infusion of a 3 per cent amino acid solution and 3 per cent glycerol solution can result in improved nitrogen balance compared with infusion of 3 per cent amino acids alone, when administered for 5 days at 40 ml/kg body weight/day. The potential adverse effects of parenteral glycerol infusion include hemolysis, hemoglobinuria, and renal failure; however, these problems have generally occurred only with administration of high concentrations of glycerol (10 per cent) given subcutaneously or intraperitoneally. No such complications have been reported with the use of 3 per cent glycerol.

ProcalAmine (American-McGaw) has been introduced as a commercial solution of 3 per cent amino acids and 3 per cent glycerin with electrolytes (Table 4–16). Each liter provides 4.6 g nitrogen and 130 nonprotein calories derived from the metabolism of glycerol. It has been suggested that this preparation may be helpful in sparing body protein and improving nitrogen balance in well-

TABLE 4–16. PROCALAMINE (AMERICAN-MCGAW)

3% Amino Acid and 3% Glycerin Solution with Electrolytes

ESSENTIAL AMINO ACIDS	MG/100 ML
Isoleucine	210
Leucine	270
Lysine (as acetate)	310
Methionine	160
Phenylalanine	170
Theonine	120
Tryptophan	46
Valine	200

NONESSENTIAL AMINO ACIDS	MG/100 ML
Alanine	210
Glycine (amino acetic acid)	420
Arginine	290
Histidine	85
Proline	340
Serine	180
Cysteine hydrochloride	< 20

Nonprotein Energy Source: 130 calories/liter
Glycerine (glycerol): 3.0 g/100 ml

ELECTROLYTE CONTENT	MEQ/L
Sodium	35
Potassium	24
Magnesium	5
Calcium	3
Chloride	41
Phosphate (HPO_4)	7
Acetate	47

nourished, mildly catabolic patients who require very short–term parenteral nutrition. Administration of this solution is not likely to achieve positive nitrogen balance under any other circumstance and, consequently, its use should be restricted. Furthermore, there is no evidence that maintenance of body protein in the well-nourished, minimally catabolic patient will in any way alter the patient's hospital course.

TOTAL PARENTERAL NUTRITION IN THE PEDIATRIC PATIENT

In addition to the problems presented earlier, infants, especially preterm infants, are particularly susceptible to calorie malnutrition. Low-birth-weight infants have a relatively lower caloric reserve, since fat deposition takes place primarily in the last trimester of pregnancy. In the 1000 g fetus only about 1 per cent of the body weight is fat, while in the term fetus (3500 g) about 16 per cent is fat. A second physiologic factor that makes infants more likely to die from caloric insufficiency is their high metabolic rate per unit of body mass compared with the adult metabolic rate. An infant has a resting metabolic rate of about 50 kcal/kg/day, to which must be added an additional 50 to 60 kcal/kg/day for response to cold stress, activity, and growth. The rate of total caloric expenditure is nearly three times the rate expected for an adult. Thus, infants faced with inadequate enteral caloric intake are at a particular disadvantage because of their low caloric reserves and high metabolic rate.

Although the calorie and water requirements for infants and children differ from those of adults, the components of total parenteral nutrition are similar. Positive nitrogen balance can be achieved regularly with the infusion of hypertonic dextrose–amino acids via techniques already described for adults. Protein, as amino acids, should approximate 2.5 g/kg/day, or about 10 per cent (range, 8 to 15 per cent) of the total calories infused per day. It must be remembered that the composition of the infusate cannot be uniform from patient to patient. Hypertonic dextrose infusion must be started at low concentrations and slowly increased while glucose tolerance is carefully monitored. A recommended composition for a pediatric infusate is given in Table 4–17. Electrolytes or minerals or both may have to be altered frequently in accordance with the clinical situation and careful monitoring of blood levels.

Since the dextrose–amino acid infusate is markedly hypertonic, it must be infused into the central venous system. Infants weighing less than 10 lb have very small subclavian veins, making percutaneous subclavian puncture both difficult and dangerous. In infants, long-term intravenous catheterization is achieved by inserting the Silastic catheter through an external or internal jugular vein cut-down and threading it into the superior vena cava. After proper placement in the superior vena cava, the proximal end of the catheter is brought through a subcutaneous tunnel to exit via a small stab wound in the parieto-occipital area of the scalp. Exit of the catheter at a point distant from the venotomy reduces the risk of infection and makes catheter care easier.

Fat emulsions should be used to supply a proportion of an infant's daily caloric requirement while on total parenteral nutrition. When fat emulsions are used in conjunction with amino acids and glucose (to obviate protein breakdown for gluconeogenesis), the tonicity is relatively isotonic. In many cases, total parenteral nutrition utilizing lipid as a calorie source can be infused through peripheral veins, a major technical advantage in neonates in which placement of central venous catheters may be difficult. The maximal lipid dosage should be no more than 4 g/kg/day or should account for no more than 40 per cent of the total calories infused. Essential fatty acid deficiency can be prevented by using lipid to meet 2 to 5 per cent of the patient's total caloric intake. The techniques for lipid infusion are described earlier.

Indications for the use of total parenteral nutrition in the pediatric patient are as follows:

1. Major anomalies of the gastrointestinal tract: congenital intestinal obstruction, major resections of the small intestine, omphalocele and gastroschisis, or necrotizing enterocolitis. (Parenteral nutrition is used in these cases as support adjunctive to surgical therapy.)

2. Chronic intractable diarrhea: These infants usually present with moder-

TABLE 4–17.   PEDIATRIC TOTAL PARENTERAL NUTRITION (RECOMMENDED COMPOSITION INFUSATE)

Constituent	Amount
Amino acids	2.5 g/kg/day
Dextrose	25–30 g/kg/day
Sodium	3–4 mEq/kg/day
Potassium	2–3 mEq/kg/day
Calcium (as gluconate)	0.5–1.0 mEq/kg/day
Magnesium (as sulfate)	0.3 mEq/kg/day
Chloride	3–4 mEq/kg/day
Phosphorus	2 mM/kg/day
Acetate	2–3 mEq/kg/day
Total volume	120–130 ml/kg/day

Vitamin Additives (per day)

Vitamin A*	5000 units	Thiamine	25 mg
Vitamin D (ergocalciferol)	500 units	Riboflavin	5 mg
Vitamin E	2.5 units	Pyridoxine	7.5 mg
Niacinamide	50 mg	Ascorbic acid	250 mg
Pantothenic acid	12.5 mg	Folic acid	500 mcg
Vitamin K$_1$	100 mcg	Vitamin B$_{12}$	10 mcg

*Not 100% available to patient because of absorption into tubing and bottle.

Trace Element Additives

Age or Weight	Zinc	Copper
5 yrs	1 mg/l Maximum of 4 mg/day	0.5 mg/l Maximum of 1.5 mg/day
> 3 kg and < 5 yrs	100 mcg/100 kcal Maximum of 100 mcg/kg/day	20 mcg/100 kcal Maximum of 20 mcg/kg/day
> 3 kg	300 mcg/100 kcal Maximum of 300 mcg/kg/day	20 mcg/100 kcal Maximum of 20 mcg/kg/day

ate or severe malnutrition secondary to protracted diarrhea, with body weight on admission often less than birth weight. Extensive diagnostic studies, including stool and urine cultures, radiographic studies, tests for cystic fibrosis, immunoglobulin determinations, and catecholamines, are negative. Usually the diarrhea is unresponsive to any type of formula feeding.

Until the advent of total parenteral nutrition this entity carried a high mortality rate. It is now possible to correct and maintain good nutritional balance in these patients. Total parenteral nutrition seems to allow gastrointestinal absorptive functions to return to normal. Although the mechanism has not been determined definitely, total parenteral nutrition seems to greatly increase the mucosal absorptive surface of the small intestine.

3. Very low-birth-weight infants: At this time, total parenteral nutrition in this group is still only an investigational tool. It may well become an established technique, as the problems and risks of establishing completely adequate

enteral intake in this group are well known. However, there is an added concern, based upon animal studies, that malnutrition at some critical point of brain growth may lead to permanent reduction of brain cell number.

BIBLIOGRAPHY

Abel, R.M., Beck, C.M., Abbott, W.M., et al.: Improved survival from acute renal failure after treatment with intravenous essential L-amino acids and glucose. N Engl J Med 288:695–699, 1973.

Aguirre, A., Fisher, J.E., and Welch, C.E.: The role of surgery and hyperalimentation in therapy of gastrointestinal cutaneous fistulae. Ann Surg 180:393–401, 1974.

Allinson, R.: Plasma trace elements during total parenteral nutrition. J Parent Ent Nutr 2:35–40, 1978.

AMA Department of Foods and Nutrition: Guidelines for essential trace element preparations for parenteral use. A statement by an expert panel. JAMA 241:2051–2054, 1979.

American Medical Association Nutrition Advisory Group: Multivitamin preparations for parenteral use. J Parent Ent Nutr 3:258–262, 1979.

Bernard, R.W., and Stahl, W.M.: Subclavian vein catheterizations: A prospective study. I. Non-infectious complications. Ann Surg 173:184–190, 1971.

Bivins, B.A., Hyde, G.L., Sachatello, C.R., and Griffen, W.O.: Physiopathology and management of hyperosmolar hyperglycemic nonketotic dehydration. Surg Gynecol Obstet 154:534–540, 1982.

Blackburn, G.L., Etter, G., and Mackenzie, T.: Criteria for choosing amino acid therapy in acute renal failure. Am J Clin Nutr 31:1841–1853, 1978.

Blackburn, G.L., Flatt, J.P., Clowes, G.H.A., Jr., et al.: Protein sparing therapy during periods of starvation with sepsis or trauma. Ann Surg 177:588–594, 1973.

Blackburn, G.L., Moldawer, L.I., Usui, S., Bothe, A., O'Keefe, S.J.D., and Bistrian, B.R.: Branched-chain amino acid administration and metabolism during starvation, injury and infection. Surgery 86:307–315, 1979.

Burke, J.F., Wolfe, R.R., Mullany, C.J., Matthews, D.E., and Bier, D.M.: Glucose requirements following burn injury. Ann Surg 190:274–285, 1979.

Buzby, G.P., Mullen, J.L., Stein, T.P., et al.: Optimal TPN caloric substrate for correction of protein malnutrition. Surg Forum 30:64–69, 1979.

Cahill, G.F., Jr.: Starvation in man. N Engl J Med 282:668–675, 1970.

Cerra, F.B., Cheung, N.K., Fischer, J.E., Kaplowitz, N., Schiff, E.R., Dienstag, J.L., Mabry, C.A., Leevy, C.M., and Kiernan, T.: A multi center trial of branched chain enriched amino acid infusion in hepatic encephalopathy. (Abstract.) Hepatology 2:699, 1982.

Copeland, E.M., MacFadyen, B.V., Lanzotti, V.J., et al.: Intravenous hyperalimentation as an adjunct to cancer chemotherapy. Am J Surg 129:167–173, 1975.

Dillon, J.D., Schaffner, W., Van Way, C.W., et al.: Septicemia and total parenteral nutrition-distinguishing catheter-related from other septic episodes. JAMA 223:1341–1344, 1975.

Dudrick, S.J., MacFadyen, B.V., Van Buren, C.T., et al.: Parenteral hyperalimentation: Metabolic problems and solutions. Ann Surg 176:259–264, 1972.

Fairfull-Smith, R.J., Stoski, D., and Freeman, J.B.: Use of glycerol in peripheral parenteral nutrition. Surgery 92:728–732, 1982.

Faulkner, W.J., and Flint, L.: Essential fatty acid deficiency associated with total parenteral nutrition. Surg Gynecol Obstet 144:665–667, 1977.

Fischer, J.E., Foster, G.S., Abel, R.M., et al.: Hyperalimentation as primary therapy for inflammatory bowel disease. Am J Surg 125:165–175, 1973.

Fischer, J.E., Yoshimura, N., Aguirre, A., James, J.H., Cummings, M.G., Abel, R.M., and Deindorfer, F.: Plasma amino acids in patients with hepatic encephalopathy. Effects of amino acid infusions. Am J Surg 127:40–47, 1974.

Freund, H., Dienstag, J., Lehrich, J., et al.: Infusion of branched-chain enriched amino acid solution in patients with hepatic encephalopathy. Ann Surg 196:209–220, 1982.

Freund, H., Hoover, H.C., Atamian, S., and Fischer, J.E.: Infusion of the branched-chain amino acids in postoperative patients. Anticatabolic properties. Ann Surg 190:18–23, 1979.

Freund, M., Yoshimura, N., Lunetta, L., and Fischer, J.E.: The role of the branched-chain amino acids in decreasing muscle catabolism in vivo. Surgery 83:611–618, 1978.

Fürst, P., Alvesstrand, A., and Bergström, J.: Effects of nutrition and catabolic stress on intracellular amino acid pools in uremia. Am J Clin Nutr 33:1387–1395, 1980.

Greenberg, G.R., Marliss, E.B., Anderson, G.H., et al.: Protein-sparing therapy in postoperative patients. N Engl J Med 294:1411–1416, 1976.

Heird, W.C., and Winters, R.W.: Total parenteral nutrition: The state of the art. J Pediatr 86:2–16, 1975.

Henderson, J.M., Millikan, W.J., and Warren, W.D.: Manipulation of the amino acid profile in cirrhosis with Hepatic-aid or F080 fails to reverse encephalopathy. Hepatology 2:706, 1982.

Holman, R.T., Johnson, S.B., and Hatch, T.F.: A case of human linolenic acid deficiency involving neurological abnormalities. Am J Clin Nutr 35:617–623, 1982.

Lowry, S.F., Goodgame, J.T., et al.: Abnormalities of zinc and copper during total parenteral nutrition. Ann Surg 189:120–128, 1979.

Mirtallo, J.M., Schneider, P.J., Mavko, K., Ruberg, R.L., and Fabri, P.J.: A comparison of essential and general amino acid infusions in the nutritional support of patients with compromised renal function. J Parent Ent Nutr 6:109–113, 1982.

Odessey, R., Khairallah, E.A., and Goldberg, A.L.: Origin and possible significance of alanine production by skeletal muscle. J Biol Chem 249:7623–7629, 1974.

Okada, A., Takagi, Y., Itakura, T., et al.: Skin lesions during intravenous hyperalimentation: Zinc deficiency. Surgery 80:629–635, 1976.

Press, M., Hartop, P.J., and Prottey, C.: Correction of essential fatty-acid deficiency in man by the cutaneous application of sunflower-seed oil. 1:597–598, 1974.

Rudman, D., Milliken, W.J., Richardson, T.J., Bixler, T.J. II, Stackhouse, W.J., and McGarrity, W.C.: Elemental balances during intravenous hyperalimentation of underweight adult subjects. J Clin Invest 55:94–104, 1975.

Ryan, J.A., Abel, R.M., Abbott, W.M., et al.: Catheter complications in total parenteral nutrition. N Engl J Med 290:757–760, 1974.

Striebel, J.P., Holm, E., Lutz, M., and Storz, L.W.: Parenteral nutrition and coma therapy with amino acids in hepatic failure. J Parent Ent Nutr 3:240–246, 1979.

Ulmer, D.D.: Trace elements. N Engl J Med 297:318–321, 1977.

5

MODIFICATIONS IN ENERGY

Weight-Gaining Diets

Arnold Andersen, M.D.,
Simeon Margolis, M.D., Ph.D. and
Helen D. Mullan, B.S., R.D.

INTRODUCTION

Weight loss is common in many medical and psychiatric disorders. When severe, weight loss itself may complicate the management of the underlying condition and can even cause death. Although it is obvious that the intake of a high caloric diet will promote weight gain in these patients, successful implementation of such diets is fraught with many difficulties.

GOAL AND RATIONALE OF THERAPY

Whatever the underlying cause, severe weight loss may increase susceptibility to infection, decrease the effectiveness of various treatments, decrease ventilatory and ambulatory reserves, retard wound healing, and even lead to death from inanition. Correction of severe weight loss will generally reverse or minimize these problems.

PATIENT SELECTION

Severe weight loss may be due to decreased nutritional intake caused by disease states, limited availability of foods, increased catabolic rate, or excessive nutrient loss resulting from intestinal malabsorption. It is essential to identify and treat, if at all possible, any disorder responsible for significant weight loss, particularly those that frequently go unrecognized for prolonged periods, such as depression, anorexia nervosa, and structural abnormalities of the gastrointestinal tract.

DIETARY PRINCIPLES

When intensive nutritional support is indicated, it must first be decided whether orally ingested foods can be tolerated and utilized or whether total parenteral nutrition or enteral feedings are necessary. Usually, orally ingested foods are preferred even in very-low-weight patients.

The rate of nutritional rehabilitation depends on the degree of malnutrition and on whether the underlying condition impairs the patient's ability to tolerate a high nutrient intake. In some situations, such as after severe burns, very high caloric loads are desirable from the outset to keep pace with the increased catabolic rate. If no contraindications are present, most patients can tolerate an initial diet of 1800 to 2000 kcal with progressive increments over 2 weeks to 4000 kcal or more per day. Some conditions may limit a patient's ability to handle increased nutrient intake comfortably—for example, the dumping syndrome that may develop after gastric resection.

Ideally, nutritional rehabilitation should be based on a balanced diet of proteins, lipids, and carbohydrates, with vitamin and mineral supplementation. However, the prescribed diet may require modifications dictated by underlying conditions. For example, in patients with nontropical sprue or intestinal lactase deficiency, poorly tolerated nutritional components must be replaced with items that do not cause symptoms. For patients who have been starved or whose intake of food has been markedly reduced for a long time, lipids and lactose should initially be restricted severely and reintroduced gradually.

Complications of refeeding may occur when the caloric intake of severely malnourished patients is increased too rapidly. Such individuals might include prisoners of war, patients in developing countries with kwashiorkor, and patients with anorexia nervosa. Crampy abdominal pain and distention may develop following institution of a high-calorie intake, because of gastric atony and decreased intestinal enzyme production, particularly of lactase. Coexistent hypoalbuminemia may contribute to the development of refeeding edema.

It may be necessary to limit intake initially to 1200 kcal/day and to utilize simple carbohydrates or dilute skim milk. Intake can usually be increased to 2000 kcal/day after 4 to 7 days of refeeding. Patients with kwashiorkor may have moderate protein intolerance; thus, protein refeeding may cause hyperammonemia and resultant symptoms.

Few drugs are helpful, and in most cases none are necessary, especially when the underlying illness is being treated appropriately. However, medications such as phenothiazines or tricyclic antidepressants, which increase the patient's sense of well-being, may promote weight gain in some situations. Cyproheptadine may increase appetite in some individuals.

TABLE 5–1.   HIGH-CALORIE SUPPLEMENTS—REGULAR FOODS

Item	Usual Serving Size (ml)	Calories (kcal)	Protein (g)	Fat (g)	Carbo-hydrate (g)	Sodium (mg)	Potassium (mg)
Custard	120	143	6.0	5.0	20	128.0	174
Eggnog	240	290	15.0	9.0	37	220.0	590
Gelatin	120	76	2.0	0.0	17	61.0	0
Ice cream	60	131	3.0	7.0	14	42.0	121
Milk	240	170	8.0	10.0	12	127.0	355
Milkshake							
Vanilla	240	320	14.0	10.0	45	200.0	590
Chocolate	240	330	14.0	10.0	47	240.0	590
Sherbet	60	138	0.8	1.6	30	9.5	21
Whipped top-ping, liquid	120	334	0.0	28.0	21	62.0	0

DIETARY IMPLEMENTATION

The calorie intake necessary to maintain present weight, considering both basal needs and level of activity, should be determined. The supplemental daily calorie requirement is determined by multiplying the desired weight gain (in lbs) by 3500 kcal and dividing the result by the number of days in the planned nutritional rehabilitation period. An increase of 500 kcal/day over maintenance requirements will usually result in a weight gain of 1 pound per week.

Six evenly spaced meals a day are recommended to improve tolerance. Care should be taken not to overfeed at any one meal, but patients should be *encouraged* to eat everything served to them. If necessary, the caloric density of the food can be increased by utilizing high-calorie supplements (Tables 5–1 and 5–2), without increasing its total volume. Sample meal plans for high-calorie diets are provided in Table 5–3. The usual procedure is to serve a normal diet to the patient using high-calorie nourishment between meals, but if the patient is very low in weight the diet should initially be low in both fat and milk products.

TABLE 5–2.   PROPRIETARY SUPPLEMENTS*

A—Modular

Item	Usual Serving Size (ml)	Calories (kcal)	Protein (g)	Fat (g)	Carbo-hydrate (g)	Sodium (mg)	Potassium (mg)
Casec (Mead Johnson)	100 g	370	88	2	0	150	0
Controlyte (Doyle)	100 g	504	Tr	24	72	10	4
MCT (Mead Johnson)	120 ml	920	0	102	0	0	0
Microlipid (Organon)	120 ml	540	0	60	0	0	0

*For additional products refer to Chapter 3, Enteral Nutrition.

TABLE 5–2.   PROPRIETARY SUPPLEMENTS (Continued)

Item	Usual Serving Size (ml)	Calories (kcal)	Protein (g)	Fat (g)	Carbo-hydrate (g)	Sodium (mg)	Potassium (mg)
Moducal (Mead Johnson)	100 g	380	0	0	95	70	5
Polycose Liquid (Ross)	100 ml	200	0	0	50	58	20
Polycose Powder (Ross)	100 g	376	0	0	94	115	39
Pro-Mix (Navaco)	100 g	376	80	4	5	150	1335
Propac (Organon)	100 g	400	77	8	5	230	512
Sumacal (Organon)	100 ml	200	0	0	50	65	7.8

B—Complete

Item	Usual Serving Size (ml)	Calories (kcal)	Protein (g)	Fat (g)	Carbo-hydrate (g)	Sodium (mg)	Potassium (mg)
Formula 2 (Cutter)	100	100	3.7	4.0	12.3	2.6	4.6
Meritene Liquid (Doyle)	100	100	6.0	3.3	11.5	3.9	4.2
Meritene Powder (Doyle) (as pre-pared with whole milk)	100	107	6.9	3.4	11.9	4.1	7.5
Nutri 1000 (Cutter)	100	106	4.0	5.6	10.1	2.3	3.9
Sustacal (Mead Johnson)	100	101	6.1	2.4	13.6	4.0	6.6
Citrotein (Doyle)	100	66	4.3	2.2	12.9	3.1	1.9
Ensure (Ross)	100	106	3.7	3.7	14.6	3.2	3.2
Ensure Plus (Ross)	100	150	5.6	5.3	20.0	4.6	4.8
Magnacal (Organon)	100	200	7.0	8.0	25.0	4.3	3.2
Nutri 1000 Lactose Free (Cutter)	100	106	4.0	5.5	10.1	2.3	3.9
Nutri-Aid (American-McGaw)	100	106	3.9	3.7	14.2	3.3	3.2
Osmolite (Ross)	100	106	3.7	3.9	14.5	2.4	2.7
Osmolite HN (Ross)	100	106	4.4	3.6	14.1	4.0	3.9
Precision High Nitrogen (Doyle)	100	105	4.3	0.13	21.6	4.2	2.3

Table continues on following page

TABLE 5–2.   PROPRIETARY SUPPLEMENTS* (Continued)

B — Complete

Item	Usual Serving Size (ml)	Calories (kcal)	Protein (g)	Fat (g)	Carbo-hydrate (g)	Sodium (mg)	Potassium (mg)
Precision Isotonic (Doyle)	100	96	2.8	3.0	14.4	3.3	2.4
Precision Isotein HN (Doyle)	100	119	6.8	3.4	15.6	2.9	2.1
Precision Low Residue (Doyle)	100	111	2.6	.16	24.8	3.0	2.2
Renu (Organon)	100	100	3.3	4.0	13.0	2.1	3.2
Sustacal (Mead Johnson)	100	100	6.0	2.3	13.8	4.0	5.2
Sustacal HC (Mead Johnson)	100	150	6.1	5.8	19.0	3.6	3.0

TABLE 5–3.   SAMPLE HIGH-CALORIE MEAL PLANS

Calorie Level	1500 P-F-C (80-50-185)	2000 P-F-C (95-80-225)	2500 P-F-C (120-100-280)	3000 P-F-C (150-115-340)	3500 P-F-C (160-135-415)	4000 P-F-C (180-155-477)
BREAKFAST						
Fruit Exchange*	1	1	1	2	2	2
Meat Exchange	1	1	2	2	2	2
Bread Exchange	2	2	2	2	3	4
Fat Exchange	1	1	1	1	2	3
Milk Exchange (whole unless noted)	1†	1	1	1	1	1
MID-AM SNACK§	—	—	—	140 kcal	220 kcal	220 kcal
Fruit Exchange*	—	—	—	—	2	2
Bread Exchange	—	—	—	2	2	2
Milk (whole)	—	—	—	—	—	—
LUNCH						
Meat Exchange	2	3	3	3	3	4
Vegetable Exchange	1	1	1	2	2	2
Bread Exchange	2	2	2	2	2	4
Fat Exchange	1	1	1	1	1	2
Fruit Exchange*	1	2	2	2	2	2
Milk (whole)	—	—	—	—	—	—

*If sweetened fruit is used, caloric value will be higher.
†Skim milk.

Table continues on following page

TABLE 5–3. SAMPLE HIGH-CALORIE MEAL PLANS (Continued)

Calorie Level	1500 P-F-C (80-50-185)	2000 P-F-C (95-80-225)	2500 P-F-C (120-100-280)	3000 P-F-C (150-115-340)	3500 P-F-C (160-135-415)	4000 P-F-C (180-155-477)
MID-PM SNACK§	—	—	310 kcal	455 kcal	455 kcal	495 kcal
Meat Exchange	—	—	—	2	2	2
Bread Exchange	—	—	2	2	2	2
Fat Exchange	—	—	—	—	—	—
Fruit Exchange*	—	—	—	—	—	1
Milk (whole)	—	—	1	1	1	1
DINNER						
Meat Exchange	3	3	3	4	4	5
Vegetable Exchange	2	2	2	2	2	2
Bread Exchange	2	2	2	3	4	4
Fat Exchange	2	2	2	2	3	3
Fruit Exchange*	1	1	2	2	2	2
Milk Exchange (whole unless noted)	1†	1	1	1	1	1
SUGAR EXCHANGE FOR WHOLE DAY‡	—	3	4	4	6	6
EVENING SNACK§	110 kcal	255 kcal	325 kcal	325 kcal	495 kcal	495 kcal
Meat Exchange	—	1	2	2	2	2
Bread Exchange	1	2	2	2	2	2
Fat Exchange	—	—	—	—	—	—
Fruit Exchange*	1	1	1	1	1	1
Milk (whole)	—	—	—	—	1	1

Sugar Exchanges: Approximately 20 kcal/serving.

FOOD	AMOUNT	FOOD	AMOUNT
Jelly, assorted	1 tsp	Molasses	1 tsp
Sugar—all types	1 tsp	Hard candy	1 piece (5 g)
Honey	1 tsp	Gumdrops	5 small (7 g)
Syrup	1 tsp	Jelly beans	3 (8 g)

Desserts/Beverages: These foods may be used singly or in combination to approximate the number of calories in the planned snacks.

FOOD	AMOUNT	CALORIES
Brownies	1 piece (2 × 2 × ¾)	150
Cake (average): angel food, fruit, or pound	1 slice (3 × 3 × ½)	150
Cookies: sugar filled, chocolate chip	2 average (total weight 1 ounce)	170
Jello	1 cup	160
Pudding (average, assorted flavors)	½ cup	180
Chocolate candy	1 oz.	150
Cola, soda, or sweetened powdered drink mix	12 oz	150
Iced cake	1 slice (⅛ of 8″ cake)	370
Pie	1 slice (⅙ of 9″ pie)	375

§Desserts in following list or selections from the high-calorie supplement list (Tables 5–1 and 5–2) may be used as isocaloric replacements for snacks. However, this could alter the protein, fat, and carbohydrate content of the plan.
‡See sugar exchanges that follow.
  Dietary calculations are based upon the Exchange Lists for Meal Planning (see Appendix).

Table continues on following page

Dietary Management of Obesity

Simeon Margolis, M.D., Ph.D. and
Helen D. Mullan, B.S., R.D.

INTRODUCTION

Obesity is defined as an excess of body fat; however, in most instances the diagnosis of obesity is made when the patient's weight exceeds the normal range for height, age, and body build (ideal body weight) given in standard tables published in 1980 (see Table A–10, in Appendix). This approach is generally acceptable, although it actually determines only whether an individual is overweight, a situation that may be due to increased muscle or bone mass as well as to excessive body fat. Aside from skinfold thickness measurements, specific methods for quantifying body fat are impractical for routine clinical use.

Skinfold thickness is a fairly reliable estimate of total body fat and the measurements are simple to perform. The triceps skinfold thickness is most commonly used; it is measured with a caliper at a point midway between the shoulder and elbow. A triceps skinfold thickness of greater than 20 mm in men or 30 mm in women defines the presence of obesity (see Chapter 1, section on nutritional assessment).

Obesity can be classified as mild, moderate, severe, or morbid when weight exceeds ideal body weight by 15 to 30, 30 to 50, 50 to 100, or more than 100 per cent, respectively. Both genetic background and environmental factors contribute to the high incidence of obesity in children of obese parents. Genetic factors are especially prominent in the more severe forms of obesity.

Although it is not usually possible to identify a specific cause for obesity, an underlying medical disorder occasionally may contribute to or be completely responsible for the obese state. Such disorders include lesions in the ventromedial nucleus of the hypothalamus, Cushing syndrome, hypothyroidism, insulinoma, and gonadal insufficiency. Weight gain may also result from treatment with certain drugs, such as the phenothiazines, butyrophenones (e.g., haloperidol), tricyclic antidepressants, corticosteroids, birth control pills, or cyproheptadine. Finally, obesity may follow the prescription of certain diets, such as the frequent feeding programs used for patients with peptic ulcer disease, gastroesophageal reflux, or reactive hypoglycemia.

In the American population, obesity is especially common in women of lower socioeconomic status. There is also a steady increase in average weight with age, until about age 50, in both sexes. Consequently, the incidence of obesity increases from about 25 per cent in both sexes between 30 and 39 years of age to 32 per cent in men and 40 per cent in women in their forties.

Excessive accumulation of fat can result from both increased numbers and increased size of fat cells. In childhood obesity, there is an increased number of fat cells (hyperplasia). The degree of hyperplasia decreases until adolescence, and available evidence suggests that the number of fat cells increases very little after puberty. During adult life, weight gain results primarily from an increase in the size of existing fat cells (hypertrophy). Thus, the relative contribution of hyperplasia and hypertrophy of fat cells is largely determined by the age of onset of the obese state.

The importance of preventing obesity in childhood is supported by animal studies suggesting that the development of severe or morbid obesity usually occurs only in the presence of fat cell hyperplasia resulting from excessive caloric intake during childhood. Obesity beginning in childhood, particularly morbid obesity, is often refractory to dietary control. Adult-onset obesity is generally more responsive to dietary measures.

Although psychologic problems often contribute to the development of obesity, obesity itself is responsible for significant psychologic difficulties. In dietary planning it is important to bear in mind that obese patients, as a group, exhibit certain characteristic eating patterns. They are more prone to stimulation by external cues and less responsive to internal physiologic stimuli for eating or satiety. Obese individuals tend to prefer sweetened foods and are more selective when given less palatable foods. They generally eat more food per meal and eat fewer meals and faster meals. They tend to skip breakfast and eat more food as the day progresses; many overeat especially at night.

GOALS AND RATIONALE OF TREATMENT

1. To decrease adipose tissue to achieve a weight within 15 per cent of ideal body weight (see Table A-10, in Appendix).

2. To improve the patient's understanding of nutritional principles and help develop more healthy dietary patterns.

3. To prevent loss of muscle mass and maintain muscle tone by increased excercise during the weight-reduction period.

4. To achieve long-term maintenance of weight loss.

Having a slim appearance has become a national fad, and many individuals seek advice on weight reduction for purely cosmetic reasons. The medical consequences of mild obesity (15 to 30 per cent overweight) are uncertain. On the other hand, more severe obesity is associated with decreased life expectancy and an increased frequency of many medical disorders, as indicated in Table 5-4.

Obesity regularly causes increased glucocorticoid production, hyperinsulinism, and diminished release of growth hormone in response to provocative stimuli. These abnormalities are usually reversed with a return to normal weight. Of particular significance are the marked increase in basal insulin levels and the increased insulin response to a carbohydrate load in obese individuals. These insulin abnormalities apparently result from tissue resistance to the

TABLE 5–4.   COMPLICATIONS OF OBESITY (> 30% OVERWEIGHT)

Cardiovascular	Hypertension
	Coronary artery disease
	Congestive heart disease
	Varicose veins
Endocrine and metabolic	Diabetes mellitus
	Amenorrhea
	Hirsutism
	Fatty liver
	Hypertriglyceridemia
Pulmonary	Pickwickian syndrome
	Respiratory tract infections
Gastrointestinal	Cholecystitis and cholelithiasis
	Dyspepsia
Psychiatric and Social Problems	
Miscellaneous	Skin infections
	Osteoarthritis
	Toxemia of pregnancy

actions of insulin, perhaps caused by a decrease in the number of cellular hormone receptors.

The stress of obesity may unmask a genetic predisposition toward diabetes mellitus and produce glucose intolerance. The insulin resistance of obesity undoubtedly accounts for the close association between obesity and adult-onset diabetes mellitus. Elevated insulin levels may also contribute significantly to the frequent development of hypertriglyceridemia seen in obese patients. Both carbohydrate intolerance and hypertriglyceridemia improve when the obese patient loses weight.

PATIENT SELECTION

The decision to initiate a weight reduction program may be based on cosmetic, social, or medical considerations. Available evidence suggests that mild obesity (15 to 30 per cent overweight) rarely causes medical problems in an otherwise healthy individual. However, weight reduction is medically indicated in mildly obese individuals who have diabetes mellitus, hypertriglyceridemia, or hypertension. Weight reduction may also be a useful preventive measure in those individuals with a strong family history of diabetes mellitus, hyperlipidemia, or coronary artery disease. Reduced weight may be helpful to individuals with lower extremity arthritis, chronic low back problems, or venous insufficiency. Weight reduction is indicated in all individuals more than 30 per cent overweight because of the multiplicity of complications associated with the more extreme forms of obesity.

As noted earlier, special attention must be given to the prevention of obesity during childhood, since the resultant adipose tissue hyperplasia apparently programs the child for the more severe and refractory forms of obesity in adult life. The importance of preventive measures is highlighted by the fact that morbid obesity is rarely correctable by dietary measures. Even in moderate obesity, the patient is more likely to succeed on a dietary regimen if he became overweight as an adult. Effective weight loss occurs most commonly when a patient has not attempted to lose weight previously and is well-adjusted emotionally. Most patients do lose weight on a diet, but only about 10 per cent maintain significant weight loss 1 year later.

MANAGEMENT PRINCIPLES

General Considerations

Medical evaluation of the obese patient should include diagnostic efforts to rule out the rare situation in which obesity is secondary to some other medical illness and to point out any medical complications of obesity that may increase motivation for weight loss.

An understanding of the psychologic history of the patient is also important. Major considerations include appreciation of their life situation; assessment of marital, familial, occupational, and financial status; and elucidation of psychologic symptoms and the possible use of food as a mechanism for dealing with psychologic stress.

Caloric intake depends on the desired rate of weight loss. Calories should not be reduced by more than 20 to 40 per cent of the usual dietary intake, to encourage compliance with the diet and promote gradual weight loss. Provision of only general advice to limit total caloric intake is seldom effective. Instead, the patient needs specific instructions: (1) an individually planned diet with instructions from a dietitian, including printed sample menus and a week of specific meal plans; and (2) encouragement to keep a diary listing foods consumed, the time of day the food was eaten, and the location of the meal. The patient's emotional state at the moment of food ingestion should also be recorded. The diary serves to increase accountability and facilitate understanding of eating patterns.

The rate of weight loss depends upon the difference between caloric intake and energy expenditure. A deficit of about 3500 kcal is required for the loss of 1 lb of fat. The rapid weight loss often noted during the initial period on a calorie-restricted diet is mostly due to the loss of water. Patients must be informed of this so that they do not get discouraged with their diet when the rate of weight loss declines or even plateaus temporarily. Even under conditions of total fasting, the steady-state weight loss does not exceed about $1/2$ lb per day.

Complete or Protein-Sparing Modified Fasting

Significant weight loss can be achieved by prolonged complete fasting. Although used with considerable initial success in many morbidly obese patients, this approach suffers from a number of problems. Prolonged starvation may cause weakness, vitamin and mineral deficiencies, renal stones, and negative nitrogen balance. Deficiencies of vitamins and minerals can be prevented by appropriate supplementation during the period of fasting. In order to overcome the negative nitrogen balance and loss of muscle mass associated with complete starvation, several research groups have added small amounts of high-quality protein during the fast. When carried out under close medical supervision, this approach achieves weight reduction and minimizes the ill effects of total fasting.

On the basis of the success of these studies, Linn described a "Last Chance Diet," consisting of strict starvation supplemented by liquid protein, noncaloric drinks, vitamins, and minerals. Unfortunately, the initial liquid protein used was deficient in essential amino acids, and at least 50 deaths, mostly in women, have been attributed to the use of this regimen. These deaths were probably caused by myocardial damage and resultant arrhythmias.

The relatively large number of deaths resulting from protein-sparing fasts, compared with that resulting from total starvation may depend on two factors: whether the regimen is physician-supervised and whether it is balanced in amino acid content. Total starvation is generally carried out under close medical supervision. In addition, there is evidence that ingestion of a limited diet whose amino acid content is grossly imbalanced causes more nutritional complications than does total starvation. Although better quality protein supplements are now available, the use of protein-sparing modified fasts, as well as other types of starvation, requires careful medical supervision.

The long-term results of prolonged starvation or semistarvation are poor. Within a year after the fast, about 80 per cent of patients return to their former weight or even exceed it. The poor success of total starvation probably results from the failure of this approach to teach and habituate improved patterns of nutrition and eating. Nevertheless, a short period of starvation, if carried out under carefully supervised inpatient conditions with attention to hydration, vitamins, and electrolyte replacement, may be a worthwhile way to initiate weight loss, particularly when obesity is associated with severe medical complications. The short-term fast must be followed by a more conventional program of dietary and behavior modification, to encourage patients to make permanent changes in their eating habits.

Fad Diets

Fad diets are identified by short-term general popularity and adherence by the individual, zealous promotion and enthusiastic use, and marked divergence from the usual diet of the individual and of the general population. The dangers, if any, of a fad diet depend on the degree of nutritional imbalance and the length of time it is followed. With a few notable exceptions, such as the aforementioned "Last Chance Diet," fad weight-loss diets are not harmful, especially since they are most often followed for a relatively short time.

A successful weight-reducing diet obviously must be based on a reduction in caloric intake. Most nutritionists recommend a balanced diet containing a decreased number of calories to attain this goal. Instead, fad diets are based on elimination or marked reduction in the intake of certain types of foods, often in conjunction with the liberal use of other specific foods. Although there is no evidence that any given distribution of calories is particularly efficacious in promoting weight loss, some foods may provide greater satiety than others at similar caloric loads. For example, protein is relatively more satisfying than carbohydrate, especially more so than the simple sugars. Fad diets also take advantage of the fact that many dieters find it more difficult to moderate the intake of their usual foods than to follow a diet that totally eliminates or emphasizes specific foods.

Although the distribution of calories from the various food categories differs widely among the fad diets for weight reduction and although a few have emphasized a high intake of complex carbohydrates, most emphasize a low carbohydrate intake. In some, the usual balance is maintained between protein and fat intake. Other low-carbohydrate diets recommend a relatively high intake of either protein or fat. The latter programs tend to raise serum cholesterol levels, but this effect may be acceptable over the usual short period of adherence. Some diets that are rich in protein and do not restrict calories produce a significant initial weight loss that is almost entirely from increased loss of water.

In summary, many obese individuals may follow the majority of weight-reducing fad diets safely and enjoy a brief period of successful weight reduction. The poor long-term palatability of these diets, especially the more nutritionally unbalanced ones that stress particular foods, such as grapefruit or rice, limit both the utility and the risks of weight-reducing fad diets. Moreover, fad diets do not promote the improved nutritional habits necessary for continuation or maintenance of weight reduction once the fad diet loses its appeal.

Exercise

It is difficult to lose significant amounts of weight through increased exercise alone. Loss of 1 lb of fat requires either a decreased caloric intake or an increased energy expenditure of about 3500 kcal, the equivalent of walking approximately 35 miles. Nonetheless, a moderate increase in exercise or encouragement to expend more calories in the course of routine activities may be a valuable adjunct to reduction of caloric intake. Exercise increases muscle tone and may prevent loss of muscle mass during weight reduction. Patterns of increased physical activity help to maintain weight loss over a long period of time.

Behavioral Changes

The use of behavioral modification in the treatment of obesity is based on the assumption that long-term weight control requires major changes in eating habits, especially in individuals whose eating is stimulated by extraneous factors such as environment or mood rather than by hunger.

Most patients can be instructed easily in a few simple behavioral techniques that often assist in weight loss. These include eating more slowly while noting the taste of each bite; eating only in a specified spot with a complete place setting; and avoiding eating while carrying out other distracting activities, such as watching television.

For other patients, a more formalized approach may be necessary. Such a program, often done with a group of patients, may consist of the following components:

1. *Self-monitoring*: A diary of the patient's eating behavior helps to pinpoint problem areas and gives feedback on progress.

2. *Stimulus control*: After a systematic examination of factors that result in extra eating, strategies are developed to eliminate these "cues" for eating.

3. *Slowed rate of eating*: This maneuver aims at helping obese patients to eat less and enjoy it more.

4. *Nutrition and exercise education*: This component includes information on energy balance, nutrient needs, low-calorie cooking methods, and the value of exercise in weight control.

5. *Reinforcement*: A system of rewards given for appropriate changes in eating behavior and sometimes for weight loss itself is based on the premise that rewards make desired behavior more likely to become a habit. Food should never be used as a reward.

Several manuals describing behavioral modifications for weight control are available for health professionals. Two particularly helpful ones are

Ferguson, J.M.: Learning to Eat: Behavioral Modification for Weight Control. Palo Alto, CA: Bull Publishing, 1975.

Stuart, R.B., and Davis, B.: Slim Chance in a Fat World: Behavioral Control of Obesity. Champaign, IL: Illinois Research Press, 1981.

Weight-Reduction Groups

Obese individuals require considerable support and encouragement during periods of weight reduction and even after the weight goal has been achieved. Most physicians cannot—or will not—spend enough time with their obese patients to meet these needs. Various group approaches have been developed to provide continued support.

Physician-organized efforts have utilized conventional psychiatric group therapy or have stressed group interactions to promote modification of behavior. However, the expense and small number of such groups have limited their impact on the treatment of obesity. A number of ethical commercial groups have employed the elements of patient support and gentle peer pressure to foster weight reduction. Although their rate of success has not been documented by careful studies, available evidence suggests that these groups are as successful as individual physicians in promoting weight loss and its long-term maintenance.

Surgery

Several surgical procedures have been used for the treatment of morbid obesity. Indications include failure of dietary management after several years of attempts and the presence of serious medical, psychiatric, or social problems that will not improve without weight loss. Small-intestinal bypass has usually proven successful in promoting effective weight loss. However, excessive long-term complications that may develop following this procedure generally outweigh the benefits of the resultant weight loss. Newer procedures such as gastric bypass and gastric partitioning can achieve significant weight loss with a lower complication rate, but longer follow-up is needed to determine their true efficacy and role in the management of morbid obesity.

MAJOR DIETARY MODIFICATIONS

CALORIC INTAKE.   The patient's intake of calories must be reduced to allow weight loss. The number of calories to be allowed depends upon the desired rate of weight loss, the present caloric intake, and the level of physical activity. A reduction of 500 kcal/day below maintenance requirements (see Tables A–11 and A–12, in Appendix) will result in a weight loss of about 1 lb per week. Ideally, a patient should lose 1 to 2 lbs per week.

DISTRIBUTION OF CALORIES.   Total calories should be distributed among proteins, fats, and carbohydrates according to proportions generally recommended for all individuals, namely, 15 to 20 per cent protein, 30 per cent fat, and 50 to 55 per cent carbohydrate. Most foods are restricted in the amounts allowed. Highly concentrated sources of calories, such as pies and pastries, are eliminated altogether. The Exchange Lists for Meal Planning (see Table A–13, in Appendix) are used to plan the diets. Exchange foods may be saved from meals and used later as snacks, or the exchange foods planned as snacks may be incorporated into the meals. A sample meal plan for a 1200-kcal reducing diet is given in Table 5–5. Table 5–6 provides sample meal patterns for weight-reduction diets ranging in energy intake from 1000 to 1800 kcal per day.

NUTRITION.   The diet should be adequate in all nutrients, since it is intended to be the basis of lifelong eating habits that will maintain the weight loss achieved.

PHYSICAL ACTIVITY.   The patient should be taught the relationship between weight control, physical activity, and caloric intake. Increased physical activity is encouraged as tolerated.

PATIENT PARTICIPATION.   The patient should participate in the planning of the diet. Setting reasonable, realistic goals and individualizing the diet to fit the patient's cultural and socioeconomic background will encourage long-term compliance.

FOLLOW-UP.   Frequent follow-up sessions should be planned to monitor the patient's progress, allow positive reinforcement, provide additional information, and make changes in the diet as needed.

TABLE 5–5.   SAMPLE MEAL PLAN FOR A 1200-CALORIE WEIGHT REDUCTION DIET*

Breakfast

½ grapefruit
½ cup bran flakes
1 slice whole wheat toast
1 tsp margarine
1 cup skim milk
Coffee or tea as desired

Lunch

2 oz sliced roast turkey
2 slices rye bread with lettuce and tomato
1 tsp mayonnaise
¼ cantaloupe
Iced tea with lemon and artificial sweetener

Supper

2 oz broiled beef pattie
½ cup broccoli with ½ tsp margarine
½ cup carrots with ½ tsp margarine
Lettuce wedge with 1 tbs French salad dressing
¾ cup fresh strawberries
2 squares of graham crackers
1 cup skim milk

Snack

1 fresh pear

The composition of this meal plan is:

Calories	1200	Calcium	873	mg
Protein	60 g	Iron	16	mg
Fat	40 g	Phosphorus	1208	mg
Carbohydrate	153 g	Potassium	2284	mg
		Sodium	1212[†]	mg

*Refer to exchange lists for meal planning.
†Sodium content of diet alone (no salt added in cooking).

TABLE 5–6. SAMPLE PATTERNS FOR REDUCTION DIETS*

	1000 Calories 20% Protein	1200 Calories 20% Protein	1500 Calories 20% Protein	1800 Calories 15% Protein
BREAKFAST				
Fruit Exchanges	1	1	1	2
Meat Exchanges	—	—	1	—
Bread Exchanges	1	2	2	3
Fat Exchanges	1	1	1	2
Milk Exchanges (skim)	1	1	1	1
LUNCH				
Meat Exchanges	2	2	2	2
Vegetable Exchanges	1	1	—	1
Bread Exchanges	1	2	2	3
Fat Exchanges	1	1	1	3
Fruit Exchanges	1	1	2	2
Milk Exchanges (skim)	—	—	—	—
DINNER				
Meat Exchanges	2	2	3	2
Vegetable Exchanges	2	2	1	1
Bread Exchanges	1	1	2	3
Fat Exchanges	1	2	2	3
Fruit Exchanges	1	1	2	2
Milk Exchanges (skim)	1	1	—	—
SNACK				
Fruit Exchanges	1	1	—	—
Bread Exchanges	—	—	1	1½
Milk Exchanges (skim)	—	—	1	1

*All meal patterns are adequate in all essential nutrients.

BIBLIOGRAPHY

Andres, R.: Effect of obesity on total mortality. Int J Obesity 4:381–386, 1980.

Berland, T.: Diets '79. Consumer Guide Magazine Health Quarterly 223:1–256, 1979.

Berland, T.: Rating the diets. Consumer Guide 53, 1974.

Bierman, E.L., and Hirsch, J.: Obesity. *In* Williams, R.H. (Ed.): Textbook of Endocrinology, 6th Ed. Philadelphia, W.B. Saunders Co., 1981, pp. 907–921.

Bray, G.A.: Treatment for obesity. *In* Brodoff, B.N., and Bleicher, S.L. (Eds.): Diabetes Mellitus and Obesity. Baltimore, Williams and Wilkins, 1982, pp. 322–332.

Bray, G.A.: Obesity in America: An overview of the second Fogarty International Center Conference on Obesity. Int J Obesity 3:363–375, 1979.

Brownell, K.D.: Obesity: Behavioral treatments for a serious, prevalent and refractory problem. *In* Goodstein, R.K. (Ed.): Eating and Weight Disorders. Advances in Treatment and Research. New York, Springer Publishing Co., 1983, pp. 41–70.

Cahill, G.F., Jr.: Starvation in Man. *In* Albrink, M.J. (Ed.): Clinics in Endocrinology and Metabolism. Vol. 5, No. 2, London, W.B. Saunders Company, Ltd., 1976.

Dally, P., Gomez, J., and Isaacs, A.J.: Anorexia Nervosa. London, William Heinemann Medical Books, Ltd., 1979.

Dickerman, R.M.: Gastric exclusion surgery in the management of morbid obesity. Ann Rev Med 33:263–270, 1982.

Drenick, E.J., and Johnson, D.: Weight reduction by fasting and semi-starvation in morbid obesity: Long-term follow-up. Int J Obesity 2:123–132, 1978.

Garner, M., and Garfinkel, P.E.: The eating attitudes test: An index of the symptoms of anorexia nervosa. Psychol Med 9:273–279, 1979.

Keys, A.: Overweight, obesity, coronary heart disease and mortality. Nutr Rev 38:297–307, 1980.

Lantigua, R.A., Amatruda, J.M., Biddle, T.L., Forbes, G.S., and Lockwood, D.H.: Cardiac arrhythmias associated with a liquid protein diet for the treatment of obesity. N Engl J Med 303:735–738, 1980.

Lew, E.A., and Garfinkel, L.: Variations in mortality by weight among 750,000 men and women. J Chron Dis 32:563–576, 1979.

Lewis, S.B., Wallin, J.D., Kane, J.P., *et al.*: Effect of diet composition on metabolic adaptations to hypocaloric nutrition: Comparison of high carbohydrate and high fat isocaloric diets. Am J Clin Nutr 30:160–170, 1977.

Pozefsky, T., and Margolis, S.: Eating disorders: Obesity and anorexia nervosa. *In* Harvey, A.M., Johns, R.J., McKusick, V.A., Owens, A.H., and Ross, R. (Eds.): The Principles and Practice of Medicine (21st Ed.). New York, Appleton-Century-Crofts, 1984, pp. 945–954.

Russell, G.F.M.: The nutritional disorder in anorexia nervosa. J Psychosom Res 11:141–149, 1967.

Sims, E.A.H.: Characterization of the syndromes of obesity. *In* Brodoff, B.N., and Bleicher, S.L. (Eds.): Diabetes Mellitus and Obesity. Baltimore, Williams and Wilkins, 1982, pp. 219–226.

Sims, E.A.H., Danforth, E., Jr., Horton, E.S., Bray, G.A., Glennon, J.A., and Salans, L.B.: Endocrine and metabolic effects of experimental obesity in man. Recent Prog Horm Res 29:457–487, 1973.

Sours, J.E., Frattali, V.P., Brand, C.D., Feldman, R.A., Forbes, A.L., Swanson, R.C., and Paris, A.L.: Sudden death associated with very low caloric weight reduction regimens. Am J Clin Nutr 34:453–461, 1981.

Stuart, R.B., and Davis, B.: Slim Chance in a Fat World: Behavioral Control of Obesity. Champaign, Illinois, Research Press, 1981.

Stunkard, A.J. (Ed.): Obesity. Philadelphia, W.B. Saunders Co., 1980.

Van Itallie, T.B., and Yang, M.U.: Diet and weight loss. N Engl J Med 297:1158–1161, 1977.

Wadden, T.A., Stunkard, A.J., and Brownell, K.D.: Very-low calorie diets: Their efficacy, safety, and future. Ann Intern Med 99:675–684, 1983.

6
CARBOHYDRATE DISORDERS

Diabetes Mellitus

K.M. Shakir, M.D.,
Simeon Margolis, M.D., Ph.D., and
Millicent T. Kelly, R.D.

INTRODUCTION

Patients with diabetes mellitus traditionally have been separated into juvenile and adult-onset types. Although this classification is based on the age of onset of the disorder, other differences also characterize the groups. Juvenile diabetics are generally lean and require insulin treatment. Adult-onset diabetics are usually obese and often can be managed without insulin. However, some young patients are obese and develop a form of diabetes quite similar to that found in mature adults; they can be managed by dietary measures alone. On the other hand, the diabetes in some normal-weight adults requires insulin for control. Accordingly, a new classification of diabetes has been recommended and will be used in this section. This classification divides patients into insulin-dependent (most juvenile) or type I and non–insulin-dependent (most adult-onset) or type II diabetics.

Although the overall goals and rationale for management are the same for all patients with diabetes, the specific dietary strategies appropriate for lean, insulin-dependent diabetics differ significantly from those for obese, non–insulin-dependent diabetics.

GOALS AND RATIONALE OF MANAGEMENT FOR ALL DIABETICS

The main goals and rationale of dietary treatment are as follows:

1. *Reverse or minimize hyperglycemia.* In obese, non–insulin-dependent diabetics, weight reduction, even when modest in degree, usually improves glucose tolerance and at times reverses the diabetes. Although diet therapy does

not improve the disease itself in insulin-dependent diabetes, dietary measures are essential for the effective use of insulin.

Hyperglycemia may cause glucosuria with concomitant polyuria, polydipsia, and weight loss. Blood glucose levels must be controlled to prevent diabetic ketoacidosis and nonketotic hyperosmolar coma. Hyperglycemia is also associated with the development of cataracts and an increased susceptibility to infection. It has not yet been proved that excellent control of blood glucose levels delays or prevents the small blood vessel changes that are largely responsible for the late retinal, renal, and neurologic complications of diabetes. Nonetheless, recent evidence suggests that excellent control minimizes these late problems. There is a growing tendency to strive for rigorous control of blood glucose levels. However, the potential long-term benefits from such rigorous control must be balanced against the increased risk of hypoglycemia. In addition, most experts agree that control of blood glucose does not reduce the accelerated progression of atherosclerosis that is commonly associated with diabetes.

2. *Avoid hypoglycemia.* All patients treated with insulin must follow dietary measures carefully in order to avoid hypoglycemic episodes.

3. *Prevent the late complications of diabetes.* As discussed earlier, the control of hyperglycemia may forestall the small blood vessel abnormalities responsible for some late complications of diabetes (retinopathy, nephropathy, and neuropathy).

Diabetics are also at high risk for premature atherosclerosis, particularly of peripheral and coronary arteries. Although diabetics with hyperlipidemia require particular attention (see Chapter 7, section on dietary modification of plasma lipid and lipoprotein levels), all diabetic patients should follow dietary measures to reduce serum lipids. Until recently, the standard diabetic diet was low in carbohydrate and relatively high in fat. However, diabetic patients from underdeveloped countries where diets are rich in starch and low in fat have a significantly lower incidence of coronary artery disease than do diabetic patients in the United States. This and other observations have led the American Diabetes Association to modify its dietary recommendations for the management of diabetes. The currently recommended diet liberalizes the intake of carbohydrates, particularly of complex carbohydrates, and stresses restriction of saturated fats and cholesterol. Control of weight and of hyperglycemia usually improves hypertriglyceridemia considerably and may modestly lower serum cholesterol and raise high-density lipoprotein (HDL) levels.

4. *Manage associated conditions.* To manage conditions associated with diabetes, such as hypertension and renal failure, additional dietary alterations may be needed, as discussed later. The management of diabetes during pregnancy is discussed in Chapter 1, section on nutrition in pregnancy and lactation.

MANAGEMENT OF NON–INSULIN-DEPENDENT DIABETES MELLITUS

Efforts are directed particularly toward achieving ideal body weight (see Appendix) in all patients, since weight loss may reverse or dramatically reduce the severity of diabetes. Attempts should be made to achieve normal serum cholesterol and triglyceride levels in hyperlipidemic patients and to lower serum cholesterol and raise HDL levels in all patients with diabetes. Hypertension or renal failure may require further dietary modifications, such as a low-sodium diet.

DIETARY PRINCIPLES AND MODIFICATIONS. Age, sex, body weight, physical activity, endogenous insulin secretion, drug therapy, and the presence of diabetic complications all influence the details of the diabetic diet. Dietary preferences based on ethnic background, eating habits, and patient attitudes are also important. A simple, practical, and palatable diet can be prescribed after taking all of these factors into consideration.

1. *Calorie requirements.* These depend on the patient's age, sex, present weight, and physical activity (see Appendix).

2. *Distribution of calories among carbohydrates, fat, and protein.* The American Diabetes Association recommends that carbohydrates should comprise 50 to 55 per cent of ingested calories, whereas fat should account for 30 to 35 per cent, with no more than one-third of the fat being saturated and the remainder being polyunsaturated or monounsaturated. Proteins should provide the remaining 15 to 20 per cent of total calories. These proportions are nearly identical with those in the average American diet. Patients should avoid excessive intake of carbohydrates at a single meal and of large amounts of simple sugars between meals, particularly as liquids and unaccompanied by other food types, because of the resultant short-term increase in blood glucose level.

3. *Caloric distribution and timing of meals.* The diet may be divided into three meals with or without a snack in the afternoon or evening. The distribution is determined by individual preferences and lifestyles; the pattern need not be constant.

4. *Alcohol.* Moderate alcohol intake can be permitted for most diabetics by exchanging fat or carbohydrate calories or both for alcohol calories. The alcohol content of various alcoholic beverages is given in Table 14–1. The caloric content of these beverages, for moderate alcohol intake, can be calculated by multiplying the alcohol content by 7 kcal/g.

In fact, moderate alcohol use may prove beneficial because it raises serum HDL levels. However, alcohol may raise triglyceride levels in patients with hypertriglyceridemia and may provoke a disulfiram-like reaction in occasional diabetics on sulfonylurea drugs.

5. *Vitamins and minerals.* Vitamin and mineral supplements are needed only when diabetes is associated with malabsorption secondary to pancreatitis or pancreatectomy; prolonged, severe caloric restriction in markedly obese patients; or chronic ingestion of nutritionally inadequate diets, usually by patients from low socioeconomic backgrounds.

6. *Modifications for exercise or illness.* Dietary modifications are usually not required for moderate exercise, missed meals, or mild intercurrent illness. Occasionally, strenuous exercise or severe illness may necessitate supplementary feedings of 15 to 50 g of a carbohydrate food source between meals.

7. *Dietary fiber.* Since recent studies indicate that fiber-rich diets may improve diabetic control, the American Diabetes Association has recommended that, whenever acceptable to the patient, natural foods containing unrefined carbohydrate fiber should be substituted for highly refined low-fiber carbohydrates. Anderson has recently published a guide for the use of high-fiber diets in the management of diabetics (see Bibliography).

MANAGEMENT OF INSULIN-DEPENDENT DIABETES MELLITUS

In patients with little or no pancreatic beta cell function, dietary management is directed toward the establishment of regular eating patterns, to maximize the effectiveness of insulin therapy and to diminish the risk of hypoglycemia. The main objective is dietary regulation rather than dietary deprivation. Management of obesity is important in the small number of insulin-dependent patients who are overweight. Control of serum lipids is also important in all insulin-dependent diabetics.

DIETARY PRINCIPLES AND MODIFICATIONS.   Dietary management is very similar to that described for non–insulin-dependent diabetes. This section describes only those features unique to insulin-dependent diabetes.

1. *Caloric distribution and timing of meals* (see Table 6–1). For patients on insulin, consistency in the timing of meals and the distribution of calories throughout the day is more important than the exact caloric intake or the proportions of carbohydrates, protein, and fat in the diet. Most patients taking intermediate-acting insulins, such as NPH or lente insulins, are advised to ingest regular midafternoon or bedtime snacks or both. Such snacks should be planned to fit the lifestyle of the patient. Although these measures diminish the risk of hypoglycemia, all patients are taught to recognize the early symptoms of hypoglycemia and always to carry with them some source of rapidly absorbed carbohydrate.

2. *Modifications for strenuous exercise or intercurrent illness.* Additional food is rarely required for mild exercise. However, to minimize the chance of developing hypoglycemia, 10 to 50 g of extra carbohydrate should be ingested prior to nonhabitual exercise occurring more that 2 hours after a meal. During intercurrent illness, consumption of 50 to 75 g of carbohydrate in any form is recommended every 6 to 8 hours to prevent starvation ketosis.

3. *Alcohol.* The basic principles concerning alcohol consumption are the same as for non–insulin-dependent diabetic patients. However, large amounts of alcohol are more likely to precipitate hypoglycemia in insulin-dependent diabetics (the symptoms of which may go unrecognized if they are mistaken for alcoholic intoxication).

MAJOR DIETARY CONSIDERATIONS

1. *Calories.* It is important for diabetic patients to achieve and maintain ideal body weight (see Appendix).

TABLE 6–1.   GUIDE FOR DISTRIBUTION OF CARBOHYDRATE INTAKE FOR PATIENTS ON INSULIN

Type of Insulin	Peak Action Time (hrs)	Duration of Blood Sugar Lowering Effect (hrs)	Distribution of Carbohydrates*					Shorthand Notation
			B	L	S_N	D	S_N	
Crystalline zinc insulin (CZI) or regular insulin prior to each meal	2–4	8	$\frac{1}{3}$	$\frac{1}{3}$		$\frac{1}{3}$		$\frac{111}{3}$
Neutral Protamine Hagedorn (NPH) insulin or Lente insulin	8–10	24	$\frac{2}{7}$	$\frac{2}{7}$	$\frac{1}{7}$	$\frac{2}{7}$		$\frac{2212}{7}$
					or			
			$\frac{2}{8}$	$\frac{2}{8}$	$\frac{1}{8}$	$\frac{2}{8}$	$\frac{1}{8}$	$\frac{22121}{8}$
					or			
			$\frac{2}{7}$	$\frac{2}{7}$		$\frac{2}{7}$	$\frac{1}{7}$	$\frac{2221}{7}$
Protamine zinc insulin (PZI)	20–22	36	$\frac{2}{7}$	$\frac{2}{7}$		$\frac{2}{7}$	$\frac{1}{7}$	$\frac{2221}{7}$

*In many diabetics treated with intermediate-acting insulins, there is a tendency for blood glucose levels to rise shortly before breakfast. As a consequence, the highest blood glucose levels of the day may occur after breakfast. In such patients it may be advisable to add regular insulin to the morning dose of NPH or to reduce the amount of carbohydrate in the breakfast.

The timing and number of snacks on NPH or lente insulin depends on the patient's response to insulin and the time of the evening meal. Since these intermediate-acting insulins tend to reach their peak action in the afternoon, a snack is usually scheduled between lunch and dinner. The afternoon snack may be replaced by an evening snack in those patients who eat an early dinner or in whom insulin action is delayed. Some patients prefer both afternoon and evening snacks.

2. *Protein.* Approximately 15 to 20 per cent of total calories should be protein. To comply with the American Diabetes Association recommendation to reduce the intake of cholesterol and saturated fats, a protein intake of no more than 15 per cent of total calories is ideal. Protein intake should be increased during pregnancy and in patients with the nephrotic syndrome, extensive weight loss, or debilitating disease. In patients receiving long-acting insulins, protein should be included in the afternoon or evening snack or both to help prevent hypoglycemia.

3. *Fat.* Fat should comprise approximately 30 to 35 per cent of total calories, partially substituting polyunsaturated fats for saturated ones. Skim or low-fat milk is recommended and whole egg intake is limited to 3 to 4 per week.

4. *Carbohydrate.* Approximately 50 to 55 per cent of total calories should be derived from carbohydrate. Complex carbohydrates should be substituted for simple sugars when feasible. Limiting the intake of simple sugars was originally suggested on the assumption that their ingestion would raise blood glucose levels to a greater degree than would ingestion of complex carbohydrates.

Subsequently, it was shown that the fiber present in complex carbohydrates slowed the rate of glucose absorption from the intestine.

More recently, studies have demonstrated that there is considerable variability in the glycemic response to various starches and sugars. For example, when equivalent amounts of carbohydrate were ingested as potatoes or rice, potatoes provoked higher blood glucose and insulin levels. Blood glucose responses were especially delayed after the ingestion of legumes and dairy products.

Simple sugars also vary in their effect on blood glucose levels. The rise in blood glucose is much greater for glucose than it is for sucrose and fructose. In fact, fruit increases blood glucose to a lesser degree than does an equivalent amount of potatoes, even though the carbohydrate in fruit is largely in the form of simple sugars while in potatoes it is in the form of starch.

The form in which a food is eaten also determines the glycemic response. The response was greater for pureed than for whole apples and greater for ground than for whole rice. The variable responses to starchy foods reflect differences not only in their fiber content but also in the digestibility of the starch.

These studies clearly show that there are great differences in the glycemic response to foods that have traditionally been considered equivalent in exchange lists. Efforts to achieve better control of postprandial glucose levels may be aided by reference to the glycemic index for various foods presented in a review by Jenkins et al. (see Bibliography).

The glycemic index is defined as

$$\frac{\text{area under the 2-hr glucose response curve for a food}}{\begin{array}{c}\text{area under the 2-hr glucose response curve for the}\\\text{equivalent amount of glucose}\end{array}} \times 100$$

5. *Distribution and timing of meals.* Distributional considerations are applicable to carbohydrates only. Their distribution depends on individual preference and on the type of insulin or oral hypoglycemic drug being used (see Table 6–1).

Sugar Substitutes and "Sugar-Free" Foods

Neither sugar substitutes nor "sugar-free" foods are essential to the dietary management of persons with diabetes. Both caloric and noncaloric sweeteners are available as substitutes for sucrose. The major nutritive sweeteners are fructose, xylitol, and sorbitol. Since these sugars are absorbed from the intestine more slowly than is glucose, they produce less postprandial hyperglycemia and a reduced insulin response compared with that evoked by sucrose ingestion. However, they do not aid in weight control, since the caloric intake (4 kcal/g) required to achieve a given level of sweetness is similar to that of sucrose. When taken in large amounts (more than 20 to 50 g), xylitol and sorbitol can cause diarrhea. Although the long-term benefit of these sugar substitutes in the management of diabetes remains unproven, replacement of sucrose with xylitol markedly reduces dental caries. Invert sugar (hydrolyzed sucrose) is sometimes used because it tastes sweeter than sugar. Aspartame (the methyl ester of L-aspartyl-L-phenylalanine) is a low-calorie, non-nutritive sweetener that is 180 times as sweet as sucrose.

Saccharin is the only noncaloric sweetener besides aspartame that is currently available in this country. Since the use of cyclamates was banned in 1969, saccharin consumption has increased substantially. Saccharin is used primarily as an additive to beverages. The reduced caloric intake resulting from the use of soft drinks and other beverages sweetened with saccharin can, at best, have a mildly beneficial effect in the maintenance of ideal weight in diabetic patients.

On the basis of reports of an increased incidence of cancer—primarily of the urinary bladder—after chronic ingestion of saccharin by animals and man, the Food and Drug Administration in April 1977 proposed that the use of saccharin be restricted. In July 1978, a Select Committee on Sugar Substitutes, sponsored by the American Diabetes Association, concluded that, "based on the evidence now available, there appears to be little justification for placing further governmental restrictions on the use of saccharin by the American public at the present time." The only restriction currently in effect is a requirement that the food label list the saccharin content of the product. The label must also indicate that saccharin may be hazardous to one's health because it has been shown to cause cancer in laboratory animals.

"Sugar-free" foods are not necessary to achieve the dietary goals generally recommended for the treatment of diabetes. Nonetheless, many companies manufacture and widely advertise for people with diabetes specially prepared (dietetic) products, such as candies and cookies, that contain sorbitol or fructose instead of sucrose. Diabetic patients are tempted to use these products because they are touted as "sugar-free." However, conversion of sorbitol to fructose and its subsequent metabolism yields the same number of calories as products containing an equal amount of sucrose. In fact, dietetic candies and cookies not only are more expensive but also contain as many calories as regular candies and cookies, if not more. There is no particular nutritional benefit despite their higher cost.

However, dietetic fruits and preserves do contain fewer calories than regular fruits and preserves. The greatest caloric savings result from the use of "water-packed" fruits rather than their counterparts packed in syrup. There may also be some advantage to the use of special puddings and gelatins that contain fewer calories and are less expensive than their regular counterparts.

Diabetic Diets for Children

Quantitative dietary recommendations are often needed for the proper treatment of diabetes in children. However, the restricted diets recommended for diabetic children in the past proved unsatisfactory for growth and emotional stability, especially during the teenage years. The objectives of dietary management of the child with diabetes mellitus are essentially the same as those for the adult with insulin-dependent diabetes, but the diet must include adequate calories for growth, development, and activity. Either measured or calorie-controlled diets are used to treat children with diabetes.

The measured dietary regimen utilizes the Exchange Lists for Meal Planning (see Appendix, Table A–13). A calorie-controlled diet is employed when it is felt that the child will not be receptive to the more rigid, measured diet. In both diets, the recommended calories and the distribution of carbohydrates (shown in Table 6–1) take into account the type and amount of insulin used and the physical activity of the child. The allowance of 1000 kcal plus 100 kcal for each year of age (up to 12 years of age) is a good approximation of daily energy requirement of the normal preadolescent child. However, this formula underestimates the needs for the active adolescent. Younger children are usually given three meals along with snacks at midmorning, midafternoon, and bedtime. The midmorning snack can generally be discontinued between the ages of 7 and 10. A source of protein is included with each feeding.

CALCULATIONS FOR DIABETIC DIETS

A sample procedure for calculation of a diabetic diet for a 70-kg man is shown in Table 6–2. A sample exchange pattern for this diet is found in Table 6–3. Table 6–4 gives sample exchange patterns to be used in planning meals for diabetic patients with a daily intake of from 1000 to 2400 kcal.

Close interactions among physician, dietitian, and patient are necessary in formulating an appropriate diet. The dietary plan, which should be simple, practical, and compatible with the patient's lifestyle, is designed after the dietitian interviews the patient for a dietary assessment. Any prior dietary restrictions must be incorporated into the diabetic diet pattern in a manner calculated

TABLE 6–2. SAMPLE PROCEDURE FOR CALCULATION OF A DIABETIC DIET

Example	A 154-lb (70-kg) 5'8" male. Normal weight, moderate activity on 50 units NPH insulin
Calories	30 kcal/kg (moderate activity) (see Appendix) $30 \times 70 = 2100$ calories/day
Protein	Approximately 15% of 2100 calories = 315 kcal/day $315 \div 4$ kcal/g = 78 g/day
Fat	Approximately 30% of 2100 calories = 630 kcal/day 630 calories $\div 9$ kcal/g = 70 g/day
Carbohydrate	Approximately 55% of 2100 calories = 1155 kcal/day 1155 calories $\div 4$ kcal/g = 288 g/day
Distribution	With NPH insulin the distribution for carbohydrate is usually 82 g breakfast, 82 g lunch, 42 g snack, 82 g dinner, $\left(\frac{2212}{7}\right)$ (see Table 6-1)
Diet Order	2100-calorie Diabetic Diet Protein–80 g, Fat–70 g, CHO–288 g, $\left(\frac{2212}{7}\right)$

TABLE 6–3.   SAMPLE MEAL PATTERN FOR 2100-CALORIE
DIABETIC DIET

	Protein (g)	Fat (g)	CHO (g)
BREAKFAST			
2 fruit exchanges	—	—	20
2 meat exchanges	—	—	—
3 bread exchanges	6	—	45
3 fat exchanges	—	15	—
1 cup skim milk	8	—	12
Coffee or tea	—	—	—
Total	14	15	77
LUNCH			
2 meat exchanges	14	10	—
1 vegetable exchange	2	—	5
4 bread exchanges	8	—	60
2 fruit exchanges	—	—	20
3 fat exchanges	—	15	—
Total	24	25	85
SNACK			
2 bread exchanges	4	—	30
1 cup skim milk	8	—	12
Total	12	—	42
DINNER			
3 meat exchanges	21	15	—
1 vegetable exchange	2	—	5
2 fruit exchanges	—	—	20
4 bread exchanges	8	—	60
3 fat exchanges	—	15	—
Noncalorie beverage as allowed	—	—	—
Total	31	30	85
Grand Totals	81	70	289

to meet the individual patient's medical and socioeconomic needs. The patient must be educated regarding the importance of adhering to the balanced and scheduled meal pattern. Regular and consistent dietary intake is stressed, particularly in insulin-dependent diabetics. The "Exchange Lists for Meal Planning," recently developed jointly by the American Diabetic Association and the American Dietetic Association, is recommended for patient use (see Appendix).

It is important to identify any problems with comprehension of the initial dietary prescription and to assess dietary compliance at subsequent visits. Adjustments in the initial recommendation may be necessary. Proper encouragement and adequate patient motivation are essential for successful dietary therapy. Behavioral modification techniques have been used with success in learning new eating habits. Initial compliance can result in lasting control.

Sample meals for 1500- and 2100-kcal diabetic diets are given in Tables 6–5 and 6–6.

TABLE 6–4. SAMPLE DIABETIC MEAL PATTERNS*

Caloric Level Gms Pro–Fat–CHO	1000 56–35–124	1200 60–40–150	1500 75–50–185	1800 68–60–250	2100 80–70–290	2400 90–80–330
BREAKFAST						
Fruit exchanges	1	1½	1	2	2	2
Meat exchanges	—	—	1	—	—	1
Bread exchanges	1	1	2	3	3	4
Fat exchanges	—	1	2	2	3	3
Milk exchanges						
(skim)	1	1	1	1	1	1
LUNCH						
Meat exchanges	2	2	2	2	2	2
Vegetable exchanges	—	2	2	1	1	2
Bread exchanges	2	2	2	3	4	4
Fat exchanges	1	1	1	3	3	3
Fruit exchanges	1	—	1	2	2	2
SNACK						
Bread exchanges	—	1	1½	1½	2	2
Fat exchanges	—	—	—	—	—	1
Fruit exchanges	—	—	—	—	—	1
Milk exchanges						
(skim)	1	1	1	1	1	1
DINNER						
Meat exchanges	2	2	2	2	3	3
Vegetable exchanges	2	2	2	1	1	2
Bread exchanges	1	1	2	3	4	4
Fat exchanges	2	2	2	3	3	3
Fruit exchanges	1	1	1	2	2	2

*Caloric distribution is 15% protein, 30% fat, and 55% CHO, except diets at calorie levels 1000 through 1500 contain 20% protein. All meal patterns are adequate in the essential nutrients.

TABLE 6–5.   SAMPLE MEALS FOR A 1500-CALORIE
DIABETIC DIET

Breakfast	½ cup unsweetened orange juice 1 poached egg or egg substitute 2 halves English muffin, toasted 2 tsp margarine 1 cup skim milk Coffee

Lunch	*Sandwich*: 2 oz sliced roast beef
	             lettuce, 2 tomato slices
	             2 slices whole wheat bread
	½ cup cole slaw (1 tsp mayonnaise + 1 tsp vinegar)
	1 medium fresh nectarine
	Iced tea with lemon and artificial sweetener

Snack	¾ cup corn flakes 1 cup skim milk
Dinner	3 oz broiled steak 1 small baked potato, 1 tsp margarine ½ cup steamed asparagus, 1 tsp margarine Tossed salad, low-calorie dressing 1 slice French bread ¼ honeydew melon Coffee

TABLE 6–6.   SAMPLE MEALS FOR A 2100-CALORIE
DIABETIC DIET

Breakfast	½ cup unsweetened grapefruit juice ½ cup bran flakes with ½ small banana 2 slices toast 3 tsp margarine 1 cup skim milk Coffee

Lunch	*Sandwich*: 2 oz broiled hamburger pattie
	             1 hamburger roll
	             lettuce
	             1 tsp mayonnaise
	½ cup carrot sticks
	4 squares of graham crackers
	24 fresh grapes
	Iced tea with lemon and artificial sweetener

Snack	6 rye wafers 1 cup skim milk
Dinner	1 broiled chicken breast (3 oz) 1 baked potato (1 cup), 1 tsp margarine ½ cup spinach, 1 tsp margarine Mixed green salad, 1 tbs French dressing 2 slices Italian bread ½ cantaloupe Coffee

Symptomatic Postprandial Hypoglycemia

Simeon Margolis, M.D., Ph.D.

INTRODUCTION

Although a low plasma glucose level (chemical hypoglycemia) is not uncommon some hours after a meal, the clinical condition of symptomatic postprandial hypoglycemia occurs far less frequently. Symptoms of hypoglycemia, which result from excessive release of catecholamines from the adrenal medulla, include sweating, nervousness, tremor, palpitations, faintness, acral and perioral numbness, and weakness. The symptoms are brief and self-limited because of the release of hormones that rapidly raises the plasma glucose level.

Patients with symptomatic postprandial hypoglycemia are divided into three major groups:

1. *Alimentary hypoglycemia.* This usually develops following procedures such as partial gastric resection, gastrojejunostomy, or vagotomy and pyloroplasty, all of which hasten the movement of gastric contents into the small intestine. The resultant rapid rise in plasma glucose triggers excessive insulin release, which may cause hypoglycemic symptoms 1 to 3 hours after a meal.

2. *Non–insulin-dependent diabetes mellitus.* In the early stages of non–insulin-dependent diabetes mellitus, the delayed release of insulin in response to a meal may result in symptomatic hypoglycemia 3 to 5 hours after eating.

3. *Idiopathic hypoglycemia.* This is most common in tense and emotionally labile young women. The plasma glucose response to either a meal or a glucose load is generally blunted in these individuals. In most of these patients, the hypoglycemia is attributed to delayed, but not excessive, insulin production.

GOALS AND RATIONALE OF TREATMENT

The goal of treatment is to prevent the development of hypoglycemic symptoms by appropriate dietary modifications. The standard approach to treatment is based on theoretic considerations and anecdotal evidence, since very few studies have addressed the effects of diet on postprandial hypoglycemia. The usual dietary prescription for symptomatic postprandial hypoglycemia, a diet high in protein and restricted in carbohydrate, may be effective in some patients, but rigid adherence to these measures may not be necessary. In fact, other factors are probably more important in the control of symptoms from all types of postprandial hypoglycemia. These include multiple small feedings, attention to the types of carbohydrate ingested, and the inclusion of some fat and fiber with each feeding.

Multiple small feedings are employed to decrease the rate at which carbohydrates are emptied from the stomach. Complex carbohydrates requiring digestion (such as starches) are recommended, whereas the intake of simple sugars should be limited. It is important to recognize, however, that the blood glucose and insulin responses vary considerably with the type of starch-containing food and its mode of preparation. Major differences have also been observed in response to the ingestion of various foods rich in simple sugars. Patients with postprandial hypoglycemia should favor foods that minimize the subsequent rise in blood glucose and insulin. The inclusion of ample dietary fiber tends to slow the rise of plasma glucose and insulin in normal subjects. The provision of dietary fat may also slow gastric emptying; a relatively high-fat diet may be employed in all types of postprandial hypoglycemia but is especially important in patients with alimentary hypoglycemia (see Chapter 11, dumping syndrome section).

In overweight patients with symptomatic hypoglycemia from diabetes, achievement of ideal body weight is an important dietary measure.

PATIENT SELECTION

The presence of postprandial hypoglycemia should be considered in patients with the typical symptoms listed earlier. Particular attention should be paid to those with a history of gastric surgery or known glucose intolerance. In addition to the development of symptoms in an appropriate relationship to meals, the definitive diagnosis requires that the typical symptoms are accompanied by low plasma glucose levels (usually less than 50 mg/dl) during a 5-hour oral glucose tolerance test. The pattern of the glucose tolerance test together with the patient's history usually permits differentiation between the various types of symptomatic postprandial hypoglycemia. It is critical that the diagnosis of symptomatic hypoglycemia be made accurately, because both physicians and patients have erroneously attributed a wide variety of common and often vague symptoms, such as lack of energy, chronic anxiety, lethargy, and mental dullness, to postprandial hypoglycemia.

DIETARY PRINCIPLES

1. Multiple small feedings
2. Preferential selection of complex carbohydrates and dietary fiber; limitation of simple sugars
3. Inclusion of some fat with each meal
4. Weight reduction in obese patients with diabetes mellitus
5. Possibly a high-protein, restricted-carbohydrate diet

BIBLIOGRAPHY

Diabetes Mellitus

American Diabetes Association: Principles of nutrition and dietary recommendations for individuals with diabetes mellitus: 1979. Diabetes 28:1027–1030, 1979.

American Diabetes Association Statement: The saccharin question re-examined. J Am Dietetic Assoc 74:574–581, 1979.

American Diabetes Association and American Dietetic Association: Guide for Professionals: The Effective Application of "Exchange Lists for Meal Planning." New York and Chicago, 1977.

Anderson, J. W.: Diabetes: A practical new guide to healthy living. London, Martin Dunitz, 1981.

Anderson, J. W., Midgley, W. R., and Wedman, B.: Fiber and diabetes. Diabetes Care 2:369–379, 1979.

Bennion, L. J., and Grundy, S. M.: Effects of diabetes mellitus on cholesterol metabolism in man. N Engl J Med 296:1365–1371, 1977.

Brunzell, J. D.: Use of fructose, sorbitol, or xylitol as a sweetener in diabetes mellitus. J Am Diet Assoc 73:499–506, 1978.

Brunzell, J. D., Lerner, R.L., Hazzard, W. R., Porte, D., Jr., and Bierman, E. L.: Improved glucose tolerance with high carbohydrate feeding in mild diabetes. N Engl J Med 284:521–524, 1971.

Crapo, P.A., Reaven, G., and Olefsky, J.: Plasma glucose and insulin responses to orally administered simple and complex carbohydrates. Diabetes 25:741–747, 1976.

Doar, J. W. H., Wilde, C. E., Thompson, M. E., and Sewell, P. F. J.: Influence of treatment with diet alone on oral glucose-tolerance test and plasma sugar and insulin levels in patients with maturity-onset diabetes mellitus. Lancet 1:1263–1266, 1975.

Hockaday, T. D. R., Hockaday, J. M., Mann, J. I., and Turner, R. C.: Prospective comparison of modified fat–high carbohydrate with standard low-carbohydrate dietary advice in the treatment of diabetes: One year follow-up study. Br J Nutr 39:357–362, 1978.

Jenkins, D. J. A., Taylor, R. H., and Wolever, T. M. S.: The diabetic diet, dietary carbohydrate and differences in digestibility. Diabetologia 23:477–484, 1982.

Kalkhoff, R. K., and Levin, M. E.: The saccharin controversy. Diabetes Care 1:211–222, 1978.

Kaufmann, R. L., Arral, J. P., Soeldner, J. S., Wilmshurst, E. G., Lemaire, J. R., Gleason, R. E., and White, P.: Plasma lipid levels in diabetic children—effects of diet restricted in cholesterol and saturated fats. Diabetes 24:677–679, 1975.

Mintz, D. H., Skyler, J. S., and Chez, R. A.: Diabetes mellitus and pregnancy. Diabetes Care 1:49–63, 1978.

Miranda, P. M., and Horwitz, D. L.: High-fiber diets in the treatment of diabetes mellitus. Ann Int Med 88:482–486, 1978.

Reaven G.M.: What is the role of high carbohydrate-low fat diets in the treatment of diabetes mellitus? Spec Topics Endo Metab 3:117–137, 1982.

Reckless, J. P. D., Betterridge, D. J., Wu, P., Payne, B., and Galton, D. J.: High-density and low-density lipoproteins and prevalence of vascular disease in diabetes mellitus. Br Med J 1:883–886, 1978.

Symptomatic Postprandial Hypoglycemia

Crapo, P.A., Reaven, G., and Olefsky, J.: Plasma glucose and insulin responses to orally administered simple and complex carbohydrates. Diabetes 25:741–747, 1976.

Ensinck, J. W., and Williams, R. H.: Disorders causing hypoglycemia. In Williams, R. (Ed.): Textbook of Endocrinology. Philadelphia, W. B. Saunders Co., 1981, pp. 844–875.

Hofeldt, F. D.: Reactive hypoglycemia. Metabolism 24:1193–1208, 1975.

Hofeldt, F. D., Lufkin, E. G., Hagler, L., et al.: Are abnormalities in insulin secretion responsible for reactive hypoglycemia? Diabetes 23:589–596, 1974.

Jenkins, D. J. A., Taylor, R. H., and Wolever, T. M. S.: The diabetic diet, dietary carbohydrate and differences in digestibility. Diabetologia 23:477–484, 1982.

Luyckx, A. S., and Lefebvre, P. J.: Plasma insulin in reactive hypoglycemia. Diabetes 20:435–442, 1971.

Margolis, S., and Georgopoulos, A.: Hypoglycemia. In Harvey, AM, Johns, J.R., McKusick, V.A. Owens, A.H., and Ross, R.S. (Eds.): The Principles and Practice of Medicine, 21 ed. New York, Appleton-Century-Crofts, 1984, pp. 904–914.

Marks, V., and Rose, F.: Hypoglycemia. St. Louis, Blackwell Scientific Publications, 1981.

Permutt, M. A.: Postprandial hypoglycemia. Diabetes 25:719–733, 1976.

Rotwein, P.S., Giddings S.J., and Permutt A.: Diagnosis and management of hypoglycemic disorders in adults. Spec Topics Endo Metab 3:87–115, 1982.

Yager, J., and Young, R. T.: Non-hypoglycemia is an epidemic condition. N Engl J Med 291:907–908, 1974.

7
MODIFICATIONS IN FAT

Fat-Restricted Diets in the Management of Gastrointestinal Disorders

Theodore M. Bayless, M.D., and
Gloria Elfert, M.S., R.D.

INTRODUCTION

Restriction of fat intake may be useful in the dietary management of patients with several gastrointestinal disorders. Limitation of dietary fat intake may decrease symptoms and prevent complications in patients with cholecystitis and cholelithiasis. Fat restriction can help control diarrhea and steatorrhea in patients with malabsorption resulting from pancreatic insufficiency, ileal resection or bypass, or intestinal lymphatic obstruction. Medium-chain triglycerides may prove a valuable adjunct in limiting losses of lymphatic proteins into the intestine in patients with lymphatic obstruction and can serve as a major source of calories in patients with the short-gut syndrome. Limitation of dietary fat may diminish oxaluria and prevent oxalate calculi from forming as a result of excessive oxalate absorption in patients with fat malabsorption from ileal abnormalities.

There is no evidence of any beneficial effects from fat restriction in patients with hepatitis, treated celiac disease, or recurrent acute pancreatitis except when the latter results from severe hypertriglyceridemia.

GOALS AND RATIONALE OF TREATMENT

CHOLECYSTITIS AND CHOLELITHIASIS. Fatty acids in the duodenum are potent stimuli for the release of the hormone cholecystokinin, which produces contraction of the gallbladder. Thus, a fatty meal causes gallbladder contraction and might force a small gallstone into the cystic or common bile duct, or it might increase pressure in a gallbladder that is already somewhat obstructed and diseased. As a result, symptoms such as upper abdominal pain, nausea, or vomiting often occur 1 to 2 hours after ingesting a fatty meal.

In general, cholecystectomy is the treatment of choice for most patients with symptoms due to gallstones; however, a fat-restricted diet may benefit patients who are poor surgical risks or in whom cholecystectomy must be deferred. Fat restriction may minimize symptoms and prevent complications of cholelithiasis.

PANCREATITIS. A fatty meal also stimulates pancreatic enzyme secretion via the same cholecystokinin (pancreozymin) pathway. Theoretically, therefore, a large fatty meal might cause pancreatitis in a patient with an obstructed pancreatic duct. However, there is little evidence that fat restriction either hastens recovery after an attack of pancreatitis or prevents acute exacerbations in patients with recurrent pancreatitis unless the attacks are secondary to hypertriglyceridemia.

MALABSORPTION. The treatment for a malabsorptive state depends on the establishment of a specific diagnosis, since effective remedies are available for certain conditions. The value of fat restriction depends on the cause of malabsorption.

Pancreatic insufficiency—Even when this problem is treated with therapeutic amounts of exogenous pancreatic extract given before and after each meal, dietary fat intake should be restricted to the amount that can be tolerated without causing diarrhea.

Celiac disease is best treated by a gluten-free diet; fat restriction is usually not necessary.

Small-bowel resection—In patients with an *ileal resection,* the loss of bile acids may cause fat malabsorption. Bile acids are necessary for fat absorption. These acids are synthesized by the liver, secreted in the bile, and reabsorbed in the terminal ileum to enter the enterohepatic circulation. Ileal resection impairs bile acid reabsorption, and excess fecal loss results. Although the liver can compensate somewhat by increasing bile acid synthesis, extensive ileal resection for disease or ileal bypass—as in the surgical treatment of morbid obesity —causes steatorrhea from inadequate bile acids for fat absorption. Since oral supplementation of bile acids is not practical, dietary fat restriction may be necessary.

Following massive small-bowel resection (short-gut syndrome), severe fat restriction may be necessary to lessen the watery diarrhea that results from the laxative-like action of some fatty acids. It is a challenge to the nutritionist to supply these patients with adequate protein and calories, while maintaining a very low fat intake. Some of these patients tolerate hyperosmolar commercial preparations poorly; lactose intolerance further complicates therapy in others.

Medium-chain triglycerides (MCT) do not require bile acids for absorption and, therefore, can be an important source of calories and essential fatty acids. MCT oil is available commercially and can be used with food or taken as a medication. Commercial nutritional supplements containing MCT are also available.

Lymphatic obstruction is caused by conditions such as lymphoma or congenital intestinal lymphangiectasia and may result in mild fat malabsorption. Even more troublesome may be the excessive intestinal protein loss that results from leakage of protein-rich lymph into the bowel. Since long-chain fatty acids are transported via the lymphatics, dietary fat restriction lessens the lymphatic flow and thus decreases gut protein loss. Since MCT are transported via the portal vein, their use as a source of calories may be helpful in these patients.

Oxaluria and oxalate renal calculi may occur in patients with fat malabsorption, especially in those with ileal disease, resection, or bypass. Apparently, calcium binding by excess fecal fat leaves dietary oxalates unbound; their increased absorption by the colon produces oxaluria and oxalate stones. Dietary management includes restriction of fat and of oxalate-containing foods (Tables 7–1 and 7–2).

FAT-RESTRICTED DIETS

The amount of fat permitted in the diet is determined by the disorder or patient tolerance to fat or both. Table 7–2 lists foods that are allowed or should be omitted from a fat-restricted diet. If polyunsaturated fats are desired, free fats in the diet may be selected from the exchange list for fats (see Table A–13, Appendix). Calories must be adjusted to meet individual needs. Other gastrointestinal problems, such as lactose or gluten intolerance, should be considered in planning the dietary regimen.

TABLE 7–1. FOODS CONTAINING MORE OXALIC ACID THAN 100 MG/100 G FRESH WEIGHT

Food	Oxalic Acid Content (mg/100 g)
Rhubarb	260–860
Spinach	356–780
Beets (root)	96.8–675
Cocoa	623
Walnuts	563
Almonds	378
Dandelions	255
Peanuts	187–210
Parsley	100–166
Turmeric	151
Chocolate	117–140
Beans, spotted	104

Compiled from Hodgkinson, A.: Oxalic Acid in Biology and Medicine. New York, Academic Press, 1977; Finch, A.M., *et al.*: Clin Sci 60:411–418, 1981; Brinkley, L., *et al.*: Urology 17:534–538, 1981; Kaul, S., and Verma, S.L.: Ind J Med Res 55:274–278, 1967; and Kasidas, G.P., and Rose, G.A.: J Hum Nutr 34:255–266, 1980.

TABLE 7–2.   FAT-RESTRICTED DIET

Foods Permitted	Foods Omitted
MEATS	
Poultry (without skins); fish (including shellfish); veal (all cuts); rabbit, venison, squirrel; organ meats* — brains, sweetbreads, liver, kidney, heart; pork — loin, ham, sirloin roast, tenderloin, Canadian bacon; lamb — leg roast, leg chops, loin roast, loin chops, arm chop, rib chop; beef — round, sirloin, arm, flank, hind shank, T-bone, tenderloin, cube or porterhouse steak, lean ground beef.	Fried or fat meat, sausage, scrapple, frankfurters, stewing hens, spareribs, salt pork, beef shortribs, duck, goose, hamhocks, pigs' feet, lamb shanks, luncheon meats, tongue, gravies (unless fat-free).
(*Note*: Prepare these by baking, broiling, stewing, or simmering without additional fat. Use the lean portion of the meat. All visible fat must be removed.)	
CHEESE	
Cottage, mysost, or Edam cheese substituted for 1 oz meat.	Cheese in excess of prescribed amounts.
EGGS*	
1 a day (with yolk) prepared without fat or with part of the fat allowed; egg whites as desired.	More than 1 egg a day unless substituted for part of the meat allowed (1 egg = 1 oz meat).
MILK	
Skim, or buttermilk made from skim milk.	Whole, chocolate, and buttermilk made from whole milk.
FRUITS	
As desired.	Avocado in excess of amount allowed under fats.
VEGETABLES	
As desired (cooked in clear, salted water and seasoned; dried beans, peas, or lentils.	Potato chips.

*High in cholesterol.

Table continues on following page

TABLE 7–2.   FAT-RESTRICTED DIET (Continued)

Foods Permitted	Foods Omitted
SOUPS	
Fat-free broth, bouillon, bouillon cubes, consommé, fat-free cream soups made with skim milk and thickening.	All others unless prepared without fat.
BREAD AND CEREAL PRODUCTS	
Any type of cereal; spaghetti, noodles, rice, macaroni; whole grain or enriched baker's bread.	Homemade breads of any kind, waffles, pancakes, doughnuts, fritters, popcorn prepared with fat.
FATS	
Choose 1 each meal: 1 tsp butter, margarine, shortening, oil, or mayonnaise; 1 tbs boiled salad dressing; 2 tbs coffee cream; 1 strip crisp bacon; 2 tsp peanut butter; 5 small ripe olives; 10 medium green olives; ⅛ avocado, 4" diameter (⅛ cup); or 6 small nuts.	Any in excess of prescribed amount.
DESSERTS	
Sherbet made with skim milk, fruit ice; gelatin; rice, bread, cornstarch, tapioca, or junket pudding made with skim milk; fruit whips with gelatin, sugar, and egg white; fruit; angel food cake; meringues; and low-fat yogurt and frozen yogurt.	Cake, pie, pastry, ice cream, or any dessert containing shortening, chocolate, or fats of any kind.
SWEETS	
Jelly, jam, marmalade, honey, syrup, molasses, sugar, hard sugar candies, fondant, gumdrops, jelly beans, marshmallows, 1–2 tbs thin chocolate syrup.	Any candy made with chocolate, nuts, butter, cream, or fat of any kind.
SEASONINGS	
As desired.	
BEVERAGES	
Skim or buttermilk made with skim milk; coffee, tea, Postum, fruit juice, soft drinks; cocoa made with cocoa powder and skim milk.	Whole milk, buttermilk made with whole milk, chocolate milk, cream in excess of amount allowed under fats.

DIETARY MANAGEMENT

The meal pattern in Table 7–3 provides a fat-restricted diet that contains approximately 40 g of fat. If tolerated, the amount of fat may be increased to 50 g by the addition of two more fat choices per day. Dietary fat can also be reduced, if necessary, to approximately 25 g by omitting all free fat and by using meat selections from the lean meat exchange list (see Table A–13, Appendix). MCT oil can be added as a source of free fat, if indicated. It can also be used in special recipes that are available from the manufacturer. Portagen, a beverage containing MCT, may be used as a supplement if extra calories are indicated. MCT oil contains 8.3 kcal/g (7.7 kcal/ml).

TABLE 7–3. FAT-RESTRICTED DIET: SAMPLE MEAL PLAN

Breakfast

1 serving fruit or juice
1 serving cereal
1 egg
2 slices toast, 1 tbs jelly
1 tsp margarine or substitute
1 cup skim milk
Beverage, with 2 tsp sugar

Lunch

3 oz lean meat
½ cup potato or equivalent
1 serving vegetable
2 slices bread
1 tsp margarine or substitute
1 serving fruit
Beverage with 2 tsp sugar

Dinner

3 oz lean meat
½ cup potato or equivalent
2 servings vegetables
2 slices bread
1 tsp margarine or substitute
1 serving dessert
1 cup skim milk
Beverage with 2 tsp sugar

Snack

1 serving fruit
1 bread or equivalent

The composition of the diet is approximately

Calories	1940	Calcium	1216 mg
Protein	92 g	Iron	17 mg
Fat	40 g	Phosphorus	1444 mg
Carbohydrate	303 g	Potassium	3913 mg
		Sodium	3176 mg*

*Sodium content of diet without added salt.

Dietary Modification of Plasma Lipid and Lipoprotein Levels

Simeon Margolis, M.D., Ph.D., and
Gloria Elfert, M.S., R.D.

INTRODUCTION

A diagnosis of hyperlipidemia is made whenever the fasting concentration of plasma cholesterol, LDL cholesterol, or triglycerides exceeds the upper limits of normal (95th percentile) for the individual's age and sex (see Table 7–4). Such abnormalities may be associated with significant medical problems. Some

TABLE 7–4. NORMAL LIMITS FOR FASTING CHOLESTEROL, TRIGLYCERIDES, AND LDL AND HDL CHOLESTEROL

| Age (yrs) | Cholesterol (mg/dl) | | | Triglycerides (mg/dl)* |
	Total*	LDL*	HDL**	
Males (white)				
10–14	202	132	37	125
15–19	197	130	30	148
20–24	218	147	30	201
25–29	244	165	31	249
30–34	254	185	28	266
35–39	270	189	29	321
40–44	268	186	27	320
45–49	276	202	30	327
50–54	277	197	28	320
55–59	276	203	28	286
60–64	276	210	30	291
Females (white)				
10–14	201	136	37	131
15–19	200	135	35	124
20–24	216	136	37	131
25–29	222	151	37	145
30–34	231	150	38	151
35–39	242	172	34	176
40–44	252	174	33	191
45–49	265	187	33	214
50–54	285	215	37	233
55–59	300	213	36	262
60–64	297	234	36	239

*95th percentile.
**5th percentile.
From U.S. Department of Health and Human Services, Public Health Service, National Institute of Health, Lipid Metabolism Branch, NHLBI: The Lipid Research Clinics. Population Studies Data Book, Vol. 1. Bethesda, NIH Publication No. 80-1527, 1980. Normal ranges for blacks have not yet been defined.

subjects with plasma cholesterol within the normal range may also have an increased risk for premature vascular disease.

Both cholesterol and triglycerides are transported by the plasma lipoproteins: chylomicrons, very low density lipoproteins (VLDL or pre-β), low density lipoproteins (LDL or β), and high density lipoproteins (HDL or α). Chylomicrons contain about 90 per cent triglycerides and are formed in the intestine to transport absorbed dietary fat. Since they are rapidly cleared from the circulation, chylomicrons are not present in the fasting blood of normal individuals. However, the other lipoproteins are always present in the blood. The VLDL, synthesized primarily by the liver and to a lesser degree by the intestine, consist of 50 to 65 per cent triglycerides. LDL, which are composed of about 50 per cent cholesterol, are formed during the metabolism of circulating VLDL. HDL, which are synthesized by both the liver and the intestine, contain about 50 per cent protein; no single class of lipids predominates in HDL. In individuals with normal plasma lipids, about 70 per cent of the total cholesterol is carried by LDL; the remaining cholesterol is divided approximately equally between VLDL and HDL.

The basis of classification of the various hyperlipidemias is the presence of increased concentrations of one or more of the plasma lipoproteins. All hyperlipidemic subjects fall into one of the six types listed in Table 7–5. Type IIA is characterized by elevated levels of plasma LDL cholesterol and usually total plasma cholesterol, but triglyceride levels are normal. The other types all exhibit increased plasma triglyceride concentrations. Identification of the specific type of hyperlipidemia is recommended before the institution of dietary measures aimed at lowering plasma lipid levels.

Two dietary approaches have been recommended for patients with hyperlipidemia. In general, they are in agreement on the major elements necessary for control of plasma lipids. In the first, originating from the National Institutes of Health (NIH), dietary management depends on the type of hyperlipidemia. The second approach (the unified diet), developed by the American Heart Association (AHA), involves a progressive, three-phase reduction in the intake of total fat and cholesterol for patients with either hypercholesterolemia or hypertriglyceridemia. In each of these phases, less than 10 per cent of the calories are from saturated fat and about 10 per cent are from polyunsaturated fat. Reduction of caloric intake to achieve ideal body weight is another general principle. In phase I, fat intake is restricted to 30 to 35 per cent of calories and cholesterol is limited to 300 mg/day. Fat intake is essentially the same in phase II, but daily cholesterol is further reduced to 100 to 250 mg. In phase III, total fat is lowered to 20 to 25 per cent of calories and cholesterol is restricted to 100 mg/day. Fat intake is further limited in patients with type I or type V hyperlipidemia.

The AHA diets have the advantage of simplifying the dietary approach for physicians and nutritionists, but phases II and III of the diet are difficult for most patients to follow. Therefore, this chapter presents a modification of the NIH diets, individualizing dietary recommendations for the various hyperlipidemia types. These recommendations are very similar to those of phase I of the

TABLE 7-5. CLASSIFICATION OF HYPERLIPIDEMIAS

Type and Prevalence	Appearance of Plasma on Overnight Refrigeration	Major Fraction Elevated — LIPID	Major Fraction Elevated — LIPOPROTEIN	Clinical Manifestations (Signs and Symptoms)	Risk of Coronary Artery Disease	Other Features
I—Rare	Creamy layer over clear infranatant	TG*	Chylomicrons	Bouts of abdominal pain, hepatosplenomegaly, eruptive xanthomas; recurrent pancreatitis	Normal	Deficient lipoprotein lipase activity causes inability to utilize dietary fat. Symptoms begin in infancy or childhood.
IIA—Common	Clear	CH	LDL	Tendinous and tuberous xanthomas; corneal arcus, xanthelasma	Very high	A small fraction of these individuals have a genetic form, familial hypercholesterolemia, which is inherited as an autosomal dominant trait and can be diagnosed at birth.
IIB—Common	Clear or cloudy	CH TG	LDL & VLDL			
III—Uncommon	Clear or cloudy	CH TG	Abnormal "broad beta" lipoprotein	Palmar xanthomas; risk of peripheral vascular disease is high	Very high	Obesity and abnormal glucose tolerance are common. Abnormal conversion of VLDL to LDL.
IV—Common	Clear or grossly cloudy	TG	VLDL		Uncertain	Obesity and abnormal glucose tolerance are common. Usually not manifested until early adulthood.
V—Uncommon	Creamy layer over cloudy infranatant	TG	Chylomicrons & VLDL	Bouts of abdominal pain, hepatomegaly, eruptive xanthomas; recurrent pancreatitis	Normal	Sensitive to dietary fat. Obesity and abnormal glucose tolerance are common. Symptoms begin in adult life.

*TG = Triglycerides; CH = cholesterol.

AHA diet. A meal plan for a diet that restricts cholesterol intake to 100 mg/day is also provided (see Table 7–10).

The dietary management of hypercholesterolemia (type IIA) and the management of the various forms of hypertriglyceridemia are described separately in this chapter. The section on hypercholesterolemia is entitled "Reduction of Plasma LDL and Cholesterol Levels," because the same dietary measures are used to lower plasma cholesterol whether or not the individual has cholesterol values within the normal range.

Dietary management (Table 7–6) is the keystone of therapy for all hyperlipidemic patients and is more likely to succeed when a trained nutritionist works with the patient. The goals of dietary management are to reduce the risks of premature vascular disease and recurrent attacks of acute pancreatitis by modifying plasma lipid and lipoprotein levels. Caloric intake should be controlled in order to achieve and maintain ideal body weight, particularly in patients with hypertriglyceridemia.

Drugs are widely and inappropriately used in initiating the treatment of hyperlipidemia. Because of both their side effects and expense, drugs should be introduced—in conjunction with dietary measures—only when diet is ineffective or cannot be followed by the patient. A 6-week period is generally long enough to determine the effectiveness of dietary therapy; drugs may be employed when plasma lipid levels fail to decrease sufficiently over this period.

RATIONALE FOR DIETARY MANAGEMENT

Prevention of Premature Vascular Disease

Prospective epidemiologic studies have shown that hypercholesterolemia is a major risk factor for coronary artery disease. In fact, complications of coronary artery disease correlate with plasma cholesterol levels even within the "normal range." There is general agreement that LDL, which ordinarily carries 60 to 75 per cent of the cholesterol in the plasma, promotes atherosclerosis. Preventive measures, therefore, are aimed at reducing plasma LDL levels. Although encouraging, dietary studies have not proven that reduction of plasma cholesterol or LDL levels slows the atherosclerotic process or increases longevity. However, a recently reported study (The Lipid Research Clinics Coronary Primary Prevention Trial) has provided strong evidence that reduction of total plasma cholesterol and LDL-cholesterol levels, using the ion-exchange resin cholestyramine, significantly lowers the occurrence of death due to coronary heart disease and of nonfatal myocardial infarction. The combination of the epidemiologic evidence and the results of the coronary prevention trial support the use of dietary measures to lower plasma LDL-cholesterol, at least in selected individuals (see Patient Selection section).

HDL protects against coronary artery disease. Therefore, efforts should be made to increase the plasma levels of HDL and to avoid dietary measures that lower HDL. Currently, it seems that vigorous exercise and modest alcohol intake raise HDL levels, whereas obesity and cigarette smoking lower HDL.

TABLE 7-6. DIETARY MANAGEMENT FOR TYPES I–V HYPERLIPIDEMIAS

	Calories	Fat	Cholesterol	Carbohydrate	Alcohol
Type I	Unrestricted	25–30 g/day; type of fat not important*	Not to exceed 500 mg/day	Unrestricted	None permitted
Type IIA	Weight control is not a major goal of treatment	30% of calories, $\frac{1}{3}$ as saturated fat; P/S = 1:1	Less than 300 mg/day	Unrestricted	No restriction
Type IIB, Type III, and Type IV	Reduce calorie intake if necessary to achieve and maintain ideal weight	35% of calories, $\frac{1}{3}$ as saturated fat; P/S = 1:1	Less than 300 mg/day, except in type IV	No limitation of total, but complex carbohydrates emphasized and concentrated sweets restricted	Restricted to 25 g/day
Type V	Reduce calorie intake if necessary to achieve and maintain ideal weight	25–30% calories; type of fat not important**	Not to exceed 500 mg/day	Same as for types IIB, III, and IV	None permitted

*To enhance the palatability of the diet medium-chain triglyceride (MCT) supplements may be prescribed.
**If patient has recurrent pancreatitis or is otherwise intolerant of the fat content of this diet, the fat level should be further reduced and MCT supplements used.

Completed studies have failed to demonstrate that elevated plasma triglycerides are an independent risk factor for premature coronary artery disease. In part, high plasma triglycerides are not an independent risk factor because hypertriglyceridemia is almost always associated with reduced HDL and often with increased plasma cholesterol, both of which are clearly major risk factors. Nonetheless, dietary measures to reduce plasma triglyceride levels seem warranted, particularly when they are above 400 mg/dl and when individuals have other significant risk factors for premature vascular disease, such as diabetes mellitus. Reduction of plasma triglycerides may lower plasma cholesterol and raise HDL levels, but this desirable effect is often not achieved.

Prevention of Acute Pancreatitis

Severe hypertriglyceridemia, especially with levels above 1000 mg/dl as seen in patients with type I or type V hyperlipidemia, may provoke attacks of acute pancreatitis. Pancreatic lipase, present in high concentration in pancreatic capillaries, may produce rapid hydrolysis of the triglyceride component of circulating chylomicrons. The resulting high concentrations of free fatty acids in pancreatic capillaries could cause microthrombi with resultant tissue ischemia or could exert a direct toxic effect on pancreatic acinar cells. Alternatively, pancreatic lipase could alter the structure of chylomicrons, causing clumping and resultant capillary occlusion. The attacks can usually be prevented by controlling the plasma triglyceride levels.

REDUCTION OF PLASMA LDL AND CHOLESTEROL LEVELS

Patient Selection

The purpose for reduction of plasma LDL and cholesterol levels is to prevent premature vascular disease. The decision of whether to lower plasma cholesterol in a given individual depends on the cholesterol level, the distribution of cholesterol among the various lipoprotein fractions, the severity of existing coronary artery disease, age, enthusiasm for preventive measures, and the treatment philosophy of the physician.

The normal ranges for plasma cholesterol and LDL cholesterol, as well as for triglycerides and HDL cholesterol, are generally defined by the 5th to 95th percentile values found in large population studies (Table 7-4). Dietary therapy is usually indicated when plasma cholesterol levels exceed the 95th percentile for an individual's age and sex. Such cholesterol values are almost always associated with an elevation of LDL cholesterol, the major atherogenic lipoprotein. However, sole reliance on plasma cholesterol levels may be misleading. In some individuals, LDL cholesterol levels may be elevated even though the plasma cholesterol is within the normal range. Conversely, a high total cholesterol may be caused by elevated levels of HDL in rare individuals.

Lipoprotein concentrations are commonly measured and expressed by the amount of cholesterol carried on each lipoprotein. HDL cholesterol (HDL$_{Ch}$) is determined after precipitation of the other lipoproteins with heparin-manganese. Since it is technically difficult to measure LDL cholesterol (LDL_{Ch}) directly, the value is calculated by subtracting the concentrations of HDL and VLDL cholesterol ($VLDL_{Ch}$) from total cholesterol. $VLDL_{Ch}$ can be estimated from the empirical observation that the amount of cholesterol carried by VLDL is approximately 20 per cent of the value for total triglycerides. The following formula can be used to estimate LDL_{Ch}:

$$LDL_{Ch} = \text{Total plasma cholesterol} - HDL_{Ch} - \frac{\text{Plasma triglycerides}}{5}$$

This formula is generally applicable when plasma triglycerides are less than 400 mg/dl.

Patients with elevated levels of LDL_{Ch} are defined as having type II hyperlipidemia, type IIA if their triglycerides are elevated, and type IIB if their triglycerides are normal. The dietary modifications described in the next sections are recommended for all patients with type IIA. for page 158

It is also desirable to consider reducing cholesterol levels in some individuals who have other major risk factors for vascular disease, such as hypertension, cigarette smoking, and diabetes mellitus, when their plasma cholesterol is above 200 mg/dl but still within the normal range. The decision for dietary modifications in such patients should be based in part on the relative contributions of LDL and HDL to the total plasma cholesterol value. Patients with a normal cholesterol level above 200 mg/dl should not be discouraged from following a modified diet when they express an interest in the prevention of premature vascular disease even though they are negative for known risk factors.

Since reduction of plasma cholesterol levels is probably more effective in preventing disease than in reversing it, dietary modifications are more likely to be beneficial in younger individuals and in those who do not exhibit significant clinical evidence of atherosclerosis. It is, therefore, advisable to identify and initiate dietary measures at the earliest possible age in high-risk subjects. Conversely, major changes in diet are probably not justified in people more than 65 years of age.

Patients commonly become interested in modifying their diet following a myocardial infarction or other major clinical manifestation of atherosclerotic disease. Nutritional advice can be justified in these circumstances as a means of supporting patients' desire to take positive steps to combat their illness. However, several studies have failed to show that any decrease in the frequency of recurrent myocardial infarction or sudden death accompanies a reduction in serum cholesterol. Such findings are consistent with the severity of atherosclerotic changes in most patients with myocardial infarction. On the other hand, in patients with coronary bypass surgery, control of plasma cholesterol levels may help to delay or prevent stenosis of the bypassed vessels.

Dietary Principles

The most effective dietary approach for lowering plasma cholesterol levels is the reduction of saturated fat intake to a maximum of 10 per cent of total calories. This goal is achieved by restricting total fats to about 30 per cent of the total caloric intake and by partially replacing saturated fats with polyunsaturated ones. The ratio of polyunsaturated to saturated fats should be about 1:1.

It is important to point out that a decrease in the total and saturated fat intake lowers both LDL and HDL levels. Since the reduction of HDL levels is undesirable, diets extremely low in total fat or high in polyunsaturated fats should be avoided. Moreover, the physician should determine the effect of any diet on both plasma cholesterol and HDL levels to ensure a favorable overall response in the patient.

Restriction of dietary saturated fat will simultaneously decrease cholesterol intake. Reduction in plasma cholesterol can be achieved by restricting the total intake of cholesterol to less than 300 mg/day. More severe restriction of dietary cholesterol to about 100 mg/day will decrease the plasma cholesterol levels even further.

These dietary measures usually reduce plasma cholesterol levels by 10 to 20 per cent. Alcohol intake has no adverse effect on plasma cholesterol levels. In fact, moderate alcohol intake may be beneficial by raising plasma HDL levels.

Much recent work has examined the effects of a high-fiber intake on plasma cholesterol levels. Certain types of dietary fiber, such as pectins and guar gum, do seem to lower the plasma cholesterol level, while others, such as cellulose and bran, do not affect it. However, further studies are necessary to establish the role of dietary fiber modification as a measure for lowering plasma cholesterol. Although many individuals have added lecithin to their diets to try to lower their cholesterol levels, there is no solid evidence that an increased intake of lecithin reduces plasma cholesterol.

Dietary Measures for the Reduction of Plasma LDL and Cholesterol Levels

The diet restricts total fat intake, partially substitutes polyunsaturated for saturated fats, and limits the intake of high-cholesterol foods. When the diet is planned to fit the patient's lifestyle, it can be followed without undue difficulty. Cholesterol and fat content for food groups is shown in Table 7–7 and for individual foods in Table 7–8. Sample 300-mg and 100-mg cholesterol diets are provided (Tables 7–9 and 7–10). The latter diet is difficult to follow, since meat, fish, and poultry must be limited to 3 oz/day.

Saturated fats, which tend to raise the serum cholesterol level, are generally solid at room temperature and are found primarily in foods of animal origin and in a few saturated vegetable fats (coconut oil, palm oil, and cocoa butter). Monounsaturated fats neither raise nor lower plasma cholesterol. Olive and peanut oils are rich in monounsaturated fats. Polyunsaturated fats, which tend to lower plasma cholesterol, are found in such vegetable oils as safflower, sunflower, corn, cottonseed, and soybean. Hydrogenation of a polyunsaturated fat increases its saturation and converts it from a liquid to a solid state. The degree of hardness is indicative of the degree of saturation.

Cholesterol is found only in foods of animal origin and is present in especially high amounts in organ meats, egg yolk, and shrimp. Limitation of these foods, especially eggs, is the main way to reduce cholesterol intake in an American diet.

When several foods are combined into one product, the individual components must be evaluated to determine whether the product can be included in the diet. The diet can be diversified by including special products, such as low-fat cheese and cheese products, nondairy cream substitutes with a favorable P/S ratio, and egg substitutes. (P/S is defined as the amount of polyunsaturated (P) fat divided by the amount of saturated (S) fat.) When carefully planned and closely followed, the diet is adequate in all nutrients with the possible exception of iron.

Calculation of the Diet

1. Assess the patient's dietary habits.
2. Determine the daily caloric requirement of the patient.
3. Determine the total fat intake (30 per cent of total calories): Required calories $\times$ 0.30 = calories from fat/day. Calories from fat/day $\div$ 9 calories per gram of fat = grams of total fat/day.

Text continues on page 171

TABLE 7–7. AVERAGE CHOLESTEROL AND FAT CONTENT OF FOOD GROUPS

Food	Amount	Cholesterol (mg)	Total Fat (g)	Saturated Fat (g)	Polyunsaturated Fat (g)
Lean meat, fish, poultry <3 g fat/oz	28 g (1 oz)	25.1	2.0	0.7	0.5
Lean and medium-fat meat, fish, poultry <5 g fat/oz	28 g (1 oz)	25.0	4.1	1.3	0.4
Low-fat cheese <3 g fat/oz	28 g (1 oz)	3.3	0.8	0.5	tr
Medium-fat cheese <5 g fat/oz	28 g (1 oz)	15.2	4.3	2.7	0.1
Bread, average	25 g	—	0.8	0.2	0.2
Cereals, pastas, fruits, and vegetables		tr	tr	tr	tr
Milk, skim	244 g (1 cup)	4.0	0.4	0.3	tr
Milk 1% fat	244 g (1 cup)	10.0	2.6	1.6	0.1
Milk 2% fat	244 g (1 cup)	18.0	4.7	2.9	0.2
Egg substitutes Egg Beaters	60 g ($\frac{1}{4}$ cup)	0.0	0.0	0.0	0.0
Scramblers	57 g ($\frac{1}{4}$ cup)	0.0	3.0	1.0	2.0
Margarines/Oils		See Table 7–9.			

The average values listed above are used in the calculation of individual diets.
The cholesterol, total fat, saturated fat, and unsaturated fat contents of specific foods are given in Table 7–9.

TABLE 7–8.   CHOLESTEROL AND FAT CONTENT OF FOODS

Food	Amount	Cholesterol (mg)	Total Fat (g)	Saturated Fat (g)	Polyun- saturated Fat (g)
Meat, Fish, Poultry (cooked)					
LOW-FAT, LESS THAN 3 G/OZ					
Beef					
Brisket, lean only	28 g (1 oz)	25.5	2.9	1.3	0.2
Flank steak	28 g (1 oz)	25.5	2.0	0.9	0.1
T-Bone steak, lean	28 g (1 oz)	25.5	2.9	1.2	0.2
Sirloin steak, lean	28 g (1 oz)	25.5	2.2	0.9	0.1
Short plate, lean	28 g (1 oz)	25.5	2.9	1.3	0.2
Round steak, lean	28 g (1 oz)	25.5	1.8	0.8	0.1
Rump, lean	28 g (1 oz)	25.5	2.6	1.1	0.2
Pork					
Leg, lean only	28 g (1 oz)	25.0	2.5	0.9	0.1
Leg, cured lean	28 g (1 oz)	25.0	2.5	0.8	0.3
Lamb					
Leg, lean only	28 g (1 oz)	27.0	2.7	1.1	0.2
Loin, lean only	28 g (1 oz)	27.0	1.7	0.7	0.1
Rib, lean only	28 g (1 oz)	27.0	2.0	0.8	0.1
Shoulder, lean only	28 g (1 oz)	27.0	1.6	0.7	0.1
Veal					
All cuts, separable lean	28 g (1 oz)	25.2	0.7	0.2	0.1
Foreshank, total edible	28 g (1 oz)	25.2	2.9	1.2	0.1
Fish (fillet)					
Anchovies	28 g (1 oz)		1.8	0.5	0.6
Bass, striped	28 g (1 oz)		0.6	0.1	0.2
Cod, Atlantic	28 g (1 oz)	14.0	0.2	tr	0.1
Flounder	28 g (1 oz)	14.0	0.3	0.1	0.1
Haddock	28 g (1 oz)	17.0	0.2	tr	0.1
Halibut, Atlantic	28 g (1 oz)	14.0	0.3	0.1	0.1
Herring, Atlantic	28 g (1 oz)	24.0	1.7	0.5	0.4
Mackerel, Atlantic	28 g (1 oz)	27.0	2.7	0.7	0.7
Perch (ocean)	28 g (1 oz)		0.7	0.1	0.2
Pike, northern	28 g (1 oz)		0.2	tr	0.1
Rockfish	28 g (1 oz)		0.4	0.1	0.2
Salmon, pink	28 g (1 oz)	9.8	1.5	0.2	0.6
Salmon, sockeye	28 g (1 oz)	9.8	2.5	0.5	1.3
Sole, lemon	28 g (1 oz)		0.2	tr	0.1
Sturgeon, common	28 g (1 oz)		0.9	0.2	0.1
Trout, rainbow	28 g (1 oz)	15.4	1.3	0.3	0.4
Tuna, albacore, water-canned, light	28 g (1 oz)	17.6	1.9	0.6	0.5
Whitefish	28 g (1 oz)		1.5	0.2	0.4
Clam (ark shell)	28 g (1 oz)	14.0	0.4	0.1	0.1
Crab, blue	28 g (1 oz)	28.0	0.4	0.1	0.2
Crab, Alaskan King	28 g (1 oz)		0.4	0.1	0.2
Oyster, Eastern	28 g (1 oz)	56.0	0.6	0.1	0.2
Oyster, Pacific	28 g (1 oz)	56.0	0.6	0.1	0.3
Mussel, California	28 g (1 oz)	42.0	0.5	0.1	0.2
Scallop	28 g (1 oz)	15.0	0.2	tr	0.1
Lobster	28 g (1 oz)	56.0	0.3	tr	0.2
Shrimp	28 g (1 oz)	42.0	0.3	tr	0.2
Lobster tail	28 g (1 oz)	56.0	0.3	tr	0.1

Table continues on following page

TABLE 7–8.   CHOLESTEROL AND FAT CONTENT OF FOODS (Continued)

Food	Amount	Cholesterol (mg)	Total Fat (g)	Saturated Fat (g)	Polyun-saturated Fat (g)
Poultry (roasted)					
Chicken, dark (no skin)	28 g (1 oz)	25.0	2.7	0.7	0.7
Chicken, light (no skin)	28 g (1 oz)	22.0	1.3	0.4	0.3
Turkey, dark (no skin)	28 g (1 oz)	28.0	2.2	0.7	0.7
Turkey, light (no skin)	28 g (1 oz)	22.0	1.0	0.3	0.3
MEDIUM-FAT, LESS THAN 5 G/OZ					
Beef					
Chuck, lean	28 g (1 oz)	25.0	3.9	1.7	0.2
Rib, lean	28 g (1 oz)	25.0	3.9	1.7	0.2
Ground beef, 15%	28 g (1 oz)	25.0	4.2	1.8	0.3
Pork					
Loin, lean only	28 g (1 oz)	25.0	3.9	1.3	0.4
Loin, cured	28 g (1 oz)	25.0	4.9	1.7	0.5
Veal					
Leg, total edible	28 g (1 oz)	25.2	3.1	1.3	0.2
Loin, total edible	28 g (1 oz)	25.2	3.8	1.6	0.2
Shoulder, total edible	28 g (1 oz)	25.2	3.6	1.5	0.2
Rib, total edible	28 g (1 oz)	25.2	4.7	2.0	0.3
HIGH-FAT, MORE THAN 5 G/OZ					
Beef					
Brisket, total edible	28 g (1 oz)	25.0	9.7	4.1	0.4
Chuck, total edible	28 g (1 oz)	25.0	10.3	4.3	0.4
Rib, whole	28 g (1 oz)	25.0	11.0	4.6	0.4
Ground beef, 20%	28 g (1 oz)	25.0	6.3	2.7	0.3
Pork					
Boston blade	28 g (1 oz)	25.0	9.2	3.3	1.0
Spareribs	28 g (1 oz)	25.0	10.9	3.8	1.2
Leg, fresh	28 g (1 oz)	25.0	5.7	2.0	0.6
Leg, cured	28 g (1 oz)	25.0	6.2	2.2	0.8
Boston blade, cured	28 g (1 oz)	25.0	7.2	2.5	0.8
Lamb					
Leg, total edible	28 g (1 oz)	28.0	5.9	2.7	0.3
Loin	28 g (1 oz)	28.0	9.1	4.2	0.5
Rib	28 g (1 oz)	28.0	10.1	4.7	0.6
Shoulder	28 g (1 oz)	28.0	7.5	3.5	0.4
Veal					
Breast, total edible	28 g (1 oz)	25.2	5.9	2.6	0.4
MISCELLANEOUS MEATS					
Organ Meats					
Brains	28 g (1 oz)	560.0	2.4	0.6	0.3
Kidneys	28 g (1 oz)	225.0	3.4	1.3	0.5
Liver, chicken	28 g (1 oz)	208.0	1.2	0.5	0.3
Liver, beef or veal	28 g (1 oz)	122.0	1.1	0.4	0.2
Sweetbreads	28 g (1 oz)	130.0	6.5	2.7	0.3
Heart	28 g (1 oz)	77.0	1.6	0.5	0.2
Giblets	28 g (1 oz)	60.0	0.9	0.3	0.2

Table continues on following page

TABLE 7–8.   CHOLESTEROL AND FAT CONTENT OF FOODS (Continued)

Food	Amount	Cholesterol (mg)	Total Fat (g)	Saturated Fat (g)	Polyun-saturated Fat (g)
Gizzard	28 g (1 oz)	55.0	0.9	0.3	0.2
Tongue	28 g (1 oz)	25.0	4.7	1.6	0.6
Variety Meats					
Cold cuts (average)	28 g (1 oz)	25.0	7.6	2.7	0.9
Frankfurter (sample)	45 g (1 avg)	18.0	13.0	4.9	1.6
Sausage, pork, cooked	28 g (1 oz)	18.2	9.1	3.3	1.1
Bacon, cooked	5 g	3.0	3.4	1.3	0.4
Egg					
Whole, one	50 g	274.0	5.6	1.7	0.7
Yolk	17 g	274.0	5.6	1.7	0.7
White	33 g	0.0	0.0	0.0	0.0
Cheese					
Low-Fat, less than 3 g/oz					
Cottage cheese, dry	28 g (1 oz)	1.9	0.1	0.1	tr
Cottage cheese, 1% fat	28 g (1 oz)	1.1	0.3	0.2	tr
Cottage cheese, 2% fat	28 g (1 oz)	2.2	0.5	0.3	tr
Cottage cheese, regular	28 g (1 oz)	4.2	1.3	0.8	tr
Ricotta, part-skim	28 g (1 oz)	8.7	2.2	1.4	0.1
Medium-Fat, Less Than 5 g/oz					
Mozzarella, low moisture, part skim	28 g (1 oz)	16.2	4.5	2.8	0.1
Mozzarella, part skim	28 g (1 oz)	15.1	4.8	3.0	0.1
Ricotta, whole milk	28 g (1 oz)	14.3	3.6	2.3	0.1
High-Fat, more than 5 g/oz					
American, processed	28 g (1 oz)	26.3	8.8	5.5	0.3
Blue	28 g (1 oz)	21.0	8.0	5.2	0.2
Camembert	28 g (1 oz)	20.0	6.8	4.3	0.2
Cheddar	28 g (1 oz)	29.4	9.3	5.9	0.3
Cheese food, American, cold-pack	28 g (1 oz)	17.9	6.4	4.3	0.2
Cheese food, American, processed	28 g (1 oz)	17.9	6.9	4.3	0.2
Cheese spread	28 g (1 oz)	15.4	5.9	3.7	0.2
Colby	28 g (1 oz)	26.6	9.0	5.7	0.3
Cream	28 g (1 oz)	30.8	9.8	6.2	0.4
Edam	28 g (1 oz)	24.9	7.8	4.9	0.2
Feta	28 g (1 oz)	24.9	6.0	4.2	0.2
Fontina	28 g (1 oz)	32.5	8.7	5.4	0.5
Gouda	28 g (1 oz)	31.9	7.7	4.9	0.2
Gruyère	28 g (1 oz)	30.8	9.1	5.3	0.5
Limburger	28 g (1 oz)	25.2	7.6	4.7	0.1
Mozzarella, whole milk	28 g (1 oz)	21.8	6.0	3.7	0.2
Mozzarella, whole milk, low-moisture	28 g (1 oz)	24.9	6.9	4.4	0.2
Muenster	28 g (1 oz)	26.9	8.4	5.4	0.2
Neufchâtel	28 g (1 oz)	21.3	6.6	4.1	0.2

Table continues on following page

TABLE 7–8.   CHOLESTEROL AND FAT CONTENT OF FOODS (Continued)

Food	Amount		Cholesterol (mg)	Total Fat (g)	Saturated Fat (g)	Polyun- saturated Fat (g)
Parmesan (hard)	28 g	(1 oz)	19.0	7.2	4.6	0.2
Port du Salut	28 g	(1 oz)	34.4	7.9	4.7	0.2
Provolone	28 g	(1 oz)	19.3	7.5	4.8	0.2
Roquefort	28 g	(1 oz)	25.2	8.6	5.4	0.4
Swiss, natural	28 g	(1 oz)	25.8	7.7	5.0	0.3
Swiss, process	28 g	(1 oz)	23.8	7.0	4.5	0.2
Tilsit, whole milk	28 g	(1 oz)	28.6	7.3	4.7	0.2
Other Dairy Products						
Butter	5 g	(1 tsp)	11.0	4.1	2.5	0.2
Milk, low-fat, 2%	244 g	(1 cup)	18.0	4.7	2.9	0.2
low-fat, 1%	244 g	(1 cup)	10.0	2.6	1.6	0.1
nonfat	245 g	(1 cup)	4.0	0.4	0.3	tr
evaporated, skim	32 g	(1 oz)	1.0	0.1	tr	tr
evaporated, whole	32 g	(1 oz)	9.0	2.4	1.5	0.1
whole	244 g	(1 cup)	33.0	8.2	5.1	0.3
low-sodium	244 g	(1 cup)	33.0	8.4	5.3	0.3
dry, nonfat	30 g	($\frac{1}{4}$ cup)	6.0	0.2	0.2	tr
condensed	38 g	(1 oz)	13.0	3.0	2.1	0.1
chocolate, whole	250 g	(1 cup)	30.0	8.5	5.3	0.3
chocolate, 1%	250 g	(1 cup)	7.0	2.5	1.5	0.1
Yogurt, plain, whole	227 g	(1 cup)	29.0	7.4	4.8	0.2
Yogurt, plain, 2% milk	227 g	(1 cup)	14.0	3.5	2.3	0.1
Yogurt, fruited, 2%	227 g	(1 cup)	10.0	2.6	1.7	0.1
Half & Half cream, 11% fat	15 g	(1 tbs)	6.0	1.7	1.1	0.1
Coffee cream, 20% fat	15 g	(1 tbs)	10.0	2.9	1.8	0.1
Medium cream, 25% fat	15 g	(1 tbs)	13.0	3.8	2.3	0.1
Light whipping cream, 30% fat	15 g	(1 tbs)	17.0	4.6	2.9	0.1
Heavy whipping cream, 37% fat	15 g	(1 tbs)	21.0	5.6	3.5	0.2
Pressurized whipping cream	3 g	(1 tbs)	2.0	0.7	0.4	tr
Eggnog	254 g	(1 cup)	149.0	19.0	11.3	0.9
Ice cream, vanilla, regular, 10% fat	133 g	(1 cup)	59.0	14.3	8.9	0.5
Ice cream, vanilla rich, 16% fat	148 g	(1 cup)	88.0	23.7	14.7	0.9
Ice milk, vanilla, 4% fat	131 g	(1 cup)	18.0	5.6	3.5	0.2
Ice milk, soft, vanilla	175 g	(1 cup)	13.0	4.6	2.9	0.2
Sherbet	193 g	(1 cup)	14.0	3.8	2.4	0.1
Sour cream, regular	24 g	(2 tbs)	10.0	5.0	3.1	0.2
Nondairy Products						
Coffee whitener	15 g	($\frac{1}{2}$ oz)	0.0	1.5	0.3	tr
Coffee whitener, powder	2 g	(1 tbs)	0.0	0.7	0.7	tr
Dessert topping, powder	1.3 g	(1 tbs)	0.0	0.5	0.5	tr
Pressurized dessert topping	4 g		0.0	0.9	0.8	tr

Table continues on following page

TABLE 7–8.   CHOLESTEROL AND FAT CONTENT OF FOODS (Continued)

Food	Amount		Cholesterol (mg)	Total Fat (g)	Saturated Fat (g)	Polyun-saturated Fat (g)
Frozen dessert topping	4 g	(1 tbs)	0.0	1.0	0.9	tr
Sour cream, imitation	28 g	(2 tbs)	0.0	5.5	5.0	tr
Fats						
Butter	5 g	(1 pat)	11.0	4.1	2.5	0.2
Coconut oil	14 g	(1 tbs)	—	13.6	11.8	0.2
Corn oil	14 g	(1 tbs)	—	13.6	1.7	8.0
Cottonseed oil	14 g	(1 tbs)	—	13.6	3.5	7.1
Olive oil	14 g	(1 tbs)	—	13.5	1.8	1.1
Palm oil	14 g	(1 tbs)	—	13.6	6.7	1.3
Peanut oil	14 g	(1 tbs)	—	13.5	2.3	4.3
Poppyseed oil	14 g	(1 tbs)	—	13.6	1.8	8.5
Safflower, linoleic	14 g	(1 tbs)	—	13.6	1.2	10.1
oleic	14 g	(1 tbs)	—	13.6	0.8	1.9
Sesame oil	14 g	(1 tbs)	—	13.6	1.9	5.7
Soybean oil	14 g	(1 tbs)	—	13.6	2.0	7.9
Sunflower oil, less than 60% linoleic	14 g	(1 tbs)	—	13.6	1.4	5.5
Sunflower oil, more than 60% linoleic	14 g	(1 tbs)	—	13.6	1.4	8.9

Margarines

STICK

Coconut, safflower (liquid) coconut and Palm (hydrogenated)	5 g	(1 tsp)	—	3.8	2.7	0.6
Corn, hydrogenated	5 g	(1 tsp)	—	3.8	0.6	0.8
liquid and hydrogenated	5 g	(1 tsp)	—	3.8	0.7	1.1
Lard	5 g	(1 tsp)	—	3.8	1.5	0.4
Soybean, liquid and hydrogenated	5 g	(1 tsp)	—	3.8	0.6	1.2
Sunflower (liquid), soybean, cottonseed (hydrogenated)	5 g	(1 tsp)	—	3.8	0.6	1.9

SOFT

Corn, liquid and hydrogenated	5 g	(1 tsp)	—	3.8	0.7	1.5
Safflower, liquid and hydrogenated	5 g	(1 tsp)	—	3.8	0.4	2.1
Soybean (liquid) and soybean and cotton-seed (hydrogenated)	5 g	(1 tsp)	—	3.8	0.8	1.4
Soybean, hydrogenated	5 g	(1 tsp)	—	3.8	0.6	1.3
Sunflower (liquid) and cottonseed and peanut (hydrogenated)	5 g	(1 tsp)	—	3.8	0.6	2.3

Table continues on following page

TABLE 7–8.   CHOLESTEROL AND FAT CONTENT OF FOODS (Continued)

Food	Amount		Cholesterol (mg)	Total Fat (g)	Saturated Fat (g)	Polyun-saturated Fat (g)
LIQUID						
Soybean (hydrogenated) and soybean and cottonseed (liquid)	5 g	(1 tsp)	—	3.8	0.6	1.7
Salad Dressing						
Blue cheese	15 g	(1 tbs)	—	8.0	1.5	4.3
Italian, low calorie	15 g	(1 tbs)	1.0	1.5	0.2	0.9
regular	15 g	(1 tbs)	—	7.1	1.0	4.1
Mayonnaise, sunflower and soybean	14 g	(1 tbs)	—	11.0	1.2	7.6
soybean	14 g	(1 tbs)	8.0	11.0	1.6	5.7
Mayonnaise, imitation (soybean)	15 g	(1 tbs)	4.0	2.9	0.5	1.6
Mayonnaise-type	15 g	(1 tbs)	4.0	4.9	0.7	2.6
Russian, low calorie	16 g	(1 tbs)	1.0	0.7	0.1	0.4
regular	15 g	(1 tbs)	—	7.8	1.1	4.5
Thousand Island, low-calorie	15 g	(1 tbs)	2.0	1.6	0.2	1.0
regular	16 g	(1 tbs)	—	5.6	0.9	3.1
French (clear)	14 g	(1 tbs)	—	9.8	1.8	4.7
Sandwich spread	15 g	(1 tbs)	12.0	5.2	0.8	3.1
Shortenings–Solid						
Soybean and cottonseed	13 g	(1 tbs)	—	12.8	3.2	3.3
Soybean and palm	13 g	(1 tbs)	—	12.8	3.9	1.8
Lard and vegetable oil	13 g	(1 tbs)	—	12.8	5.2	1.4
Nuts						
Almonds	15 g	($\frac{1}{2}$ oz)	—	8.1	0.6	1.5
Brazil nuts	15 g	($\frac{1}{2}$ oz)	—	10.2	2.6	3.8
Cashews	15 g	($\frac{1}{2}$ oz)	—	6.8	1.4	1.1
Chestnuts	15 g	($\frac{1}{2}$ oz)	—	0.4	tr	0.2
Filberts	15 g	($\frac{1}{2}$ oz)	—	9.7	0.7	1.0
Macadamia	15 g	($\frac{1}{2}$ oz)	—	11.4	1.6	0.3
Peanuts (average)	15 g	($\frac{1}{2}$ oz)	—	7.5	1.4	2.2
Pecans	15 g	($\frac{1}{2}$ oz)	—	10.7	0.9	2.7
Pistachio	15 g	($\frac{1}{2}$ oz)	—	8.0	1.1	1.1
Walnuts, English	15 g	($\frac{1}{2}$ oz)	—	9.5	1.0	6.3
Walnuts, black	15 g	($\frac{1}{2}$ oz)	—	8.9	0.8	6.1
Peanut butter, unhydrogenated	60 g	(2 tbs)	—	13.8	2.5	4.1
Peanut butter, hydrogenated	60 g	(2 tbs)	—	14.4	2.9	4.2
Miscellaneous						
Avocado	50 g	($\frac{1}{4}$)	—	8.2	1.2	0.9
Coconut, shredded	7.5 g	(1 tbs)	—	5.3	4.7	1.0
Olives, black	15 g	($\frac{1}{2}$ oz)	—	3.9	0.5	0.3
Olives, green	15 g	($\frac{1}{2}$ oz)	—	3.6	0.5	0.3

Table continues on following page

TABLE 7–8. CHOLESTEROL AND FAT CONTENT OF FOODS (Continued)

Food	Amount	Cholesterol (mg)	Total Fat (g)	Saturated Fat (g)	Polyun- saturated Fat (g)
Cereal Products					
Bread, all varieties	25 g (1 slice)	0	0.8	0.2	0.3
Bagel	28 g (½ bagel)	0	2.0	0.3	0.9
English muffin	28 g (½ muffin)	0	0.0	0.2	tr
Roll, dinner type	28 g (1 roll)	0	1.6	0.4	0.4
Bun, frankfurter or hamburger	30 g (1 roll)	0	3.0	1.2	0.4
Crackers: saltine-type	11 g (4 crackers)	0	1.3	0.3	0.3
butter-type	16 g (5 crackers)	3.0	2.9	1.0	0.5
Cereals, hot and cold		tr	tr	tr	tr
Pasta products, plain		tr	tr	tr	tr
Wheat germ	10 g (1 tbs)	0	1.1	0.2	0.7
Specialty Products					
Cheezola (Fisher)	28 g (1 oz)	5.0	6.0	1.0	4.0
Golden Image, Mild Imitation Cheddar (Kraft)	28 g (1 oz)	10.0	9.0	2.0	4.0
Golden Image American Flavored Imitation Pasteurized Process Cheese Food (Kraft)	28 g (1 oz)	5.0	6.0	1.0	2.0
Count Down, 99% fat-free	28 g (1 oz)	1.4	0.3	—	—
Egg Substitutes					
Egg Beaters	60 g (¼ cup)	0.0	0.0	0.0	0.0
Scramblers	57 g (¼ cup)	0.0	3.0	1.0	2.0

TABLE 7–9. SAMPLE MEAL PLAN—300-MG
CHOLESTEROL DIET

Breakfast

½ cup orange juice
¾ cup raisin bran with ½ sliced banana
1 English muffin
2 tsp margarine*
1 cup skim milk
Coffee or tea as desired
2 tsp sugar

Lunch

Sandwich: ½ cup tuna fish
    lettuce and tomato
    2 slices whole wheat bread
    1 tbs mayonnaise or margarine*
Fresh apple
1 cup skim milk

Dinner

4 oz broiled sirloin
1 baked potato (1 cup)
½ cup French-style green beans
Sliced tomato salad with 1 tbs Italian dressing
1 dinner roll
3 tsp margarine*
¼ cantaloupe
Coffee or tea as desired

Snack

1 cup skim milk
2 graham crackers
1 pear

Composition: The above plan is adequate in all nutrients.

The analysis of the above sample meal is:

Calories	2000		Phosphorus	1550	
Protein	95	g	Potassium	3700	
Carbohydrate	255	g	Saturated fat	16.5	g
Calcium	1300	mg	Polyunsaturated fat	16.5	g
Iron	18.3	mg	P/S	1:1	

*Margarine used for calculation purposes was 100% corn oil margarine (stick).

TABLE 7–10.   SAMPLE MEAL PLAN — 100-MG CHOLESTEROL DIET

Breakfast

½ cantaloupe
¼ cup Egg Beaters, scrambled
2 slices whole wheat toast
2 tsp margarine*
1 cup skim milk
2 tsp sugar
Coffee or tea as desired

Lunch

½ cup tomato juice and 6 saltines
Salad plate: ½ cup low-fat cottage cheese
              ½ cup citrus fruit sections
1 slice rye bread
3 tsp mayonnaise or margarine*
1 fresh pear

Dinner

3 oz broiled flounder
1 baked potato (1 cup)
½ cup asparagus spears
Tossed salad with 1 tbs Italian dressing
1 slice whole wheat bread
3 tsp margarine*
Fruit cocktail
Coffee or tea as desired

Snack

1 cup skim milk
2 graham crackers
12 grapes

Composition: The above plan is adequate in all nutrients, with the exception of iron for groups at risk.
The analysis of the above sample meal is:

Calories	1800		Phosphorus	1219	mg
Protein	80	g	Potassium	2929	mg
Fat	61	g	Cholesterol	91.4	mg
Carbohydrate	230	g	Saturated fat	13.4	g
Calcium	1033	mg	Polyunsaturated fat	19.9	g
Iron	14.3	mg	P/S	1.5:1	

*Margarine used for calculation purposes was 100% corn oil (stick).

4. Determine maximal intake of saturated fat (10 per cent of total calories). Intake of saturated fat/day = grams of total fat/day $\times \frac{1}{3}$.

5. Eliminate or restrict foods such as eggs that are especially high in cholesterol content.

REDUCTION OF PLASMA TRIGLYCERIDE LEVELS

The dietary goals of these regimens are as follows:

1. To prevent recurrent attacks of acute pancreatitis in patients with severe hypertriglyceridemia (types I and V)
2. To prevent premature vascular disease (types IIB, III, and IV)

Patient Selection

In patients with type I or V hyperlipidemia, efforts should be initiated to maintain triglyceride levels below 1000 mg/dl in order to prevent recurrent attacks of acute pancreatitis.

The value of lowering plasma triglyceride levels for the prevention of premature vascular disease is uncertain. Nonetheless, dietary treatment can be justified in an effort to raise HDL levels in any individual whose triglyceride levels exceed the normal range (see Table 7–4). Dietary management especially is recommended in all patients under the age of 60 when their triglyceride levels exceed 400 mg/dl, there is a strong family history of premature vascular disease, or they have other major risk factors such as hypertension, cigarette smoking, or diabetes mellitus.

Diabetes is often associated with types IIB, III, IV, and V hyperlipidemia. In these patients, insulin treatment may help to control the condition. If any degree of hypertriglyceridemia persists despite routine measures to treat diabetes, dietary measures are then indicated to lower the plasma triglycerides. When insulin deficiency is profound—for example, after prolonged treatment with oral hypoglycemic agents—diabetics may accumulate excess chylomicrons and convert from a type IV to a type V pattern. Many diabetics also have an inherited predisposition to primary hypertriglyceridemia (type IV).

Dietary Principles

Weight reduction and maintenance of ideal weight are the *most important* dietary measures for the treatment of all types of hypertriglyceridemia except type I. As shown in Table 7–6, specific dietary measures depend on the type of hyperlipidemia present.

DIETARY MEASURES FOR TYPES I AND V HYPERLIPIDEMIA

Since restriction of dietary fat minimizes chylomicron formation, the diet in type I limits total fat intake to 25 to 30 g per day. There is no restriction on the type of fat. Alcohol increases plasma triglycerides and should not be ingested. A sample meal plan is presented in Table 7–11.

TABLE 7–11. SAMPLE MEAL PLAN FOR TYPE I
HYPERLIPIDEMIA

Breakfast

½ cup orange juice
1 cup bran flakes
½ banana
1 cup skim milk
Coffee or tea, 2 tsp sugar

Lunch

Sandwich: 2 oz sliced roast turkey
           2 slices rye bread
           lettuce and tomato
1 tbs MCT oil (made into mayonnaise)
1 fresh apple
1 cup skim milk

Dinner

4 oz broiled flounder, lemon wedge
1 cup parslied boiled potatoes
½ cup asparagus
Tossed salad
1 tbs MCT oil (for salad, vegetable, and potato)
¼ honeydew melon
Coffee or tea, 2 tsp sugar

Snack

1 fresh pear
2 graham crackers
1 cup skim milk

This plan is adequate in all essential nutrients.
An approximate composition of this sample plan is:

Calories	1800		Calcium	1200	mg
Protein	85	g	Iron	15	mg
Fat-MCT	28	g	Phosphorus	1300	mg
Dietary Fat	26.9	g	Potassium	4500	mg
Carbohydrate	250	g	Sodium	1500	mg

Efforts should be made to encourage patient adherence to the severe fat restriction and to enhance the palatability of the diet. MCT oil may be used to enhance palatability and supply extra calories (8.3 kcal/g). MCT oil is absorbed directly into the bloodstream, bypassing the lymphatics, and does not result in chylomicron formation (see Chapter 11, section on cystic fibrosis diet). Portagen, a powdered, milk-based product made from MCT, may also be used. It supplies 30 kcal/oz when reconstituted and is lactose-free. The patient should be provided with recipes utilizing these products.

Since the diet is so severely fat restricted, the fat content of *all* ingested foods must be assessed in order not to exceed the defined limits:

1. *Protein*: Only lean meats or substitutes are allowed. Refer to Tables 7–7 and 7–8 for planning individual diets.

2. *Fats*: All free fats, such as butter, margarine, mayonnaise, and so on, are eliminated. MCT oil may be used to provide extra calories. Small amounts of

fat are present in basic food items such as skim milk, plain bread, cereal, vegetables, and fruits. The amount of fat permitted from these sources will be from 10 g to 30 g, depending on the caloric intake and food selection.

3. *Carbohydrates*: Plain breads, cereals, pastas, fruits, and vegetables are used as desired.

When foods are properly selected and all items are consumed, the diet should be adequate in all the essential nutrients, with the possible exception of iron.

Weight reduction, in overweight individuals, is the most important therapeutic measure in patients with type V hyperlipidemia. The guidelines for dietary measures aimed at decreasing serum triglyceride levels are followed. In order to decrease chylomicron levels, fat is limited to 25 to 30 per cent of total calories. Concentrated sweets are restricted to occasional use. Alcohol is not permitted. MCT oil may be used to provide calories, if necessary. A sample meal plan is presented in Table 7–12.

TABLE 7–12.   SAMPLE MEAL PLAN FOR TYPE V HYPERLIPIDEMIA

Breakfast

½ grapefruit
¾ cup bran flakes
2 slices toast
1 tsp margarine
1 cup skim milk
Coffee or tea as desired

Lunch

Sandwich: 2 oz sliced roast turkey
                  lettuce
                  2 slices whole wheat bread
Carrot sticks
Fresh apple
Iced tea

Dinner

3 oz broiled porterhouse steak
1 small baked potato
½ cup French-style green beans
Cucumber salad with vinegar
1 slice rye bread
2 tsp margarine
¼ cantaloupe with lemon wedge
Coffee or tea as desired

Snack

1 cup skim milk
1 graham cracker

The diet provides all essential nutrients in adequate amounts.
Analysis of this sample meal plan yields:

Calories	1500	Calcium	859	mg
Protein (20%)	75 g	Iron	21.1	mg
Fat (27%)	45 g	Potassium	3107	mg
Carbohydrate (53%)	198 g	Phosphorus	1306	mg

DIETARY MEASURES FOR TYPES IIB, III, AND IV HYPERLIPIDEMIA

Description of Diet

If the patient is overweight, weight reduction and maintenance of ideal body weight are essential. The diet should limit fat intake to 35 per cent of calories, with a P/S of 1:1. Cholesterol should be restricted to 300 mg/day, except in type IV hyperlipidemia. Alcohol is either avoided or limited to 25 g/day. Although total carbohydrate intake is not controlled, the diet emphasizes the use of complex carbohydrates in preference to simple sugars for several reasons, including the fact that restriction of simple sugars can aid in weight control. Dietary fiber reduces the insulin response to ingested carbohydrate, thereby decreasing triglyceride synthesis in the liver, and may exert some cholesterol-

TABLE 7–13.   SAMPLE MEAL PLAN FOR TYPES IIB, III,
AND IV HYPERLIPIDEMIA

Breakfast

½ grapefruit
¾ cup bran flakes
1 slice toast
2 tsp margarine*
1 cup skim milk
Coffee or tea as desired

Lunch

Sandwich: 2 oz sliced roast turkey
            lettuce and tomato
            3 tsp mayonnaise
            2 slices rye bread
Fresh apple
Iced tea

Dinner

4 oz broiled sirloin steak
1 baked potato (1 cup)
½ cup broccoli
Tossed salad with 1 tbs Italian dressing
2 tsp margarine*
¼ cantaloupe
Coffee or tea

Snack

1 cup skim milk
2 graham crackers

This menu provides all essential nutrients in adequate amounts.
Analysis of this sample meal plan yields:

Calories	1500		Iron	23 mg
Protein (20%)	74 g		Phosphorus	1350 mg
Fat (35%)	58 g		Cholesterol	150 mg
Carbohydrate (45%)	174 g		Polyunsaturated fat	14.3 mg
Calcium	822 mg		Saturated fat	14.3 mg
Potassium	3554 mg		P/S ratio	1:1

*Margarine used for calculation purposes was corn oil (stick).

lowering effect. Fructose, a component of table sugar and some fruits, tends to have a greater stimulatory effect on triglyceride synthesis than does glucose. Table 7–13 provides a sample meal plan.

When foods are properly selected and all items are consumed, the diet is adequate in all essential nutrients, with the possible exception of iron.

General Dietary Considerations

Tables 7–7 and 7–8 may be used to prepare individual diet plans. The following high-cholesterol foods are allowed in the dietary management of type IV hyperlipidemia, whereas patients with types IIB and III must be limited to 300 mg/day of cholesterol.

1. *Eggs*: 3 whole eggs (or 3 egg yolks) per week, including those used in cooking

2. *Organ meats*: 2 oz liver, sweetbreads, or heart may be substituted for 1 egg yolk

3. *Cheese*: 2 oz of regular cheese per week (cheddar, American, and so forth)

Simple desserts that do not include fat may be used, *i.e.,* gelatin (plain or fruited), angel food cake, puddings prepared with skim milk, fruit ices, and sherbets. Sweetened soft drinks, plain candies (made without fat), sugar, syrups, honey, and so on, may be used on occasion.

Alcohol adds extra calories and may increase serum triglyceride levels. Its intake should be restricted to less than 25 g/day. Even this quantity may be deleterious in some patients.

Calculation of the Diet

1. Assess the patient's dietary habits.

2. Determine the daily caloric requirement of the patient to achieve or maintain ideal body weight (see Appendix).

3. Do not restrict total carbohydrate intake, but limit intake of simple sugars.

4. Restrict cholesterol to 300 mg/day except in type IV.

5. Substitute sufficient polyunsaturated fat for saturated fat to achieve a P/S ratio of 1:1.

6. Restrict fat to 35 per cent of the total calories.

7. Eliminate or severely restrict alcoholic intake.

REFERENCES FOR CHOLESTEROL AND FAT CONTENT OF FOODS (TABLES 7–7 and 7–8)

BEEF PRODUCTS (Anderson, B. A., Kinsella, J. E., and Watts, B. K.): JADA 67:35–41, 1975.
CEREAL PRODUCTS (Weihrauch, J. L., Kinsella, J. E., and Watts, B. K.): JADA 68:335–340, 1976.
COMPOSITION OF FOODS: Dairy and Egg Products; Raw, Processed, Prepared. Agriculture Handbook No. 8-1. United States Department of Agriculture, Agricultural Research Service, 1976.
COMPOSITION OF FOODS: Fats and Oils; Raw, Processed and Prepared. Agriculture Handbook No. 8-4. United States Department of Agriculture, Agricultural Research Service, 1979.
COMPOSITION OF FOODS: Poultry Products; Raw, Processed, Prepared. Agriculture Handbook No. 8-5. United States Department of Agriculture, Agricultural Research Service, 1979.
FINFISH (Exler, J., and Weihrauch, J. L.): JADA 69:243–248, 1976.
LAMB AND VEAL (Anderson, B. A., Fristrom, G. A., and Weihrauch, J. D.): JADA 70:53–58, 1977.

NUTRITIVE VALUE OF AMERICAN FOODS IN COMMON UNITS: Agriculture Handbook No. 456. United States Department of Agriculture, Agricultural Research Service, 1975.
PORK PRODUCTS (Anderson, B. A.): JADA 69:44–49, 1976.
SHELLFISH (Exler, J., and Weihrauch, J. L.): JADA 71:518–521, 1977.

BIBLIOGRAPHY

Fat-Restricted Diets in the Management of Gastrointestinal Disorder

Bochenek, W., Rodgers, J. B., and Balint, J. A.: Effects of changes in dietary lipids on intestinal fluid loss in the short-bowel syndrome. Ann Intern Med 72:205–213, 1970.
Dobbins, J. W., and Binder, M. J.: Importance of the colon in enteric hyperoxaluria. N Engl J Med 296:298–301 , 1977.
Holt, P.: Dietary treatment of protein loss in intestinal lymphangiectasia. Pediatrics 34:629–635, 1964.

Dietary Modifications of Plasma Lipid and Lipoprotein Levels

Ahrens, E. H.: Dietary fats and coronary heart disease: Unfinished business. Lancet 2:1345–1348, 1979.
Connor, W. E., Hodges, R. E., and Bleiler, R. D.: Effect of dietary cholesterol upon serum cholesterol in man. J Clin Invest 57:331–342, 1961.
Connor, W. E., and Connor, S. L.: Dietary treatment of hyperlipidemia. In Rifkind, B. S., and Levy, R. I. (Eds.): Hyperlipidemia: Diagnosis and Therapy. New York, Grune and Stratton, 1977, pp. 281–326.
Ernst, N., Bower, P., Fisher, M., Schaefer, E. J., and Levy, R. I.: Changes in plasma lipids and lipoproteins after a modified fat diet. Lancet 2:111–112, 1980.
Gordon, T., Castelli, W. P., Hjortland, M. C., Kannell, W. B., and Dawber, T. R.: High density lipoprotein as a protective factor against coronary heart disease. Am J Med 62:707–714, 1977.
Gotto, A. M., Shepherd, J., Levy, R., Rifkind, L. D., Dennis, B., and Ernst, E. (Eds.): Nutrition, Lipids and Coronary Heart Disease. New York, Raven Press, 1979.
Keys, A., Anderson, J. T., and Grande, F.: Prediction of serum cholesterol responses of man to changes in fats in the diet. Lancet 2:959–966, 1957.
Keys, A., Anderson, J. T., and Grande, F.: Serum cholesterol response to changes in the diet. II. The effect of cholesterol in the diet. Metabolism 14:759–765, 1965.
LaRosa, J. C., Fry, A. G., Muesing, R., and Rosing, D. R.: Effects of high-protein, low-carbohydrate diets on plasma lipoproteins and body weight. JADA 77:264–270, 1980.
Leren, P.: The effect of plasma cholesterol lowering diet in male survivors of myocardial infarction: A controlled trial. Acta Med Scand 466(Suppl 5):26–82, 1966.
Lewis, B., Kahan, M., et al.: Toward an improved lipid-lowering diet: Additive effects of changes in nutrient intake. Lancet 2:1310–1313, 1981.
Lipid Research Clinics Program: The Lipid Research Clinics coronary primary prevention trial results: I. Reduction in incidence of coronary heart disease. JAMA 251:351–364, 1984.
Margolis, S.: Disorders of plasma lipids and lipoproteins. In Harvey, A. M., Johns, R. J., McKusick, V. A., Owens, A. H., and Ross, R. S., (Eds.): The Principles and Practice of Medicine, 21 ed. New York, Appleton-Century-Crofts, 1984, pp. 914–927.
McGill, H. C., Jr, McMahan, C. A., and Wene, J. D.: Unresolved problems in the diet—heart issue. Arteriosclerosis 1:164–176, 1981.
Mistry, P., Miller, N. C., Hazzard, W. R., and Lewis, B.: Individual variation in the effects of dietary cholesterol on plasma lipoproteins and cellular cholesterol hemostasis in man. J Clin Invest 67:493–503, 1981.
Oliver, M. F.: Diet and coronary heart disease. Br Med Bull 37:49–58, 1982.
Shepherd, J., Packard, C. J., Patsch, J. R., Gotto, A. M., and Taunton, O.: Effects of dietary polyunsaturated and saturated fat on the properties of high density lipoproteins and the metabolism of apolipoprotein A-1. J Clin Invest 61:1581–1591, 1978.
U.S. Department of Health and Human Services, Public Health Service, National Institutes of Health, Lipid Metabolism Branch, NHLBI: The Lipid Research Clinics, Population Studies, Data Book, Vol. 1, Bethesda, NIH Publication No. 80-1527, 1980.
Vessby, B., Boberg, J., Gustafsson, I-B., Karlström, B., Lithell, H., and Östlund-Lindquist, A.: Reduction of high density lipoprotein cholesterol and apolipoprotein A-I concentrations by a lipid-lowering diet. Atherosclerosis 35:21–27, 1980.

8
MODIFICATIONS IN PROTEIN

Nutritional Aspects of Renal Failure

Mackenzie Walser, M.D.,
Helen D. Mullan, B.S., R.D.,
Judith Z. Walker, M.P.H., R.D., and
Elizabeth C. Chandler, B.Sc., R.D.,

INTRODUCTION

Nutritional regimens designed specifically to reduce the need for urinary excretion of waste products can greatly attenuate the biochemical consequences of renal insufficiency and are indicated in both acute and chronic renal failure.

ACUTE RENAL FAILURE, INCLUDING THE OLIGURIC PHASE OF ACUTE GLOMERULONEPHRITIS

Goals and Rationale of Treatment

The primary goals of nutritional management of acute renal failure are to minimize azotemia and fluid retention. Catabolism of body proteins can be reduced by provision of nonprotein energy sources and of sufficient essential amino acids to meet daily requirements. Expansion of extracellular fluid volume with attendant peripheral edema and in some cases, pulmonary edema can be prevented by permitting ingestion of sodium in amounts sufficient only to compensate for urinary and extrarenal sodium losses. Water retention with consequent hyponatremia can be avoided by allowing only sufficient water to compensate for urinary and insensible water losses.

Patients with acute renal failure of either the oliguric or nonoliguric type are candidates for nutritional therapy. Patients in the oliguric stage of acute glomerulonephritis may also benefit from such management.

Dietary Principles

The first principle in the nutritional management of acute renal failure is that sufficient carbohydrate must be provided, either with or without fat, to prevent the utilization of body protein as an energy source. When sufficient nonprotein calories are ingested, catabolism of endogenous protein, with resultant azotemia and accumulation of acid and potassium, can often be decreased or minimized. However, those patients who are hypercatabolic in response to trauma, infection, or surgery may continue to catabolize endogenous protein at an excessive rate despite such caloric supplements.

The second principle, an area requiring still further study, is the attempt to reduce net catabolism of endogenous protein even further by providing exogenous essential amino acids, with or without nonessential amino acids, in addition to nonprotein calories. In this way, deficiencies of specific amino acids are prevented from becoming rate-limiting for protein synthesis. Otherwise, protein degradation would continue and protein synthesis would be significantly impaired.

The final dietary management principle is that extracellular fluid volume and body fluid osmolarity should be kept as close to normal as possible. This can be accomplished only by closely controlling the intake of salt and water, since the renal capacity to regulate their excretion is impaired in patients with acute renal failure.

Major Dietary Modifications

Because of varying degrees of anorexia, nausea, and vomiting, patients with acute renal failure are usually unable to ingest adequate calories, and parenteral nutrition is therefore often necessary. Peripheral infusions may supply sufficient carbohydrate and amino acids to achieve protein-sparing, despite supplying far fewer carbohydrate calories than are necessary to meet total energy needs. Since patients with acute renal failure commonly require treatment for only a short time, in most cases partial caloric deprivation probably poses less of a hazard than do the potential complications of central venous alimentation. (The risk of catheter sepsis is often increased in patients with acute renal failure, owing to impaired immune responses.) Therefore, peripheral infusion of 5 or 10 per cent dextrose solutions and/or 10 or 20 per cent lipid emulsion in sufficient quantities to provide at least 400 kcal/day is the mainstay of therapy (unless oral or enteral feeding is possible).

Essential amino acids can be provided as oral tablets or as powders if tolerated, but they are more commonly administered as a peripheral intravenous infusion (Table 8–1). The total daily dosage by either route is 10 to 20 g. Although such treatment tends to reduce urea accumulation, it does not affect mortality, contrary to initial reports. Recent evidence suggests that complete

TABLE 8–1. AMINO ACID SUPPLEMENTS FOR ORAL OR INTRAVENOUS USE IN RENAL FAILURE

	Oral Products			IV Products		
	Aminess (Cutter) g/ 30 tabs	Travasorb Renal (Travenol) g/ 3 packets	Amin-Aid (American-McGaw) g/ 3 packets	Nephramine (American-McGaw) g/ 250 ml	Aminosyn-RF (Abbott) g/ 300 ml	RenAmin (Travenol) g/ 100 ml
Histidine	1.65	1.56	0.75	0.62	1.28	0.42
Isoleucine	2.10	1.86	2.10	1.40	1.39	0.50
Leucine	3.30	2.22	3.30	2.20	2.18	0.60
Lysine	2.40	1.65	2.37	1.60	1.60	0.45
Methionine	3.30	2.10	3.30	2.20	2.18	0.50
Phenylalanine	3.30	1.80	3.30	2.20	2.18	0.49
Threonine	1.50	1.39	1.50	1.00	0.99	0.38
Tryptophan	0.75	0.60	0.75	0.50	0.50	0.16
Valine	2.40	2.76	2.40	1.60	1.58	0.82
Arginine		1.92			1.80	0.63
Proline		1.38				0.35
Glycine		1.29				0.30
Alanine		2.04				0.56
Serine		1.29				0.30
Tyrosine		0.18				0.04
Total amino acids	20.70	24.00	19.77	13.32	15.68	6.50
Carbohydrate	1.50	378.60	372.90	0	0	0
Fat	0.50	25.00	47.10	0	0	0

amino acid mixtures may be as effective as solutions containing only essential amino acids.

Sodium intake, in the patient who is neither dehydrated nor edematous, is adjusted to equal urinary sodium losses. In nonoliguric renal failure or in the diuretic phase following acute tubular necrosis, such losses may be considerable. On the other hand, in the patient with severe oliguria, sodium excretion may virtually cease, and sodium intake must be severely curtailed. Water intake should be limited to the previous day's urinary volume plus about 500 ml to allow for insensible losses. In the hyponatremic subject, water intake should be further curtailed.

Potassium-binding resins such as Kayexalate may be necessary to manage hyperkalemia. Potassium supplements are rarely needed in the early phases of acute renal failure. However, development of hypokalemia later in acute renal failure, especially during the diuretic phase, may result in the need for supplemental potassium.

CHRONIC RENAL FAILURE, PREDIALYSIS

Goals of Treatment

The goals of treatment of chronic renal failure in the predialysis stage include maintaining protein nutrition, while keeping serum urea nitrogen concentration below the level at which azotemia induces symptoms; maintaining or attaining ideal body weight; and controlling hyperphosphatemia, hypocalcemia, and the conditions stemming from these disorders—namely, secondary hyperparathyroidism, renal osteodystrophy, and metastatic calcification. Additional goals of treatment are maintenance of normal extracellular fluid volume, pH, osmolarity, and potassium content, and retardation of the progression of renal insufficiency, if possible.

Rationale of Treatment

PROTEIN NUTRITION AND AZOTEMIA.   Most signs and symptoms of chronic renal failure are attributable to the impaired excretion of waste products of protein catabolism. These products include urea and other nitrogenous compounds derived from the catabolism of ingested or endogenous protein. The nonprotein nitrogen in protein-containing foods amounts to no more than 10 per cent of their total nitrogen content and is a relatively minor nitrogenous source. High-protein foods are also major sources of potassium, sulfate, phosphate, and acid, all of which are excreted with difficulty by patients with chronic renal failure.

Overzealous restriction of protein may result in negative nitrogen balance and protein deficiency. In general, this occurs only when the intake of essential amino acids is reduced below the patient's minimal daily requirement. Normal individuals require at least 7 g of essential amino acids per day, a quantity provided by as little as 15 g of protein of high biologic value (egg protein, for example) or 25 g of protein of low or mixed biologic value. The biologic value of a protein measures the extent to which it can be utilized to maintain nitrogen balance and reflects the ratio of essential to nonessential amino acids, as well as the relative quantities of each essential amino acid.

Although essential amino acid requirements in chronic renal failure are not known with certainty, it appears that a total of 10 g of essential amino acids per day is adequate in most cases. The total nitrogen requirement in patients with renal failure is also unknown; recent studies have disproved past suggestions that these patients reutilize urea nitrogen for synthetic purposes and that, therefore, the requirement is less than that of normal subjects.

ENERGY.   Adequate caloric intake is important to minimize protein catabolism in the patient with chronic renal failure. In some obese patients, however, attainment of a desirable weight is a sufficiently important goal to take precedence. Weight reduction should be gradual, because renal failure impairs nitrogen conservation during starvation. Although the importance of adequate energy intake has been emphasized in the management of children with chronic renal failure, protein and mineral nutrition may be of equal importance in achieving normal or near-normal growth.

CALCIUM, PHOSPHORUS, AND MAGNESIUM BALANCE.   Secondary hyperparathyroidism usually begins to develop in the earliest stages of chronic renal failure for reasons that are, as yet, not fully elucidated. This condition may occur even before phosphate retention, hypocalcemia, or vitamin D deficiency is noted, although all of these abnormalities appear later in the course of the disease. Severe renal osteodystrophy, metastatic calcification (particularly in blood vessels), and troublesome itching can result from secondary hyperparathyroidism. It may also contribute to other features of the uremic syndrome, including anemia and impotence. Metastatic calcification in the kidney, caused not only by secondary hyperparathyroidism but also by elevation of the Ca × P product in the serum, further damages the kidney independently of hyperparathyroidism, and may accelerate the progression of renal insufficiency.

Reduction of phosphate intake or interference with its intestinal absorption, supplementation of calcium intake, and treatment with selected forms of vitamin D may be useful measures in managing the effects of secondary hyperparathyroidism even in the early stages of chronic renal failure. Reduced phosphate intake, achieved by avoiding foods high in phosphorus, is indicated in every case of moderate or severe renal failure (see Chapter 9). There is also suggestive evidence that phosphate restriction may help to slow the progression of renal failure even in its early stages.

Another approach effective in decreasing the body burden of phosphate is the oral administration of aluminum hydroxide or aluminum carbonate, substances that retard phosphate absorption by forming insoluble aluminum phosphate in the gut. However, the absorption of some aluminum from these compounds may have deleterious consequences in the patient with renal failure, because renal clearance of aluminum is subnormal. In dialysis patients, aluminum may cause the syndrome known as dialysis dementia. Although there is, at present, no definitive proof that toxic effects are induced by oral aluminum compounds in predialysis patients, it is possible that their prolonged use may cause osteomalacia. Aluminum salts may induce hypophosphatemia if given in excessive quantities. They are also difficult for some to take and may cause severe constipation.

Calcium supplementation is advisable in most cases of chronic renal failure, because calcium intake from food is reduced by the need to avoid milk, milk products, and cheese in order to lower phosphorus intake and because intestinal absorption of calcium is impaired even in the early stages of renal failure. Furthermore, calcium supplements tend to inhibit phosphate absorption from the gut and to suppress parathyroid hormone secretion. A total calcium intake of 1200 to 1600 mg/day is desirable. It is important, however, to control hyperphosphatemia (if present) before giving calcium supplements; otherwise renal function may deteriorate further because of renal calcification.

Even though vitamin D increases phosphorus absorption, various forms of this vitamin have been used in chronic renal failure to increase intestinal calcium absorption, suppress secondary hyperparathyroidism, and prevent or treat renal osteodystrophy. Since the kidney is the principal organ responsible for activating vitamin D (by hydroxylation at the 1 position), one would expect a deficiency of the active form of vitamin D early in chronic renal failure. According to most reports, however, such deficiency develops only in the later stages. Nevertheless, the active form of vitamin D (1,25-dihydroxycholecalciferol), other 1-hydroxylated derivatives, or dihydrotachysterol (which has a similar structure) are sometimes employed in these patients. Early in renal failure, before hyperphosphatemia appears, these compounds may suppress secondary hyperparathyroidism and, possibly, slow progression of renal insufficiency. However, after hyperphosphatemia appears, they may increase the serum $Ca \times P$ product and thereby promote soft-tissue calcification, especially in the kidney. Accelerated progression of renal insufficiency may result even if hypercalcemia does not develop. Consequently, these compounds should be used in hyperphosphatemic patients only after phosphorus restriction and calcium supplementation have failed to correct hypocalcemia or symptomatic osteodystrophy, and even then their use may not be worth the associated risk.

Magnesium balance is not usually a problem in chronic renal failure. However, the use of magnesium-containing antacids may cause dangerous hypermagnesemia owing to reduced renal clearance of magnesium. This is manifested by nausea, hypotension, lethargy, muscle weakness, and respiratory depression.

SODIUM, WATER, POTASSIUM, AND ACID-BASE BALANCE.   As chronic renal failure progresses, the ability of the kidney to adjust sodium excretion to the varying needs of the patient becomes progressively impaired, and eventually sodium excretion becomes nearly fixed. Hence, either sodium depletion (when intake is less than urinary output) or sodium retention (when intake exceeds output) may occur. The latter is considerably more common. It is, of course, more frequent in patients with hypoalbuminemia or congestive failure but may occur in the absence of these problems.

The optimal dietary sodium intake for any patient is determined by the rate of urinary sodium excretion minus the daily intake of $NaHCO_3$. Sodium bicarbonate is required by some, but not all, patients for the prevention of metabolic acidosis. The optimal daily dose varies widely. When $NaHCO_3$ intake plus dietary sodium matches urinary sodium output, sodium balance will be achieved. As renal failure progresses, regulation of sodium balance in this manner becomes critically important to avoid dangerous consequences of sodium retention or depletion.

Calcium carbonate or other calcium salts are sometimes used instead of $NaHCO_3$ in the treatment of renal acidosis, especially in Europe. However, this measure is of limited efficacy. Correction of acidosis requires that the bicarbonate concentration of the extracellular fluid be increased. Therefore, the concentration of some cation must increase simultaneously. Neither the calcium nor the potassium concentration can increase more than a few mEq/l without fatal consequences. So the only mechanisms by which calcium salts could augment the bicarbonate content of the extracellular fluid are (1) by Ca-Na exchange in bone, a process that is inherently limited in magnitude and duration, or (2) by suppression of secondary hyperparathyroidism, a condition that may contribute to renal wastage of bicarbonate. The latter effect is conjectural and has not been demonstrated to occur in renal failure patients receiving calcium salts. Thus, the rationale for using calcium salts to treat the acidosis of renal failure is weak.

Since the thirst mechanism is generally intact in chronic renal failure patients, water intake is usually appropriate for maintenance of normal serum osmolarity, despite the reduced ability of the diseased kidney to concentrate or dilute the urine. In occasional patients, excessive water intake may lead to dilutional hyponatremia. Water restriction will soon correct this disturbance, and less severe water restriction will prevent its recurrence.

Potassium excess does not usually become a problem in early or moderate renal failure, owing to increased tubular secretion and fecal excretion of potassium. Hypokalemia also rarely occurs. But in later stages of renal failure, hyperkalemia is seen often. Although dietary restriction of potassium is useful in the management of hyperkalemia, many patients prefer to take a potassium-exchange resin (such as Kayexalate) rather than accept the dietary restrictions.

PROGRESSION OF RENAL FAILURE.   High-protein diets accelerate progression of experimental chronic renal insufficiency in animals. Phosphorus restriction has recently been shown to slow progression in these models. Patients given supplements of essential amino acids or their ketoanalogues, along with protein and phosphorus restriction, have been reported to exhibit slowed or arrested progression of chronic renal failure in several recent studies. Some of these protocols, however, were not well controlled. The relative importance of protein and phosphate restriction in accounting for the observed retardation remains to be established, as does the likelihood of success of this treatment in all forms of renal disease. However, this goal of therapy is well worth pursuing because of its potential importance to the patient.

SPECIAL CONSIDERATIONS IN THE MANAGEMENT OF DIABETICS WITH RENAL FAILURE.   Since the diets prescribed in chronic renal failure are typically low in protein and high in carbohydrate, concern has been expressed about their use for the patient who is also diabetic. However, as noted in Chapter 6, carbohydrate restriction is no longer recommended in the treatment of diabetes. A more significant problem results from the need to restrict protein; a substantial fraction of carbohydrate intake may then be in the form of simple sugars. The use of simple sugars should be limited to avoid excessive fluctuation of blood glucose levels.

The insulin requirement of insulin-dependent diabetics characteristically declines as renal failure progresses, and problems with blood glucose regulation attributable to dietary carbohydrate are rare. Since the results of both chronic dialysis and transplantation are relatively poor in diabetics, nutritional therapy for renal failure becomes especially important in managing these patients.

Patient Selection

There are no contraindications to the use of nutritional therapy in the management of chronic renal failure. Since such treatment may slow or even halt progression of the underlying disease in individual patients, it is worthwhile to try this approach in every patient before accepting dialysis as inevitable. There is no evidence that the conservative management described here induces progressive protein malnutrition or makes eventual dialysis therapy or transplantation more difficult.

Dietary Principles

Management of Protein Nutrition and Azotemia

Generally, protein quantity is restricted, without altering its quality, when symptoms first develop on a normal diet, but some contend that earlier protein restriction may retard progression of renal damage. Approximately 0.6 g/kg/day of protein is required to maintain nitrogen balance when the biologic quality of protein is not regulated. As renal failure progresses, the following approaches can be used to restrict dietary protein still further:

1. Use of only protein with high biologic value. When the diet is restricted to those proteins containing high proportions of essential amino acids, as little protein as 0.35 g/kg/day will usually maintain nitrogen balance.

2. Use of 20 to 25 g/day of mixed-quality protein, supplemented by essential amino acids or their ketoanalogues. This diet is indicated in moderate or severe renal failure. Essential amino acids can be provided in doses of 10 to 20 g/day (see Table 8–1). Ketoacid supplements are not yet available commercially in the United States. Despite their low protein content, such diets are readily accepted by most patients, because the absence of any restriction on protein quality permits great variety in the choice of foods, compared with a diet containing only protein with high biologic value. The palatability of these diets is increased if a substantial fraction of the energy needs is met through the use of an electrolyte-free, nitrogen-free oligosaccharide preparation or nondairy creamers or both. Enhanced palatability then results from the nearly normal proportion of protein calories in the ingested foods. The oligosaccharide products are almost tasteless, cause diarrhea only when ingested rapidly, and are not expensive.

Protein-restricted diets may be deficient in vitamins, depending upon the choice of foods. Supplements of the B vitamins and of vitamin C and folic acid are recommended. Vitamin A should not be given, since it is commonly already present in excess. The use of vitamin D has already been discussed.

Management of Energy Balance

A caloric intake of at least 30 kcal/kg is desirable in patients who are not obese. The higher energy requirements of children are given in the section in Chapter 1 on pediatric nutrition. Most adults will consume sufficient calories if the diet is palatable, but this should be confirmed by a careful dietary history. Children may require special encouragement to consume the required amount of calories.

Management of Divalent Ion Balance

Phosphorus-restricted diets will be discussed in detail in Chapter 9. Aluminum preparations useful in reducing phosphate absorption in chronic renal failure are listed in Table 8–2. Long-term use of these preparations may cause some risk of osteomalacia in predialysis patients. The "equivalent" doses shown contain the same amount of aluminum but may have widely different

TABLE 8–2. COMMONLY USED PHOSPHATE-BINDING
ANTACIDS NOT BASED ON MAGNESIUM

Preparation	Unit Dose	Equivalent Al(OH)$_3$ Content of Unit Dose, mg
Aluminum hydroxide		
Alternagel	5 ml	600
Amphogel		
Liquid	5 ml	320
Tablet, 0.3 g	1 tab	300
Alutabs	1 tab	210
Alucaps	1 cap	126
Dialume	1 cap	175
Aluminum carbonate		
Basaljel		
Liquid	5 ml	400
Tablet	1 tab	500
Capsule	1 cap	500
Extra-strength		
liquid	5 ml	1000

phosphate-binding capacity. Unfortunately these products are not at present assayed for phosphate-binding capacity.

Calcium supplementation is most practically and economically achieved through the use of calcium carbonate, which contains 40 per cent by weight of elemental calcium. Other calcium salts that may be used include calcium gluconate (9 per cent calcium) and calcium lactate (13 per cent calcium).

Management of Sodium, Potassium, Acid-Base, and Water Balance

Optimal sodium intake is determined by the 24-hour urinary sodium excretion, in mEq/day (which tends to be relatively fixed in patients with renal failure) minus the required NaHCO$_3$ intake, in mEq/day. The latter is adjusted to maintain serum CO$_2$ content between 18 and 26 mM. Obviously, edema or sodium depletion should be corrected before the optimal sodium intake is determined.

Potassium intake need not be regulated in most patients. Some, however, will require either Kayexalate or dietary potassium restriction to prevent hyperkalemia.

Likewise, water intake may be *ad libitum* in most patients. A minority of patients, particularly those with edema or congestive heart failure or both, may develop hyponatremia and require restriction of water intake to 1 l/day or less.

Major Dietary Modifications

The protein intakes recommended here are for 70-kg patients; these should be adjusted for individuals who weigh more or less than that amount. To make the dietary modifications, the appropriate diet is first selected in Table 8–3, which gives the number of exchanges included from each food group. Sample menus are given in Table 8–4. Table 8–5 lists average compositions for each ex-

Text continues on page 194

TABLE 8–3.   SAMPLE MEAL PATTERNS FOR PREDIALYSIS, HEMODIALYSIS, AND
PERITONEAL DIALYSIS[†]
(BASED ON 70-KG PERSON)

Foods	25 g Protein; 500 mg Phosphorus[‡]	40 g Protein; 600 mg Phosphorus	70 g Protein; 2 g Sodium	105 g Protein; 2 g Sodium
BREAKFAST				
Meat Exchanges	—	1	1	2
Bread Exchanges A or B	2	2	2	2
Fruit Exchange A or B	1	1	1	1
Fat Exchanges	2	3	3	3
Milk Exchanges	—	—	2	2
Calorie Supplements				
Group A	2	1	1	—
Group B	1	1	1	1
Group C	2	2	—	—
Group D	*	*	*	*
LUNCH				
Meat Exchanges	1	1	2	3
Bread Exchanges A or B	2	2	2	2
Vegetable Exchange A or B	—	1	1	1
Fruit Exchange A or B	1	1	1	1
Fat Exchanges	3	3	3	3
Calorie Supplements				
Group A	1	1	1	—
Group B	1	1	1	$\frac{1}{2}$
Group D	*	*	*	*
Group E	1	1	—	—
MIDAFTERNOON SNACK				
Calorie Supplement				
Group A	1	2	1	—
Fruit Exchange A or B	1	—	—	—
DINNER				
Meat Exchanges	—	1	2	4
Bread Exchanges A or B	—	1	2	2
Vegetable Exchange A or B	2	1	1	1
Fruit Exchange A or B	1	1	1	1
Milk Exchanges	—	—	2	—
Fat Exchanges	4	3	3	3
Calorie Supplements				
Group A	2	1	1	—
Group B	1	1	1	$\frac{1}{2}$
Group D	*	*	*	*
Group E	1	1	—	—
EVENING SNACK				
Milk Exchange	—	—	—	1
Meat Exchange	—	—	—	1
Bread Exchanges A or B	1	1	—	2
Fruit Exchange A or B	—	—	1	1
EVENING SNACK				
Fat Exchange	1	—	—	1
Calorie Supplements				
Group A	1	1	2	—
Group B	1	1	—	—
Group D	*	*	*	*

*As desired.
[†]Exchanges are given in Table 8–6.
[‡]To be used only with supplemental essential amino acids and/or ketoacids.

TABLE 8–4.   SAMPLE MENU—25 G PROTEIN (MIXED BIOLOGIC VALUE), 500 MG PHOSPHORUS

Breakfast

½ cup grapefruit sections
¾ cup sugar-coated cold cereal
1 slice toast
2 tsp margarine
1 tbs honey
6 tbs liquid nondairy creamer
2 tbs sugar
Coffee

Lunch

Sandwich:
  1 oz sliced salt-free roast turkey
  2 slices bread
  1 tbs mayonnaise
¼ cup cranberry sauce
½ cup canned sweetened peaches
3 tbs maltodextrin
3.5 oz wine

Snack

1 oz jelly beans
1 fresh pear

Dinner

Casserole:
  1 cup rigatoni (cooked without salt)
  ½ cup cooked salt-free tomatoes
  ½ cup cooked salt-free green beans
  3 tsp margarine
1 slice French bread
1 tsp margarine
½ cup diced sweetened pineapple
iced tea
3 tbs maltodextrin
3.5 oz wine

Evening Snack

Cinnamon toast:
  1 slice bread
  2 tbs sugar
  1 tsp margarine
8 oz cranberry juice

The meal plan is adequate in all essential nutrients except iron, certain vitamins, calcium, and essential amino acids. Its composition is:

Calories	2500		Phosphorus	500	mg
Protein	25	g	Potassium	1600	mg
Calcium	27	mg	Sodium	1000	mg
Iron	6.0	mg			

SAMPLE MENU—25 G PROTEIN (MIXED BIOLOGIC VALUE), 500 MG PHOSPHORUS (Continued)

Breakfast

½ cup grapefruit sections
¾ cup sugar-coated cold cereal
1 egg fried in 1 tsp margarine
1 slice toast
2 tsp margarine
2 tbs jelly
6 tbs liquid nondairy creamer
2 tbs sugar
Coffee

Lunch

Sandwich:
  1 oz sliced salt-free roast turkey
  2 slices bread
  1 tbs mayonnaise
  lettuce and tomato (1 slice)
¼ cup cranberry sauce

Dinner

1 oz sliced, salt-free roast beef
½ cup salt-free green beans
1 slice French bread
3 tsp margarine
½ cup diced sweetened pineapple
6 oz ginger ale
3 tbs maltodextrin
3½ oz wine
½ cup canned sweetened peaches
3 tbs maltodextrin
3½ oz wine

Snack

2 oz jelly beans

Table continues on following page

SAMPLE MENU—25 G PROTEIN (MIXED BIOLOGIC VALUE), 500 MG PHOSPHORUS (Continued)

Evening Snack

Cinnamon toast:
  1 slice bread
  2 tbs sugar
  1 tsp margarine
8 oz cranberry juice

The meal plan is adequate in all essential nutrients except iron and calcium. Its composition is:

Calories	2500		Phosphorus	600	mg
Protein	40	g	Potassium	1640	mg
Calcium	350	mg	Sodium	1400	mg
Iron	8.5	mg			

SAMPLE MENU—HEMODIALYSIS, 70 G PROTEIN, 2000 MG SODIUM

Breakfast

½ cup grapefruit sections, drained
¾ cup sugar-coated cereal
1 egg fried in 1 tsp margarine
1 slice toast
2 tsp margarine
2 tbs jelly
1 cup regular milk
2 tbs sugar
½ cup coffee

Lunch

Sandwich:
  2 oz sliced, salt-free roast turkey
  2 slices regular bread
  1 tbs mayonnaise
  lettuce and tomato
¼ cup cranberry sauce
½ cup canned sweetened peaches, drained
1 cup iced tea
3 tbs maltodextrin

Snack

1 oz jelly beans

Dinner

2 oz sliced, salt-free roast beef
½ cup salt-free green beans
2 slices French bread
3 tsp margarine
½ cup diced sweetened pineapple, drained
2 tbs jelly
3 tbs maltodextrin
1 cup milk

Evening Snack

1 fresh apple (medium)
2 oz hard candy

Fluid requirement: 10 ml/kg of body weight + urine output
Diet contains: 720 ml fluid

The meal plan is adequate in all essential nutrients except iron. Its composition is:

Calories	2600		Phosphorus	1175	mg
Protein	70	g	Potassium	2750	mg
Calcium	906	mg	Sodium	2000	mg
Iron	13	mg			

SAMPLE MENU—PERITONEAL DIALYSIS, 105 G PROTEIN, 2 G SODIUM

Breakfast

½ cup grapefruit sections, drained
¾ cup sugar-coated cereal
2 eggs fried in 1 tsp margarine
1 slice regular toast
2 tsp margarine
1 cup regular milk
2 tbs sugar
½ cup coffee

Lunch

Sandwich:
  3 oz sliced, salt-free roast turkey
  2 slices regular bread
  1 tbs mayonnaise
  lettuce and tomato
½ cup canned sweetened peaches, drained
1 cup iced tea
1 tbs sugar

Dinner

4 oz sliced, salt-free roast beef
½ cup salt-free green beans
2 slices French bread
3 tsp margarine
½ cup canned sweetened pineapple tid-
  bits, drained
1 cup iced tea
1 tbs sugar

Evening Snack

Tuna salad:
  ¼ cup salt-free tuna
  1 tsp regular mayonnaise
2 slices regular bread
1 fresh pear
½ cup milk

Diet contains: 1000 ml fluid
The meal plan is adequate in all essential nutrients. Its composition is:

Calories	2500		Phosphorus	1485	mg
Protein	105	g	Potassium	3000	mg
Calcium	876	mg	Sodium	2000	mg
Iron	18	mg			

TABLE 8–5. SUMMARY TABLE FOR RENAL CALCULATIONS

Food Group	Calories	Protein, g	Sodium, mg	Potassium, mg	Phosphorus, mg	Calcium, mg
1 Milk Exchange	varies	4.0	60.0	170.0	110.0	140.0
1 Meat Exchange	75.0	6.9	30.0	95.0	75.0	15.0
1 Fruit Exchange						
Group A	40–80	0.5	1.5	110.0	12.0	15.0
Group B	40–80	0.7	3.5	215.0	18.0	18.0
1 Bread/Cereal Ex-change						
Group A	70.0	2.0	1.0	38.0	27.0	5.0
Group B	70.0+	2.0	125.0	35.0	31.0	16.0
1 Vegetable Exchange						
Group A	25.0	1.0	9.0	113.0	25.0	29.0
Group B	35.0	1.7	18.0	196.0	34.0	35.0
1 Fat Exchange	45.0	tr	50.0	1.0	1.0	1.0
1 Calorie Supplement						
Group A	100.0	0.1	9.0	9.0	4.0	4.0
Group B	93.0	0.0	19.0	tr	tr	tr
Group C	100.0	0.3	24.0	23.0	24.0	17.0
Group D	115.0	tr	tr	tr	tr	tr
Group E	80.0	0.2	8.0	95.0	0.3	18.0

TABLE 8–6.   EXCHANGE LISTS FOR RENAL DIETS*

Milk Exchanges

AVERAGE ANALYSIS: Protein   4.0 g
                   Sodium   60.0 mg
                   Potassium   170.0 mg
                   Phosphorus   110.0 mg
                   Calcium   140.0 mg
                   Calories   varies

Chocolate milk (whole milk)	½ cup	Ice milk, hard	¾ cup
Cream, half and half	½ cup	Skim milk	½ cup
Evaporated whole milk, canned	¼ cup	Whole milk	½ cup

Meat Exchanges

AVERAGE ANALYSIS: Protein   6.9 g
                   Sodium   30.0 mg
                   Potassium   95.0 mg
                   Phosphorus   75.0 mg
                   Calcium   15.0 mg
                   Calories   75

SEAFOOD

		MEAT	
Bluefish, cooked	1 oz	Beef, lean, cooked, rump	1 oz
Clams, soft, raw, fresh	¼ cup	Chicken, cooked	1 oz
Cod, fresh, cooked	1 oz	Lamb, lean, cooked, shoulder	1 oz
Flounder, cooked	1 oz	Liver (chicken), cooked	1 oz
Haddock, cooked	1 oz	Pork, lean, cooked, loin	1 oz
Halibut, cooked	1 oz	Turkey, cooked	1 oz
Lobster, cooked	1 oz	Veal, cooked, loin	1 oz
Ocean perch, cooked	1 oz		
Oysters, raw	1 oz		
Salmon, canned, cooked	1 oz	Egg	2 oz
Shrimp, cooked	1 oz		
Tuna, canned, low sodium	1 oz		

Fruit Exchanges

GROUP A

AVERAGE ANALYSIS: Protein   0.5 g
                   Sodium   1.5 mg
                   Potassium   115.0 mg
                   Phosphorus   12.0 mg
                   Calcium   15.0 mg
                   Calories   40–80

Apple, fresh (2½″diam.)	1	Raspberries, red, fresh, canned or frozen	½ cup
Applesauce, sweetened	½ cup	Strawberries, fresh, canned, unsweetened	½ cup
Apricot, fresh	1 cup		
Blackberries, fresh or frozen	½ cup		
Blueberries, fresh or frozen	½ cup	Strawberries, frozen, whole, sweetened	½ cup
Cherries, fresh	½ cup		
Figs, fresh, medium	1 cup	Tangerine, fresh, medium	1
Grapefruit, fresh, sections	½ cup	Pineapple, fresh or canned, sweetened	½ cup
Mandarin orange sections	½ cup		
Pears, canned, sweetened	½ cup	Plum, fresh, prune type	2 cups

*For specific foods not included in the "Exchange Lists for Renal Diets" refer to Table 8–7—protein, sodium, potassium, phosphorus, and calcium contents of foods.

Table continues on following page

TABLE 8–6.   EXCHANGE LISTS FOR RENAL DIETS (Continued)

Watermelon, diced	½ cup	Birdseye Awake	½ cup
JUICES		Grape juice	½ cup
		Peach nectar	½ cup
Apple juice	½ cup	Pear nectar	½ cup
GROUP B			

AVERAGE ANALYSIS:
Protein	0.7 g
Sodium	3.5 mg
Potassium	215.0 mg
Phosphorus	18.0 mg
Calcium	18.0 mg
Calories	40–80

Apricots, canned, halves, sweetened	½ cup	Peach, fresh	1 medium
Banana, sliced	½ cup	Peach, canned, sweetened	½ cup
Cantaloupe, cubed, fresh	½ cup	Pear, fresh, Bartlett	1 medium
Casaba, cubed, fresh	½ cup	Plums, canned, sweetened	½ cup
Cherries, red, canned	½ cup	Rhubarb, cooked, sweetened	½ cup
Figs, canned, sweetened	½ cup	JUICES	
Fruit cocktail, canned, sweetened	½ cup	Apricot nectar	½ cup
Grapefruit sections, canned, unsweetened	½ cup	Blackberry juice	½ cup
		Grapefruit juice	½ cup
Grapes, fresh	1 cup	Orange juice	½ cup
Honeydew, cubed, fresh	½ cup	Pineapple juice	½ cup
Melon balls, frozen	½ cup	Prune juice	½ cup
Orange sections, fresh	½ cup	Tomato juice, low sodium	½ cup
Papaya, fresh, cubed	½ cup		

Bread/Cereals Exchanges

GROUP A

AVERAGE ANALYSIS:
Protein	2.0 g
Sodium	1.0 mg
Potassium	38.0 mg
Phosphorus	27.0 mg
Calcium	5.0 mg
Calories	70

Bread, salt-free	1 slice	Cornflakes, salt-free	1 cup
Grits	½ cup	Oatmeal, regular, cooked	½ cup
Flour, wheat	2 tbs	Puffed rice (Quaker Oats)	1 cup
Matzo	1 piece	Cream of wheat, regular, enriched	½ cup
Pasta, macaroni, spaghetti, noodles, etc	½ cup	Puffed wheat (Quaker Oats)	1 cup
		Shredded wheat, spoon size, (Kellogg's)	½ cup
Popcorn, popped in oil	1 cup		
Rice, white enriched, cooked	½ cup		

GROUP B

AVERAGE ANALYSIS:
Protein	2.0 g
Sodium	125.0 mg
Potassium	35.0 mg
Phosphorus	31.0 mg
Calcium	16.0 mg
Calories	70 or more

Table continues on following page

TABLE 8–6.   EXCHANGE LISTS FOR RENAL DIETS (Continued)

Biscuit, homemade (2″ diameter—¼″ high)	1	Bran flakes, 40% (Kellogg's)	¾ cup
Bread, white, whole wheat, rye, or raisin	1 slice	Cap'n Crunch (Quaker Oats)	¾ cup
Bread, French	¾ slice	Cocoa Krispies (Kellogg's)	¾ cup
Doughnut, raised	1 small	Rice Chex (Ralston)	¾ cup
Muffin, plain	1	Special K (Kellogg's)	¾ cup
English muffin (Thomas)	½	Sugar Corn Pops (Kellogg's)	1½ cup
Pancake, homemade 1–4″ diam	1	Sugar Smacks (Kellogg's)	1 cup
Roll, dinner 1–2½″ diam	1	Crackers, animal	10
Roll, hamburger, hotdog, or kaiser	1 or ½	Cracker, graham, plain (5″ × 2½″)	1
		Crackers, unsalted (Nabisco)	4

Fat Exchanges

AVERAGE ANALYSIS:
Protein	trace
Sodium	50.0 mg
Potassium	1.0 mg
Phosphorus	1.0 mg
Calcium	1.0 mg
Calories	45

Butter	1 tsp	Mayonnaise	1 tsp
Margarine	1 tsp	Salad dressing (mayonnaise type)	1 tsp

Vegetable Exchanges

GROUP A

AVERAGE ANALYSIS:
Protein	1.0 g
Sodium	9.0 mg
Potassium	113.0 mg
Phosphorus	25.0 mg
Calcium	29.0 mg
Calories	25

Beans, cooked, green, fresh or frozen, or low sodium, canned	½ cup	Cucumber, fresh peeled	½ cup
Beans, cooked wax, fresh, or low sodium, canned	½ cup	Eggplant, cooked diced	½ cup
		Endive/Escarole, fresh, cut	½ cup
Beans, French cut, frozen, cooked	½ cup	Kale, fresh or frozen, cooked	½ cup
Beets, canned, low sodium	½ cup	Lettuce, iceberg, chopped	½ cup
Cabbage, fresh or cooked	½ cup	Mushrooms, fresh	½ cup
Carrots, raw	½ cup	Mustard greens, frozen, cooked	½ cup
Carrots, canned, low sodium	½ cup	Okra, fresh, cooked, sliced	½ cup
Cauliflower, raw or fresh, cooked	½ cup	Onions, fresh, or cooked	½ cup
Celery, raw or cooked	¼ cup	Peppers, green, fresh, cooked	½ cup
Corn, kernels, fresh, cooked	½ cup	Spinach, fresh, chopped, raw	½ cup
Corn on cob, fresh, cooked	5″ cob	Squash, summer, fresh, cooked	½ cup
Corn, canned, low sodium	½ cup	Tomato, medium, fresh	1 slice
		Turnips, fresh, cooked, diced	½ cup
		Turnip greens, frozen, cooked	½ cup

GROUP B

AVERAGE ANALYSIS:
Protein	1.7 g
Sodium	18.0 mg
Potassium	196.0 mg

Table continues on following page

TABLE 8–6.   EXCHANGE LISTS FOR RENAL DIETS (Continued)

Phosphorus	34.0 mg
Calcium	35.0 mg
Calories	35

Asparagus, fresh, frozen or low sodium canned, cooked	½ cup	Kohlrabi, fresh, raw or cooked	½ cup
Beets, fresh, sliced, cooked	½ cup	Mustard greens, fresh, cooked	½ cup
Broccoli, fresh or frozen, cooked	½ cup	Peppers, green, fresh, cooked	½ cup
Brussels sprouts, fresh or frozen	½ cup	Potato, boiled without skin, diced	½ cup
Carrots, fresh, cooked	½ cup	Radishes, sliced	½ cup
Cauliflower, frozen, cooked	½ cup	Squash, winter, frozen, cooked	½ cup
Chard, Swiss, cooked	½ cup	Sweet potato, canned	½ cup
Collards, fresh, cooked	½ cup	Tomato, fresh, 2" diameter	1 slice
Corn, frozen, cooked	½ cup	Tomato, canned, low sodium	½ cup
Dandelion greens, fresh, cooked	½ cup	Vegetables, mixed, frozen	½ cup
French-fried potatoes	5 sticks		

Calorie Supplements

Each of the foods listed in the amounts indicated yields approximately 100 calories.

CARBOHYDRATES

AVERAGE ANALYSIS:		
	Protein	0.1 g
	Sodium	9.0 mg
	Potassium	9.0 mg
	Phosphorus	4.0 mg
	Calcium	4.0 mg
	Calories	100

Low-protein porridge	¾ cup	Hard candy	1 oz
Low-protein noodles:		Table syrup	2 tbs
anellini, cooked	½ cup	Marshmallows	4 large
rigatoni, cooked	½ cup	Fruit ice	½ cup
tagliatelle, cooked	½ cup	Bright 'N' Early	8 oz
Low-protein bread	1 slice	Cranberry juice	8 oz
Cranberry sauce	¼ cup	Hi-C	8 oz
Honey	1½ tsp	Ginger ale	10 oz
Jelly	2 tbs	Grape soda	8 oz
Jam	3 tbs	Root beer	8 oz
Mints	37 pcs	Orange soda	8 oz
Jelly beans	1 oz		

MALTODEXTRIN SUPPLEMENTS (3 TBS)

AVERAGE ANALYSIS:		
	Protein	0.0 g
	Sodium	19.0 mg
	Potassium	trace
	Phosphorus	trace
	Calcium	trace
	Calories	93

Polycose liquid	Controlyte
Polycose powder	Moducal liquid
Hy-Cal	Moducal powder
Cal Plus	Sumacal

Table continues on following page

TABLE 8–6. EXCHANGE LISTS FOR RENAL DIETS (Concluded)

DAIRY SUBSTITUTES

AVERAGE ANALYSIS:	Protein	0.3 g
	Sodium	24.0 mg
	Potassium	23.0 mg
	Phosphorus	24.0 mg
	Calcium	17.0 mg
	Calories	100

Dessert topping, pressurized can	¾ cup		Powdered dessert topping	1 cup
Frozen dessert topping	½ cup		Rich's liquid	3 tbs

FAT — SALT-FREE (1 TBS)

AVERAGE ANALYSIS:	Protein	trace
	Sodium	trace
	Potassium	trace
	Phosphorus	trace
	Calcium	trace
	Calories	115

Unsalted butter	Vegetable oils
Unsalted margarine	Vegetable shortenings

ALCOHOLIC BEVERAGES

AVERAGE ANALYSIS:	Protein	tr
	Sodium	5.0 mg
	Potassium	1.0 mg
	Phosphorus	0.0 mg
	Calcium	0.0 mg
	Calories	100

Cordials and liqueurs	1 oz		Gin, rum, vodka, whiskey	1½ oz

WINES (3½ OZ)

AVERAGE ANALYSIS:	Protein	1.5 g
	Sodium	8.0 mg
	Potassium	1.0 mg
	Phosphorus	13.0 mg
	Calcium	0.0 mg
	Calories	78

White wine (Chablis)	3½ oz		Burgundy	3½ oz

change group. Exchanges within each group are then selected from Table 8–6. The exact protein, carbohydrate, fat, sodium, potassium, phosphorus, and calcium contents of any given meal plan can be obtained from the data in Table 8–7.

RESTRICTED PROTEIN, 40 G/DAY. This diet includes 3 oz of meat or its equivalent, so that 60 per cent of the daily protein intake is of high biologic value. Fruits and vegetables, with a few exceptions, can usually be taken as desired. Caloric intake must meet energy requirements. Special calorie supplements are not usually required.

RESTRICTED PROTEIN, 20 TO 25 G/DAY, HIGH BIOLOGIC VALUE. This diet is achieved by the following manipulations:

1. Select two of the following to meet the requirement for essential amino acids: 1 egg; 1 oz of meat, fish, or poultry.

Text continues on page 204

TABLE 8–7.   PROTEIN, SODIUM, POTASSIUM, PHOSPHORUS, AND CALCIUM CONTENT OF FOODS

Food Group	Amount	WT (g)	KCAL	CHO (g)	FAT (g)	PRO (g)	NA (mg)	K (mg)	PHOS (mg)	CA (mg)
MILK AND DAIRY										
Buttermilk	½ cup	123	44	6.3	0.1	4.4	159	172	117	1
Chocolate milk, made with whole milk	½ cup	125	101	13.8	4.3	4.3	59	183	118	1
Cream, half and half	½ cup	121	165	5.6	14.2	3.8	55	156	103	1
Evaporated whole milk, canned	¼ cup	63	87	6.1	5.0	4.3	74	191	129	1
Ice cream (10% fat)	¾ cup	100	196	20.8	10.5	4.5	63	181	115	1
Ice cream, rich (16% fat)	¾ cup	111	292	20.0	17.8	2.9	37	106	68	
Ice milk, hard	¾ cup	98	152	22.0	5.0	4.7	67	192	121	1
Low sodium milk	½ cup	122	75	5.4	4.2	3.8	6	307	105	1
Pudding, homemade	½ cup	128	171	26.8	5.5	4.3	78	199	122	1
Skim milk	½ cup	123	44	6.3	0.1	4.4	64	178	117	1
Sour cream	2 tbs	24	52	1.0	5.0	0.8	12	34	20	
Whipping cream, heavy, unwhipped	1 tbs	15	54	0.5	5.6	0.3	5	13	9	
Whole milk	½ cup	122	80	6.0	4.3	4.3	61	176	114	1
Yogurt, fruited, low-fat	½ cup	113	117	21.6	1.2	4.9	67	221	135	1
Yogurt, plain, low-fat	½ cup	113	71	8.0	1.7	5.9	79	265	163	2
NONDAIRY PRODUCTS										
Coffee-mate, Carnation	1 tsp	2	11	1.1	0.7	0.1	4	14	6	
Coffee whiteners, powder	1 tbs	6	33	3.3	2.0	0.3	12	48	24	
Dessert topping, frozen	1 tbs	5	13	1.0	1.0	0.0	1	1	1	
Dessert topping, powdered	1 tbs	1	6	0.5	0.4	tr	1	2	1	
Dessert topping, pressurized	1 tbs	3	8	0.4	0.7	0.1	4	4	2	
D-Zerta whipped topping	1 tbs	15	9	0.0	1.0	0.0	(2)	(0)	—	
Imitation sour cream	¼ cup	60	130	4.0	12.0	1.6	60	96	28	
Liquid cream substitute, frozen, average	¼ cup	60	85	7.0	6.0	0.8	48	116	40	
Polyrich liquid	¼ cup	56	87	8.0	6.0	0.2	12	44	20	
Rich's whipped topping	¼ cup	28	77	4.8	6.4	0.0	16	tr	0	
FATS										
Bacon, fried crisp	1 slice	8	44	0.2	4.0	1.9	77	18	17	
Butter	1 tsp	5	37	tr	4.1	tr	49	1	1	
Butter, unsalted	1 tsp	5	37	tr	4.1	tr	tr	1	1	
Cream cheese	2 tbs	28	107	0.6	10.6	2.2	70	20	26	
French dressing	1 tbs	16	67	2.8	6.2	0.1	219	13	2	
Lard, regular	1 tbs	13	117	0.0	13.0	0.0	0	0	0	
Margarine	1 tsp	5	37	tr	4.1	tr	49	1	1	
Margarine, unsalted	1 tsp	5	37	tr	4.0	tr	1	1	1	
Mayonnaise	2 tbs	10	71	0.2	7.7	0.1	56	3	2	
Salad dressing (mayonnaise type)	2 tsp	10	44	1.4	4.2	0.1	59	1	2	
Vegetable oil	1 tbs	14	122	0.0	13.6	0.0	0	0	0	
PEANUT BUTTER										
Peanut butter	2 tbs	36	202	6.0	16.2	8.0	194	200	122	
Peanut butter, low-sodium	2 tbs	36	183	4.0	15.0	8.0	2	174	110	

—Denotes lack of reliable data for a constituent believed to be present in a measurable amount.

Table continues on following page

TABLE 8–7.   PROTEIN, SODIUM, POTASSIUM, PHOSPHORUS AND CALCIUM CONTENT OF FOODS (Continued)

Food Group	Amount	WT (g)	KCAL	CHO (g)	FAT (g)	PRO (mg)	NA (mg)	K (mg)	PHOS (mg)	CA (mg)
BREAD										
Biscuit, baking powder, 1–2" diameter	1	28	103	12.8	4.8	2.1	175	33	49	34
Bread, French, ¾" slice	1 slice	25	72	14.0	0.8	2.3	144	23	21	11
raisin	1 slice	25	67	13.4	0.7	1.7	91	58	22	18
rye	1 slice	25	64	13.0	0.3	2.3	139	36	27	19
white	1 slice	25	68	12.6	0.8	2.2	127	26	24	21
whole wheat, cracked	1 slice	25	64	11.9	0.8	2.6	132	68	57	25
Bread, salt-free	1 slice	25	62	11.0	1.0	2.2	6	—	—	2
Corn grits	½ cup	123	61	13.5	0.1	1.4	1	14	13	1
Crackers, animal,	10	26	112	20.8	2.4	1.7	79	25	30	14
unsalted (Nabisco)	4	12	49	8.6	1.2	0.8	100	10	10	20
graham, plain (5" × 2½")	1	14	46	10.4	1.3	1.1	95	55	21	6
Doughnut, raised (small)	1	42	174	16.0	11.3	2.7	99	34	32	16
with icing (small)	1	37	154	21.7	6.5	2.1	160	29	61	13
Flour, wheat	2 tbs	17	61	13.0	0.1	1.8	1	16	15	3
Matzo	1 piece	30	116	25.4	0.3	3.0	tr	—	—	—
Muffin, corn	1	40	124	19.2	4.0	2.8	192	54	68	42
plain	1	40	116	16.9	4.0	3.1	176	50	60	42
Noodles, cooked	½ cup	80	99	18.7	1.2	3.3	1	35	47	8
Pancakes, from mix, 4" diameter	1	27	61	8.7	2.0	1.9	152	42	70	58
Pasta (macaroni, spaghetti)	½ cup	70	77	16.1	0.3	2.4	0.5	43	35	6
Popcorn, popped in oil	1 cup	6–12	42	5.0	2.0	0.9	1	36	17	1
Rice, white enriched, cooked	½ cup	102	109	24.8	0.1	2.1	tr	28	28	10
Roll, dinner, 2½" diameter	1	28	75	14.8	1.6	2.3	142	27	24	21
hamburger or hot dog bun	½	20	59	10.6	1.1	1.7	101	19	17	15
kaiser	½	25	77	14.9	0.8	2.5	157	25	23	12
Waffle, frozen (4" × 4" × ½")	1	34	86	14.3	2.1	2.4	219	54	71	41
English muffin	½	28	74	14.3	0.7	2.7	102	—	—	—
CEREALS										
Bran Flakes, Kellogg's	¾ cup	26	80	21.0	0.4	2.7	155	103	94	14
Captain Crunch, Quaker Oats	¾ cup	21	89	17.0	2.0	1.0	143	26	15	4
Cheerios, General Mills	¾ cup	19	73	13.2	1.3	2.6	195	62	86	26
Cocoa Krispies, Kellogg's	¾ cup	21	83	19.0	0.0	1.0	149	24	15	6
Corn Chex, Ralston	¾ cup	20	66	15.4	0.4	1.2	222	17	—	50
Corn Flakes, Kellogg's	¾ cup	16	73	14.3	0.0	1.1	162	20	6	1
Corn Flakes, salt-free	¾ cup	28	107	25.0	0.0	1.7	2	31	—	1
Frosted Flakes, Kellogg's	¾ cup	28	107	25.3	0.0	1.4	181	22	8	1
Kix, General Mills	¾ cup	19	79	16.1	1.0	1.4	—	—	—	2
Oatmeal, regular, cooked	½ cup	120	67	11.7	1.2	2.4	tr	73	68	11
Product 19, Kellogg's	¾ cup	21	80	17.8	0.2	1.8	310	17	30	4
Rice Chex, Ralston	¾ cup	19	74	16.7	0.3	1.0	161	21	19	3
Rice Krispies, Kellogg's	¾ cup	21	80	18.4	0.0	1.5	188	22	29	2
Rice, puffed, Quaker Oats	1 cup	14	54	12.6	0.1	0.9	1	15	25	3
Special K, Kellogg's	¾ cup	15	57	11.0	0.0	3.2	116	30	21	5
Sugar Corn Pops, Kellogg's	1½ cup	42	165	39.0	0.0	2.1	94	30	12	3
Sugar Smacks, Kellogg's	1 cup	28	110	24.5	0.3	2.2	34	45	40	5
Wheat, cream of, regular, enriched	½ cup	122	50	10.7	0.1	1.6	tr	11	14	5
puffed, Quaker Oats	1 cup	14	54	10.7	0.2	2.3	1	46	48	3
shredded, spoon-size, Kellogg's	½ cup	23	90	18.2	0.8	2.4	2	87	79	11
Wheaties, General Mills	¾ cup	21	83	17.0	0.7	2.2	236	—	77	10

Table continues on following page

TABLE 8–7.   PROTEIN, SODIUM, POTASSIUM, PHOSPHORUS AND CALCIUM CONTENT OF FOODS (Continued)

Food Group	Amount	WT (g)	KCAL	CHO (g)	FAT (g)	PRO (g)	NA (mg)	K (mg)	PHOS (mg)	CA (mg)
MEAT										
Beef, lean, cooked, rump	1 oz	28	56	0.0	2.6	8.1	20	91	68	3
Bologna	1 oz	28	85	0.3	7.8	3.4	369	65	36	2
Chicken, cooked	1 oz	28	52	0.0	2.2	8.0	23	113	77	4
Egg (large)	1	57	80	0.5	5.8	6.5	61	65	103	27
Frankfurter	1	45	137	0.8	12.4	5.6	495	99	60	3
Ham, lean	1 oz	28	51	0.0	2.5	7.1	254	79	56	1
Kidneys, cooked	1 oz	28	69	0.4	3.9	9.2	71	91	68	5
Lamb, lean, cooked, shoulder	1 oz	28	55	0.0	2.8	7.5	18	84	62	1
Liver, beef, cooked	1 oz	28	58	0.4	3.0	7.4	51	114	133	3
chicken, cooked	1 oz	28	44	0.9	1.2	7.4	17	43	42	3
Pork, lean, cooked, loin	1 oz	28	69	0.0	4.0	8.2	20	92	87	1
Sausage pattie	1 oz	28	127	tr	11.9	4.9	259	73	44	2
Turkey, cooked	1 oz	28	55	0.0	1.9	9.5	27	121	67	4
Veal, cooked, loin	1 oz	28	63	0.0	3.7	7.4	18	83	63	3
SEAFOOD										
Bluefish, cooked	1 oz	28	43	0.0	1.5	7.4	29	—	81	8
Clams, soft, raw, fresh, 4–5 small	¼ cup	37	29	0.5	0.7	5.1	13	85	66	—
Cod, fresh, cooked	1 oz	28	46	0.0	1.5	8.1	31	115	78	9
Flounder, cooked	1 oz	28	41	0.0	2.3	8.5	67	166	98	7
Haddock, cooked	1 oz	28	45	1.6	1.8	5.6	50	99	70	11
Halibut, cooked	1 oz	28	16	0.0	2.0	7.1	38	149	70	5
Lobster, cooked	1 oz	28	29	1.0	0.5	5.2	59	50	54	18
Ocean perch, cooked	1 oz	28	63	1.9	3.8	5.4	43	81	64	9
Oysters, raw, Eastern, 3–4 small, fresh	1 oz	28	18	1.0	0.5	2.4	21	34	91	27
Salmon, canned, low-sodium	1 oz	28	44	0.0	2.0	6.4	20	79	96	69
fresh, cooked	1 oz	28	50	0.0	2.1	7.7	33	126	117	—
Sardines	1 oz	28	56	0.2	3.1	6.8	233	167	141	124
Scallops, fresh, cooked	1 oz	28	30	0.0	0.4	6.5	74	133	95	32
Shrimp, cooked	1 oz	28	62	2.8	3.1	5.8	53	65	54	20
Tuna, canned, low-sodium	1 oz	28	35	0.0	0.2	8.4	12	80	57	5
oil-packed, drained	1 oz	28	39	0.0	0.7	8.1	174	55	66	2
Salmon, pink, canned	1 oz	28	37	0.0	1.6	5.3	188	101	80	55
CHEESE										
American cheese	1 oz	28	105	0.5	8.5	6.6	322	23	219	198
Cheddar (cellu) low-sodium	1 oz	28	109	0.0	9.0	7.0	10	150	140	12
Cheddar cheese	1 oz	28	113	0.6	9.1	7.1	198	23	136	213
Cheez-ola, reduced-sodium, low-cholesterol	1 oz	28	85	0.6	6.2	6.7	154	235	112	174
low-cholesterol	1 oz	28	85	0.6	6.2	6.7	412	30	277	174
Cottage cheese, creamed	¼ cup	61	64	1.8	2.6	8.3	140	52	93	58
dry-curd, unpacked	¼ cup	36	30	0.7	0.2	6.3	5	12	38	12
Swiss cheese	1 oz	28	104	0.5	7.9	7.8	201	29	160	262
Colby (cellu) low-sodium	1 oz	28	109	0.0	9.0	7.0	5	150	140	12
VEGETABLES										
Artichokes, cooked	1	250	52	9.9	0.2	2.8	30	301	69	51
Asparagus, canned, spears	½ cup	121	33	3.0	0.5	4.1	286	201	64	23
fresh, cooked	½ cup	90	23	3.3	0.2	2.0	1	165	45	19
canned, low-sodium	½ cup	118	30	3.6	0.4	3.1	4	195	63	23
frozen, cooked	½ cup	94	29	3.6	0.2	3.1	1	226	64	21

Table continues on following page

TABLE 8–7.   PROTEIN, SODIUM, POTASSIUM, PHOSPHORUS AND CALCIUM CONTENT OF
FOODS (Continued)

Food Group	Amount	WT (g)	KCAL	CHO (g)	FAT (g)	PRO (g)	NA (mg)	K (mg)	PHOS (mg)	CA (mg)
Beans, green, fresh, cooked	½ cup	62	19	3.4	0.2	1.0	3	95	23	32
canned, low-sodium	½ cup	68	18	3.3	0.1	1.0	2	64	17	31
frozen, cooked	½ cup	68	20	3.8	0.1	1.1	1	103	22	27
wax, canned	½ cup	68	20	3.5	0.2	1.0	160	64	17	31
wax, fresh, cooked	½ cup	63	17	2.9	0.2	0.9	2	95	23	33
canned, low-sodium	½ cup	68	17	3.2	0.1	0.8	2	64	17	31
French-cut, frozen, cooked	½ cup	65	21	3.9	0.1	1.0	1	88	20	25
Beets, canned, low-sodium	½ cup	85	34	7.4	0.1	0.8	39	142	16	16
fresh, sliced, cooked	½ cup	85	29	6.1	0.1	1.0	37	177	20	12
sliced, canned	½ cup	85	35	7.5	0.1	0.9	201	142	16	16
Beet greens, fresh, cooked	½ cup	73	18	2.4	0.2	1.6	55	242	18	72
Broccoli, fresh, cooked	½ cup	78	26	3.5	0.3	2.4	8	207	48	68
frozen, cooked	½ cup	93	31	4.3	0.3	2.7	14	196	52	50
Brussels sprouts, fresh, cooked	½ cup	78	34	4.5	0.3	3.3	8	212	56	25
frozen, cooked	½ cup	78	32	5.1	0.2	2.5	11	229	48	17
Cabbage, fresh, shredded fine	½ cup	45	12	2.5	0.1	0.6	9	105	13	22
fresh, cooked, wedge	½ cup	85	18	3.4	0.1	0.9	11	129	15	35
red, fresh, shredded fine	½ cup	45	17	3.1	0.1	0.9	12	121	16	19
Carrots, canned, low-sodium	½ cup	78	21	4.4	0.1	0.6	30	93	17	24
fresh, cooked	½ cup	78	27	5.5	0.2	0.7	26	172	24	26
raw	½ cup	28	13	2.7	0.1	0.3	13	97	10	10
sliced, canned	½ cup	78	26	5.2	0.3	0.6	183	93	17	24
Cauliflower, fresh	½ cup	50	71	2.6	0.1	1.4	6	148	28	13
Cauliflower, fresh, cooked	½ cup	63	18	2.5	0.2	1.5	6	129	27	13
Cauliflower, frozen, cooked	½ cup	90	21	3.0	0.2	1.7	9	186	34	16
Celery, raw or cooked	¼ cup	30	6	1.2	0.0	0.3	35	102	9	12
Chard, Swiss, cooked	½ cup	73	17	2.4	0.2	1.3	63	233	18	53
Collards, fresh, cooked	½ cup	73	27	3.6	0.5	2.0	18	169	28	110
Corn, canned	½ cup	83	81	16.4	0.7	2.2	195	80	41	4
canned, low-sodium	½ cup	83	73	14.9	0.6	2.1	2	80	41	4
fresh, cooked, cob 5″	1	140	82	16.2	0.8	2.5	tr	151	69	2
kernels, cooked	½ cup	83	81	15.5	0.9	2.7	tr	136	74	3
frozen, cooked	½ cup	82	76	15.5	0.4	2.5	1	152	60	3
Cucumber, fresh, peeled	½ cup	70	12	2.3	0.1	0.4	4	112	13	12
Dandelion greens, fresh, cooked	½ cup	105	41	6.7	0.6	2.1	46	244	44	147
Eggplant, cooked, diced	½ cup	100	22	4.1	0.2	1.0	1	150	21	11
Endive/Escarole, fresh, cut	½ cup	25	7	1.1	0.1	0.5	4	74	14	21
Great Northern beans, cooked, no salt	½ cup	90	109	19.1	0.5	7.0	7	375	133	45
Kale, fresh, cooked	½ cup	55	29	3.8	0.4	2.5	24	122	32	103
frozen, cooked	½ cup	65	24	3.5	0.3	1.9	14	125	31	78
Kidney beans, cooked	½ cup	128	117	21.0	0.5	7.2	4	336	139	37
dry, cooked	½ cup	93	113	19.8	0.5	7.2	3	315	130	35
Kohlrabi, fresh, raw	½ cup	70	25	4.6	0.1	1.4	6	261	36	28
fresh, cooked	½ cup	83	24	4.4	0.1	1.4	5	215	34	27
Lentils, dry, cooked	½ cup	100	108	19.3	tr	7.8	—	249	119	25
Lettuce, iceberg, chopped	½ cup	28	5	0.8	0.1	0.2	3	48	6	5
Lima beans, canned	½ cup	85	83	15.6	0.2	4.6	201	189	59	24
canned, low-sodium	½ cup	85	82	15.1	0.2	4.9	4	180	59	24
baby, frozen	½ cup	90	108	20.0	0.2	6.6	116	352	114	32

Table continues on following page

TABLE 8–7.   PROTEIN, SODIUM, POTASSIUM, PHOSPHORUS AND CALCIUM CONTENT OF FOODS (Continued)

Food Group	Amount	WT (g)	KCAL	CHO (g)	FAT (g)	PRO (g)	NA (mg)	K (mg)	PHOS (mg)	CA (mg)
Lima beans (*Continued*)										
fresh, cooked	½ cup	85	96	16.8	0.4	6.4	1	359	103	40
frozen, cooked	½ cup	85	86	16.2	0.1	5.1	86	362	76	17
Mushrooms, fresh	½ cup	35	10	1.6	0.1	1.0	5	145	41	2
Mustard greens, fresh, cooked	½ cup	70	20	2.8	0.3	1.5	13	154	23	97
frozen, cooked	½ cup	75	19	2.4	0.3	1.7	8	118	33	78
Okra, fresh, cooked, sliced	½ cup	80	28	4.8	0.3	1.6	2	139	33	74
Onions, fresh, chopped	½ cup	85	36	7.4	0.1	1.3	8	134	31	23
cooked	½ cup	105	33	6.9	0.1	1.3	8	116	31	25
green, fresh	½ cup	50	21	4.1	0.1	0.8	2	116	20	26
Peas, blackeye, canned	½ cup	128	92	15.8	0.4	6.4	301	449	143	23
blackeye, dry, cooked	½ cup	82	92	15.0	0.6	6.7	1	312	120	20
blackeye, frozen, cooked	½ cup	85	114	20.0	0.4	7.6	33	286	143	22
green, canned	½ cup	85	77	14.3	0.4	4.0	201	82	65	22
green, canned, low-sodium	½ cup	85	69	12.2	0.4	4.1	3	82	65	22
green, fresh, cooked	½ cup	80	59	9.7	0.3	4.3	1	157	79	19
green, frozen	½ cup	80	57	9.5	0.3	4.1	92	108	69	15
Peppers, green, fresh, cooked	½ cup	67	15	2.5	0.2	0.7	6	101	11	6
green, fresh, raw, diced	½ cup	75	20	3.6	0.2	0.9	10	160	17	7
Parsnips, fresh, cooked, diced	½ cup	78	55	11.6	0.4	1.2	6	294	48	35
Potato, baked	1 small	101	75	16.4	0.1	2.0	3	391	51	7
boiled in skin	½ cup	78	61	13.3	0.1	1.7	3	316	41	6
boiled without skin, diced	½ cup	78	52	11.3	0.1	1.5	2	221	33	5
French-fried	10 pcs.	50	140	18.0	6.6	2.2	3	427	56	8
Radishes, sliced	½ cup	58	11	2.0	0.1	0.6	10	185	18	18
Soybeans, dry, cooked	½ cup	90	125	9.7	5.2	9.9	2	486	161	66
Spinach, canned	½ cup	103	31	3.7	0.6	2.8	242	257	27	121
canned, low-sodium	½ cup	116	32	3.9	0.5	2.9	40	290	30	98
fresh, chopped, raw	½ cup	28	9	1.2	0.1	0.9	20	130	14	26
fresh, cooked	½ cup	90	24	3.3	0.3	2.1	45	292	34	84
frozen, cooked	½ cup	103	30	3.8	0.3	3.1	54	342	45	116
Squash, summer, fresh, cooked	½ cup	90	15	2.8	0.1	0.8	1	127	23	23
winter, fresh, cooked, mashed	½ cup	123	54	11.3	0.4	1.3	1	316	39	25
winter, frozen, cooked	½ cup	120	54	11.1	0.4	1.5	1	249	39	30
Succotash, frozen, cooked	½ cup	85	88	17.5	0.4	3.6	33	209	73	11
Sweet potato, canned	½ cup	100	109	24.9	0.2	2.0	48	200	41	25
fresh, cooked, mashed	½ cup	128	148	33.6	0.5	2.2	13	310	60	41
Tomato, fresh, cooked	½ cup	121	38	6.7	0.3	1.5	5	346	39	18
2" diameter	1	100	23	4.3	0.2	1.0	3	222	25	12
canned, low-sodium	½ cup	121	28	5.1	0.3	1.2	4	262	23	7
medium, fresh	1 slice	50	12	2.2	0.1	0.5	2	111	13	6
canned	½ cup	120	28	5.2	0.3	1.2	157	262	23	7
Turnip greens, frozen	½ cup	83	24	3.2	0.3	2.1	14	123	32	98
canned	½ cup	116	26	3.7	0.4	1.8	274	282	35	116
Turnips, fresh, cooked, diced	½ cup	78	19	3.8	0.2	0.6	27	146	19	27
Vegetables, mixed, frozen, cooked	½ cup	91	63	12.2	0.3	2.9	48	174	38	23
FRUITS										
Apple, fresh, medium, 2½" diameter	1	115	67	15.3	0.6	0.2	1.0	116	11	7

Table continues on following page

TABLE 8–7.   PROTEIN, SODIUM, POTASSIUM, PHOSPHORUS AND CALCIUM CONTENT OF FOODS (Continued)

Food Group	Amount	WT (g)	KCAL	CHO (g)	FAT (g)	PRO (g)	NA (mg)	K (mg)	PHOS (mg)	CA (mg)
FRUITS (*Continued*)										
Applesauce, sweetened	½ cup	128	125	30.4	0.3	0.3	3.0	83	6	5
Apricots, canned, halves, sweetened	½ cup	129	119	28.4	0.2	0.8	2.0	302	20	14
dried	½ cup	65	190	43.2	0.4	3.3	17.0	637	70	44
fresh	1	38	29	4.6	0.1	0.4	tr	100	8	6
Avocado, diced	½ cup	75	136	4.8	12.3	1.6	3.0	453	32	8
Banana, medium	1	175	113	26.4	0.2	1.3	1.0	440	10	5
sliced	½ cup	75	72	16.7	0.2	0.8	1.0	278	20	6
Blackberries, fresh	½ cup	72	47	9.3	0.7	0.9	0.5	123	14	23
canned	½ cup	128	125	28.4	0.8	1.0	1.5	140	16	27
Blueberries, fresh	½ cup	73	50	11.1	0.4	0.5	0.5	59	10	11
frozen	½ cup	83	51	11.2	0.4	0.6	1.0	67	11	9
Cantaloupe, cubed, fresh	½ cup	80	27	6.0	0.1	0.6	10.0	201	13	11
Casaba, cubed, fresh	½ cup	85	26	5.6	tr	1.0	10.0	214	14	12
Cherries, fresh, red sour, pitted	½ cup	78	51	11.1	0.3	1.0	1.5	148	15	17
fresh, sweet, pitted	½ cup	73	56	12.6	0.2	1.0	1.5	138	14	16
red sour, canned, pitted	½ cup	122	59	13.1	0.3	1.0	2.0	159	16	19
red sweet, canned, pitted	½ cup	113	113	26.4	0.3	1.2	2.0	162	17	20
Dates, chopped	½ cup	89	272	64.9	0.5	2.0	1.0	577	56	53
Figs, canned, sweetened	½ cup	129	119	28.4	0.3	0.7	3.0	193	17	17
fresh, medium	1	50	45	10.2	0.2	0.6	1.0	97	11	18
Fruit cocktail, canned, sweetened	½ cup	128	104	25.1	0.2	0.5	6.0	206	16	12
Grapefruit, fresh sections	½ cup	100	45	10.6	0.1	0.5	1.0	135	16	16
Grapefruit sections, canned, unsweetened	½ cup	127	95	22.6	0.2	0.8	1.5	172	18	14
Grapes, fresh (European —Muscat, Thompson, Emperor, Flame, Tokay)	1 cup	160	109	26.3	0.5	0.9	5.0	263	30	18
Grapes, fresh (American —Concord, Delaware, Niagara, Catawba)	1 cup	153	78	15.9	1.0	1.3	3.0	160	12	16
Honeydew, cubed, fresh	½ cup	85	32	6.6	0.3	0.7	10.0	214	14	12
Mandarin orange sections	½ cup	98	50	11.3	0.2	0.8	2.0	123	18	39
Melon balls, frozen	½ cup	115	76	18.1	0.1	0.7	11.0	216	14	12
Nectarine, fresh, medium	1	150	98	23.6	tr	0.8	8.0	406	33	6
Orange sections, fresh	½ cup	90	49	11.0	0.2	0.9	1.0	180	18	37
Papaya, fresh, cubed	½ cup	70	31	7.0	0.1	0.4	2.0	164	11	14
Peach, medium, fresh	1	115	42	9.7	0.1	0.6	1.0	202	19	9
canned, sweetened	½ cup	128	107	25.8	0.2	0.5	2.5	167	16	5
Pears, canned, sweetened	½ cup	128	104	25.0	0.3	0.3	1.5	107	9	7
fresh, medium, Bartlett	1	180	111	25.1	0.7	1.1	3.0	213	18	13
Pineapple, fresh	½ cup	78	45	10.6	0.2	0.3	1.0	113	6	13
canned, sweetened	½ cup	128	103	25.0	0.2	0.4	1.5	123	7	14
Plums, canned, sweetened	½ cup	136	119	28.9	0.2	0.5	1.5	184	13	12
fresh, prune type	2	60	48	11.2	0.2	0.4	tr	96	10	6
Prunes, pitted	½ cup	90	256	60.7	0.6	1.9	7.0	625	71	46
Raisins, packed	½ cup	83	266	63.9	0.2	2.1	23.0	630	84	51
Raspberries, red, fresh	½ cup	62	40	8.4	0.3	0.8	0.5	104	14	14
black, fresh	½ cup	67	55	10.5	1.0	1.0	0.5	134	15	20
red, canned	½ cup	121	47	10.7	0.1	0.8	1.0	138	18	18
red, frozen	½ cup	125	130	30.8	0.3	0.9	1.5	125	22	17
Rhubarb, cooked, sweetened	½ cup	135	199	48.6	0.2	0.7	2.5	274	21	106
Strawberries, fresh	½ cup	75	31	6.3	0.4	0.5	0.5	122	16	16
canned, unsweetened	½ cup	121	30	6.8	0.1	0.5	1.0	134	17	17

Table continues on following page

TABLE 8–7.   PROTEIN, SODIUM, POTASSIUM, PHOSPHORUS AND CALCIUM CONTENT OF FOODS (Continued)

Food Group	Amount	WT (g)	KCAL	CHO (g)	FAT (g)	PRO (g)	NA (mg)	K (mg)	PHOS (mg)	CA (mg)
Strawberries (*Continued*)										
frozen, whole, sweetened	½ cup	128	125	30.0	0.3	0.5	1.5	133	21	17
Tangerine, fresh, medium	1	116	45	10.0	0.2	0.7	2.0	108	15	34
Watermelon, diced	½ cup	80	24	5.1	0.2	0.4	1.0	80	8	6
FRUIT JUICES										
Apple juice	½ cup	124	60	15.0	tr	0.1	1.0	125	11	8
Apricot nectar	½ cup	125	77	18.3	0.2	0.4	tr	139	15	12
Blackberry juice	½ cup	122	49	10.0	0.8	0.4	1.0	208	15	15
Grape juice	½ cup	127	85	21.0	tr	0.3	2.5	147	15	14
Grapefruit juice	½ cup	123	49	11.3	0.1	0.6	1.0	200	19	11
Orange juice	½ cup	124	58	12.9	0.3	0.9	1.0	248	21	14
Peach nectar	½ cup	124	63	15.5	tr	0.3	1.0	97	14	5
Pear nectar	½ cup	125	52	12.0	0.3	0.4	2.0	49	7	4
Pineapple juice	½ cup	125	71	16.9	0.2	0.5	2.0	187	12	19
Prune juice	½ cup	123	101	24.3	0.2	0.5	2.5	301	26	18
Tomato juice, low-sodium	½ cup	121	23	5.2	0.1	1.0	3.5	275	22	9
regular	½ cup	121	23	5.2	0.1	1.1	243.0	275	22	9
SWEETS										
Cake, angel, 1½″ slice	1 slice	40	106	23.5	0.1	2.8	110.0	34	9	4
Cake, sponge, 2″ slice	1 slice	44	131	23.8	2.5	3.3	73.0	38	49	13
Chocolate chips, semi-sweet	1 oz	28	149	17.2	8.2	1.7	64.0	81	50	8
Chocolate squares, bitter	1 square	28	161	13.1	11.1	2.2	1.0	172	80	16
Cookies										
butter	5	25	116	17.8	4.3	1.6	105.0	15	24	32
gingersnaps	5	35	147	27.9	3.1	1.9	200.0	162	17	25
sugar	5	40	179	27.2	6.7	2.4	127.0	30	41	31
sugar wafers	5	48	232	35	9.2	2.3	90.0	28	38	17
vanilla wafers	10	30	139	22.3	4.8	1.6	76.0	22	19	12
Cranberry sauce	1 tbs	14	21	5.3	tr	tr	tr	4	1	1
Cupcake	1	47	175	29.8	5.5	1.6	107.0	29	35	24
Fruit ice, composite	½ cup	97	127	31.0	tr	0.4	tr	3	tr	tr
Gelatin, low-sodium, D-Zerta	½ cup	120	8.0	0	0	2.0	8	50	0	0
Gelatin, regular, flavored	½ cup	120	100	23.3	tr	1.7	55.0	91	5	2
Gumdrops	1 oz	28	100	24.5	0.2	tr	10.0	1	0	2
Hard candy	1 oz	28	110	27.6	0.3	0	9.0	1	2	6
Hershey's chocolate products										
Chocolate bar, almonds	1	32	182	15.7	11.9	3.1	28.0	137	80	68
Chocolate bar, plain, milk-chocolate	1	28	159	15.9	9.5	2.4	30.0	105	60	55
Chocolate kisses	6 pieces	28	148	14.6	9.0	2.2	22.0	112	87	56
Chocolate syrup	1 tbs	20	50	11.5	0.2	0.6	14.0	34	26	33
Cocoa powder	1 tbs	6	25	2.8	0.8	1.6	8.0	105	47	9
Krackel bar	1	40	197	21.1	11.4	2.6	64.0	146	96	72
Mr. Goodbar	1	50	281	26.0	16.5	7.2	30.0	225	145	65
Honey	1 tbs	21	70	17.3	0.0	0.1	1.0	11	1	1
Jams and preserves	1 tbs	20	56	14.0	tr	0.1	2.0	18	2	4
Jellies	1 tbs	18	51	12.7	tr	tr	3.0	14	1	4
Jelly beans	1 oz	28	106	26.4	0.1	tr	3.0	tr	1	3
Maple syrup, regular	1 tbs	20	51	12.8	0.0	0.0	3.0	26	3	33
Marshmallows, white	4 large	30	94	23.0	tr	0.4	12.0	tr	tr	4
Mints	10 pieces	7.3	27	6.5	0.1	tr	15.0	tr	tr	1
Table syrup (cane and maple)	1 tbs	20	52	13.0	0.0	0.0	tr	5	tr	3

Table continues on following page

TABLE 8–7. PROTEIN, SODIUM, POTASSIUM, PHOSPHORUS AND CALCIUM CONTENT OF FOODS (Continued)

Food Group	Amount	WT (g)	KCAL	CHO (g)	FAT (g)	PRO (g)	NA (mg)	K (mg)	PHOS (mg)	CA (mg)
SPICES, SEASONINGS, AND FLAVORINGS										
A-1 sauce	1 tbs	15	13	3.0	tr	0.3	246.0	51	—	3
Catsup, regular	3 tbs	30	35	7.6	0.2	0.6	312.0	108	16	6
Chili sauce, regular	2 tbs	34	38	8.0	0.2	1.0	456.0	126	6	4
Horseradish, prepared	1 tsp	6	2	0.5	tr	0.1	5.0	17	2	4
Lemon juice, fresh	1 tbs	15	5	1.2	tr	0.1	tr	21	2	1
Lime juice, fresh	1 tbs	15	4	1.0	tr	0.1	tr	16	2	1
Mustard, yellow	1 tsp	5	4	0.3	0.2	0.2	63.0	7	4	4
Vinegar, cider	2 tbs	30	6	1.6	0.0	0.0	0.0	30	4	2
Worcestershire sauce	1 tsp	5	4	0.9	0.0	0.1	49.0	40	3	5
LOW PROTEIN										
Arrowroot	1 tbs	8	28	7.0	0.0	0.0	4	1	0	0
Cornstarch	1 tbs	8	28	7.0	tr	tr	tr	tr	0	0
Low protein, anellini, Henkel, cooked	½ cup	110	92	22.8	tr	0.1	9	2	6	2
Low protein baking mix, Paygel, Henkel	¾ cup	100	405	83.0	8.0	0.3	55	10	48	5
Low protein bread, Henkel	½ cup	30	118	18.0	5.0	0.3	14	13	9	2
Low protein jellied dessert, Prono, Henkel	½ cup	120	56	14.0	0.0	0.0	5	77	0	29
Low protein porridge, semolina, Henkel, cooked	½ cup	100	68	17.0	tr	0.1	5	4	5	5
Low protein rigatoni, cooked	1 cup	130	108	26.9	tr	0.1	10	3	10	3
Low protein tagliatelle, cooked	½ cup	120	100	24.8	tr	0.1	10	2	11	4
ALCOHOLIC BEVERAGES										
Beer, average	12 oz	360	148	13.2	0	0.9	18	115	50	14
Cordials and liqueurs (54 proof)	1 oz	34	97	11.5	0	—	0	1	0	0
Wines										
Chablis	3½ oz	102	80	3.4	0	0.2	7	84	13	7
Rosé	3½ oz									
Burgundy	3½ oz	102	76	2.5	0	0.2	10	116	13	8
Sweet dessert	3½ oz	103	153	11.4	0	0.1	7	102		9
Gin, vodka, rum, whiskey	1 oz	28	70	—	0	—	0	1	0	0
BEVERAGES										
Coca-Cola	8 oz	240	96	24.0	—	—	20[†]	—	40	—
Sprite	8 oz	240	95	24.0	—	—	42	—	0	—
Mr. PiBB	8 oz	240	93	25.0	—	—	23	—	28	—
Fanta orange	8 oz	240	117	30.0	—	—	21	—	0	—
grape	8 oz	240	114	29.0	—	—	21	—	0	—
root beer	8 oz	240	103	27.0	—	—	23	—	0	—
ginger ale	8 oz	240	84	21.0	—	—	30	—	0	—
Sprite, sugar-free	8 oz	240	3	0.0	—	—	42	—	0	—
Mr. PiBB, sugar-free	8 oz	240	1	0.2	—	—	37	—	28	—
Fresca	8 oz	240	3	0.0	—	—	38	—	0	—
Tab	8 oz	240	0.5	0.1	—	—	30	—	30	—
Tab, black cherry	8 oz	240	2	tr	—	—	48	—	0	—
root beer	8 oz	240	1	0.2	—	—	42	—	0	—
ginger ale	8 oz	240	3	tr	—	—	47	—	0	—
orange	8 oz	240	1	0.0	—	—	43	—	0	—

[†]Value when bottling water with average sodium content is used (12 mg per 8 oz).

Table continues on following page

TABLE 8–7.   PROTEIN, SODIUM, POTASSIUM, PHOSPHORUS AND CALCIUM CONTENT OF FOODS (Concluded)

Food Group	Amount	WT (g)	KCAL	CHO (g)	FAT (g)	PRO (g)	NA (mg)	K (mg)	PHOS (mg)	CA (mg)
grape	8 oz	240	2	0.0	—	—	44	—	0	—
lemon/lime	8 oz	240	3	0.0	—	—	42	—	0	—
strawberry	8 oz	240	2	0.0	—	—	39	—	0	—
Shasta, cola	8 oz	240	95	26.0	0	0	4	2	26	*
lemon/lime	8 oz	240	93	26.0	0	0	37	2	*	*
root beer	8 oz	240	101	24.5	0	0	17	1	*	*
ginger ale	8 oz	240	78	21.3	0	0	14	—	*	*
cola	12 oz	360	143	39.0	0	0	7	4	39	*
black cherry	12 oz	360	158	43.0	0	0	36	—	*	*
cherry cola	12 oz	360	136	37.0	0	0	29	—	39	*
creme	12 oz	360	150	41.0	0	0	24	—	*	*
fruit punch	12 oz	360	168	46.0	0	0	30	—	*	*
ginger ale	12 oz	360	117	32.0	0	0	21	—	*	*
grape	12 oz	360	172	47.0	0	0	27	2	*	*
grapefruit	12 oz	360	158	43.0	0	0	21	—	*	*
lemonade	12 oz	360	142	38.0	0	0	—	—	*	*
lemon/lime	12 oz	360	139	38.0	0	0	55	4	*	*
orange	12 oz	360	172	47.0	0	0	30	10	*	*
root beer	12 oz	360	150	41.0	0	0	29	1	*	*
strawberry	12 oz	360	143	39.0	0	0	46	—	*	*
Diet Shasta, cola	12 oz	360	0.1	—	0	0	44	9	55	*
black cherry	12 oz	360	0.7	—	0	0	48	—	*	*
cherry cola	12 oz	360	0.7	—	0	0	53	—	55	*
creme	12 oz	360	0.1	—	0	0	50	—	*	*
ginger ale	12 oz	360	0.4	—	0	0	35	—	*	*
grape	12 oz	360	0.9	—	0	0	60	10	*	*
grapefruit	12 oz	360	1.9	0.5	0	0	50	—	*	*
lemon/lime	12 oz	360	0.2	—	0	0	49	18	*	*
orange	12 oz	360	0.3	—	0	0	52	13	*	*
root beer	12 oz	360	0.8	—	0	0	54	7	*	*
strawberry	12 oz	360	0.2	—	0	0	50	—	*	*
cola	8 oz	240	0.1	—	0	0	30	6	37	*
ginger ale	8 oz	240	0.3	—	0	0	24	—	*	*
root beer	8 oz	240	0.6	—	0	0	36	5	*	*
Pepsi	8 oz	240	105	26.4	—	—	6	9	37	tr
Diet Pepsi	8 oz	240	0.6	0.1	—	—	42	8	34	tr
Pepsi Light	8 oz	240	0.6	tr	—	—	28	8	18	tr
Mountain Dew	8 oz	240	118	29.6	—	—	21	6	0	tr
Teem	8 oz	240	107	24.8	—	—	21	tr	0	tr
Dr. Pepper	8 oz	240	96	24.8	—	—	18	2	27	6
sugar-free	8 oz	240	2	4.8	—	—	24	2	28	tr
Club soda	12 oz	360	0	0.0	0	0	78	1	0	18
Mineral water, Perrier	8 oz	240	0	0.0	0	0	5	0	0	33
Coffee, brewed	6 oz	180	3	0.5	tr	—	2	117	4	13
powdered instant	2 tsp	2	3	0.8	tr	—	1	72	7	3
Coffee substitute, powder	1 rd tsp	1.5	5	1.2	tr	0.1	1	24	7	1
Cranberry-apple juice drink	6 oz	190	135	34.5	1.0	0.1	13	53	4	10
Fruit punch drink	6 oz	190	99	25.2	tr	0.1	27	36	0	6
Pineapple-grapefruit juice drink	6 oz	187	95	23.8	0.1	0.4	41	103	7	11
Pineapple-orange juice drink	6 oz	187	99	23.9	0	0.4	6	90	7	9
Tea, brewed	8 oz	240	0	0.1	tr	—	19	58	10	5
instant, unsweetened, powdered	1 tsp	1	0	0.1	tr	—	1	50	4	0
instant, unsweetened, prepared	8 oz	241	0	0.1	tr	—	1	50	4	0

*Contains less than 2% of the U.S. recommended daily allowances of these nutrients.

Table continues on following page

TABLE 8–7. PROTEIN, SODIUM, POTASSIUM, PHOSPHORUS AND CALCIUM CONTENT OF FOODS (Continued)

Food Group	Amount	WT (g)	KCAL	CHO (g)	FAT (g)	PRO (g)	NA (mg)	K (mg)	PHOS (mg)	CA (mg)
Tea (*Continued*)										
instant, sweetened, powdered	3 tsp	22	86	22.1	0.1	—	13	49	3	1
instant, sweetened, prepared	8 oz	262	86	22.1	0.1	—	13	49	3	1
Awake, imitation orange juice	4 oz	125	67	16.7	0	0	7	63	—	—
Bright'N'Early	8 oz	240	133	29	1.0	0.1	1	1	—	—
Cranberry juice cocktail	8 oz	253	71	41.7	0.3	0.3	3	25	8	13
Grape Tang	8 oz	270	75	42.1	0.7	0.1	156	3	140	—
Hi-C (cherry, grape, orange, pineapple, or wild berry)	8 oz	240	130	32	0	0.4	2	3	—	—
Kool-Aid, regular	8 oz	240	100	25	0	0	1	1	18	1
Lemon Tang	8 oz	240	104	26	0	0	30	2	—	—
Lemonade, frozen, diluted	8 oz	248	114	28.3	tr	0.1	1	40	3	2
Limeade, frozen, diluted	8 oz	248	108	27	tr	0.1	tr	32	3	3
Orange Tang	8 oz	240	136	33.8	0.1	0	17	100	150	5
Start (instant breakfast drink)	8 oz	240	104	26	0	0	(47)	(47)	—	—

2. Use special low-protein products, *e.g.*, bread or pasta. These products can be difficult to obtain.

3. Use oligosaccharide products, such as Maltrin, Controlyte, HyCal, Polycose, Cal-Plus, Moducal, or Sumacal, or nondairy creamers to satisfy calorie requirements.

Unless considerable ingenuity and culinary skills are used, the diet is extremely monotonous and will not be discussed further.

RESTRICTED PROTEIN, 20 TO 25 G, MIXED BIOLOGIC VALUE. This diet is used with supplements containing essential amino acids, ketoacids, or both. It permits a wide variety of foods and is readily accepted by most patients. However, to be sure that caloric intake meets energy requirements, the aforementioned oligosaccharide supplements, special low-protein products, and nondairy creamers are employed. A moderate intake of alcohol is also a useful source of calories. Since both carbohydrate and fat intake tend to be high on this diet, margarine and vegetable oils are recommended to prevent excessive intake of saturated fats. Phosphorus intake is reduced by avoiding milk, milk products, and cheese. "Instant" beverages sold as powders and certain carbonated beverages are high in phosphorus and should be avoided. Adaptation of these restrictions to the patient's meal pattern and lifestyle, with continuing supportive education by a dietitian, will generally achieve excellent patient compliance.

CHRONIC RENAL FAILURE ON MAINTENANCE DIALYSIS

Goals and Rationale of Treatment

All patients with chronic renal failure who are on maintenance dialysis should receive dietary instructions. The goal of nutritional therapy for these patients is to minimize uremic symptoms and complications while maintaining a good nutritional status. Much of the rationale for dietary management of the predialysis patient, discussed earlier, also applies to the patient on regular dialysis; however, there are some important differences. Dialysis inevitably entails the loss of amino acids, peptides, and, in the case of peritoneal dialysis, protein. A single hemodialysis removes about 14 g of amino acids and peptides. During continuous ambulatory peritoneal dialysis, about 12 g of protein is lost daily. Furthermore, all forms of dialysis seem to increase protein requirements by an amount even larger than that accounted for by the external losses. Therefore, the protein intake of the dialysis patient must not be restricted. Another difference between predialysis and dialysis patients is that electrolyte intake, particularly sodium and potassium, becomes a critical factor in the management of dialysis patients.

Dietary Principles

For the patient on regular hemodialysis treatment, the usual recommendation for protein intake is 1 g/kg of "ideal" body weight/day (see Table A–10 in Appendix). Patients on continuous peritoneal dialysis should receive still more protein, usually 1.2 to 1.5 g protein/kg ideal body weight/day. Sodium restriction to less than 2000 mg/day is usually necessary in both groups. Tables 8–1 through 8–7 are used to guide dietary principles for the dialysis patient.

Energy intake should be encouraged in the underweight subject and restricted in the overweight subject, but severe caloric restriction is inadvisable. It should also be borne in mind that glucose is absorbed in substantial quantities during peritoneal dialysis (about 160 g/day).

Protein Modifications in Other Disorders

Mackenzie Walser, M.D.

HIGH-PROTEIN DIETS

Introduction

A protein intake above usual levels is indicated in several groups of patients, among them individuals suffering protein deficiencies of various origins, those undergoing weight reduction, those in hypercatabolic states, and those at risk to develop liver damage after jejunoileal bypass.

Goals and Rationale of Therapy

The major goal of a high-protein diet is correction or prevention of protein-deficiency states. Protein deficiency impairs many vital functions, including the maintenance of plasma colloid osmotic pressure, immune mechanisms, wound healing, coagulation, and erythropoiesis. Therefore, it is important to correct an existing protein deficiency as expeditiously as possible or to prevent its occurrence in patients at risk.

Patient Selection

High-protein diets are used in the prevention of protein deficiencies caused by external losses. In patients with the nephrotic syndrome, protein-losing enteropathy, and continuous ambulatory peritoneal dialysis and in some with enterocutaneous fistulas, significant quantities of protein are continuously lost externally. Protein deficiency may, therefore, develop. In such cases, protein intake should generally be augmented by an amount estimated to equal the external loss.

Another use for this diet is for the correction of protein deficiency. In protein-calorie malnutrition, as well as in isolated protein-deficiency states such as kwashiorkor, patients commonly require a high intake of calories along with protein replenishment.

Subjects undergoing weight reduction may also benefit from a diet containing a high proportion of protein. The use of the "protein-sparing modified fast" is discussed in Chapter 5.

Hypercatabolic subjects at risk of developing protein deficiencies may require a high-protein diet. Sepsis, trauma, burns, malignancy, and several related disorders are associated with increased catabolism of body protein as well as with increased energy utilization. Therapeutic strategies to limit protein catabolism, as well as the indications for employing these strategies, are still controversial. In these situations, the use of high-protein diets alone has not been generally advocated, since available evidence indicates that additional protein administered under such circumstances fails to correct the negative nitrogen balance. Furthermore, such patients are often anorexic or unable to eat. Enteral or total parenteral nutritional support is often utilized instead.

Finally, the diet may be indicated in subjects at risk of developing liver damage secondary to jejunoileal bypass. There is suggestive evidence that the hepatic dysfunction often seen after intestinal bypass operations for morbid obesity may be prevented or ameliorated by a high-protein intake in some individuals.

Dietary Principles

A high-protein diet is defined here as one in which protein intake is 20 per cent or more of the total caloric intake or is greater than 1.5 g/kg/day. This can be achieved either by increasing the proportion of protein foods in the diet or by adding a proprietary high-protein supplement (Table 8–8). The use of these protein supplements generally allows for lesser increases in salt, potassium, and acid loads than would the use of ordinary foods. The latter consideration is particularly important in patients with impaired renal function.

Severely protein-deficient patients often develop diarrhea or hyperammonemia when given diets containing high *proportions* of protein. Therefore, it is necessary to increase protein intake gradually, and diets containing a high percentage of protein are not commonly used.

TABLE 8–8. COMPOSITION OF ORAL AND INTRAVENOUS SUPPLEMENTS FOR THE TREATMENT OF PORTOSYSTEMIC ENCEPHALOPATHY

	Oral		Intravenous
	HEPATIC-AID (AMERICAN-McGAW) (G/PKG)	TRAVASORB-HEPATIC (TRAVENOL) (G/PKG)	HEPATAMINE (AMERICAN-McGAW) (G/500 ML)
Leucine	2.01	2.00	5.50
Isoleucine	1.04	1.67	4.50
Glycine	1.64	0.33	4.50
Valine	1.53	1.33	4.20
Proline	1.46	0.73	4.20
Alanine	1.40	0.57	3.85
Lysine (as acetate)	1.12	1.17	3.05
Arginine	1.10	1.17	3.00
Serine	0.91	0.00	2.50
Threonine	0.82	0.37	2.25
Histidine	0.44	0.33	2.20
Methionine	0.18	0.13	0.50
Phenylalanine	0.18	0.10	0.50
Tryptophan	0.12	0.10	0.33
Cysteine	0.00	0.00	0.10
Total amino acids	14.55	10.00	41.10
Carbohydrate	98.1	73.2	0.00
Fat	12.3	5.0	0.00
Calories	560.0	378.0	164.00

Major Dietary Modifications

In order for such diets to achieve a nitrogen-sparing effect, caloric intake must be adequate to meet energy needs. When neither salt retention nor renal dysfunction is present, this goal is best achieved by the use of ordinary foods. However, it may be necessary to approach the prescribed level of protein intake gradually, particularly in patients with poor appetites or protein malnutrition. In patients with salt retention or renal dysfunction, it may be preferable to employ an elemental diet in order to avoid excessive loads of sodium, potassium, phosphorus, or acid (see Chapter 3).

LOW-PROTEIN DIETS

Introduction

Protein intolerance and protein deficiency are both common in severe liver disease. Newer approaches to management of these patients include specific amino acid formulations.

Goal of Treatment

The primary goal of a low-protein diet is to control symptoms attributable to protein intolerance in patients with hyperammonemia or hepatic encephalopathy or both, without inducing protein deficiency.

Rationale for Treatment

Hyperammonemia may be caused by portosystemic shunting (most commonly due to cirrhosis) or by defective hepatic synthesis of urea. Impaired ureagenesis occurs chiefly with hereditary defects of the urea cycle enzymes, which are discussed in Chapter 13, and occasionally in acquired liver disease such as severe hepatitis or Reye's syndrome. Patients with the latter conditions generally cannot eat and must receive hypocaloric nutrition with glucose; they are rarely candidates for central venous alimentation.

Patients with portosystemic shunting are characteristically protein-intolerant. Protein loads increase the ammonia concentration of the portal blood; the ammonia load is shunted into the systemic circulation and then crosses the blood-brain barrier. Other substances derived from protein-containing foods during digestion, including aromatic amino acids, sulfur-containing amino acids, and amines—all of which are normally metabolized in the liver—contribute to the symptoms of protein intolerance in these patients. The symptoms include headache, flapping tremor, nausea, vomiting, confusion, lethargy, coma, and convulsions. Characteristic electroencephalographic changes are common. Blood in the gut (arising from bleeding esophageal varices, gastritis, or duodenal ulcer) is a common precipitating cause; blood has a high protein content of about 200 g/l. The fraction of gastrointestinal blood loss that is ultimately digested and absorbed depends on both the site and rate of bleeding.

Whether studied during acute episodes of encephalopathy or when relatively asymptomatic, patients with portosystemic shunts exhibit characteristic abnormalities of plasma amino acid concentrations. These changes include reduced branched-chain amino acid levels and increased levels of tyrosine, nonprotein-bound tryptophan, and methionine. Animals with experimental portosystemic shunts exhibit similar abnormalities in both the blood and the central nervous system.

The cause and exact significance of these abnormalities are uncertain. However, since branched-chain amino acids compete with aromatic and sulfur-containing amino acids for transport into the brain, it is rational to attempt to augment selectively circulating branched-chain amino acids in the hope of restoring brain amino acid levels toward normal.

To date, five well-controlled studies have reported on the use of parenteral branched-chain amino acids (or branched-chain amino acid–enriched solutions) in hepatic encephalopathy; each used different types of controls. Three studies demonstrated improvement (though the improvement in one was no greater than that seen in controls receiving lactulose). Only two of four well-controlled studies using oral branched-chain amino acids in chronic encephalopathy reported improvement after therapy.

The decision regarding whether to employ this mode of therapy, in the face of these contradictory results, is difficult. A short-term trial is probably justified, but long-term use, especially intravenously, may overcorrect the plasma amino acid pattern and should not be pursued unless there is clear benefit.

According to one report, administration of branched-chain ketoacids (as ornithine salts) can induce still greater benefit. Conversion of these ketoacids to branched-chain amino acids by transamination reduces the circulating levels of such urea precursors as alanine, glutamine, and glutamate. The ketoanalogue of leucine, α-ketoisocaproate, may also act directly on muscle to attenuate the accelerated rate of muscle protein degradation characteristic of these patients.

Usually, arginine levels are not decreased in the blood of encephalopathic patients. Nevertheless, because arginine and its precursor, ornithine, stimulate urea synthesis, supplementation with these amino acids has also been advocated in the therapy of portosystemic encephalopathy. While evidence of benefit from arginine or ornithine administration alone is lacking, mixtures containing high proportions of either of these amino acids, along with branched-chain amino acids or their ketoanalogues, have been helpful in some initial studies.

Patient Selection

Patients with hyperammonemia or acute or chronic portosystemic encephalopathy are candidates for treatment whether or not they are receiving other therapy, such as lactulose.

Dietary Principles

Provision of carbohydrate is important to minimize the catabolism of endogenous protein. In patients who are unable to eat, parenteral glucose infusion via a peripheral vein will serve this purpose in the short term. Nasogastric enteral alimentation via a small-bore tube has also been employed, evidently without risk of inducing hemorrhage from esophageal varices.

In patients who are able to eat, a low-protein diet is useful. The quantity of protein given should be as large as can be readily tolerated. In some cases this may be as little as 30 g per day, an amount that is inadequate to maintain nitrogen balance but that will help maintain energy balance. Vegetable protein is better tolerated than meat protein, which contains relatively high proportions of tryptophan and sulfur-containing amino acids. Patients who cannot tolerate a diet that contains adequate amounts of protein are candidates for amino acid or ketoacid supplements containing high proportions of branched-chain compounds and of arginine or ornithine.

Vitamin supplements are indicated for these patients. They are often vitamin deficient and also utilize vitamins poorly owing to defects in absorption and metabolic activation.

Major Dietary Modifications

40-G PROTEIN DIET.   A detailed description of this diet is given in Table 8–4. Substitution of vegetable protein for meat protein may be advantageous in patients with liver disease.

AMINO ACID AND KETOACID SUPPLEMENTS.   Three branched-chain amino acid–enriched products are currently marketed in the United States. Their composition is given in Table 8–1. According to the package inserts, recommended dosages are 15 to 60 g of amino acids (1 to 6 packages) daily for the oral products and 80 to 120 g (2 to 3 bottles) daily for the intravenous product. These doses are probably too high. It is essential that adequate carbohydrate calories be administered in conjunction with the intravenous product. Ketoacid-containing products are not yet available in the United States.

BIBLIOGRAPHY

Abel, R. M., Beck, C. H., and Abbot, W. M.: Improved survival from acute renal failure after treatment with intravenous essential L-amino acids and glucose. N Engl J Med 288:695–697, 1973.

Alfrey, A. C., Hegg, A., and Craswell, P.: Metabolism and toxicity of aluminum in renal failure. Am J Clin Nutr 33:1509–1516, 1980.

Alvestrand, A., Ahlberg, M., Bergström, J., and Fürst, P.: Clinical results of long-term treatment with low protein diet and a new amino acid preparation in chronic uremia patients. Clin Nephrol 19:67–73, 1983.

Anon.: 20-gram protein diet: 7-day menu for use with Aminess TM tablets. Cutter Laboratories, Berkeley, California, 1983.

Barsotti, G., Guiducci, A., Ciardella, F., and Giovannetti, S.: Effects on renal function of a low-nitrogen diet supplemented with essential amino acids and ketoanalogues and of hemodialysis and free protein supply in patients with chronic renal failure. Nephron 27:113–117, 1981.

Bergström, J., Fürst, P., and Noreé, L-O: Treatment of chronic uremic patients with protein-poor diet and oral supply of essential amino acids. I. Nitrogen balance studies. Clin Nephrol 3:187–194, 1975.

Blackburn, G. L., Grant, J. P., Young, V. R., and Wright, P. S. G. (Eds.): Amino Acids: Metabolism and Medical Applications. Boston: John Wright/PSG Inc., 1983.

Blumenkrantz, M. J., Kopple, J. D., Moran, J. K., Grodstein, G. P., and Coburn, J. W.: Nitrogen and urea metabolism during continuous ambulatory peritoneal dialysis. Kidney Int 20:78–82, 1981.

Brenner, B. M., Meyer, T. W., and Hostetter, T. H.: Dietary protein intake and the progressive nature of kidney disease: The role of hemodynamically mediated glomerular injury in the pathogenesis of progressive glomerular sclerosis in aging, renal ablation, and intrinsic renal disease. N Engl J Med 307:652–659, 1982.

Cerra, F. B., Cheung, N. K., Fischer, J. E., Kaplowitz, N., Schiff, E. R., Dienstag, J. L., Mabry, C. D., Leevy, C. M., and Kiernan, T.: A multicenter trial of branched chain enriched amino acid infusion (F080) in hepatic encephalopathy (HE). Hepatology 2:699, 1982.

Coburn, J. W., Hartenbower, D. L., Brickman, A. S., Massry, S. G., and Kopple, J. D.: Intestinal absorption of calcium, magnesium, and phosphorus in chronic renal insufficiency. In David, D. S. (Ed.): Calcium Metabolism in Renal Failure and Nephrolithiasis. New York, John Wiley and Sons, 1977, pp. 77–109.

Egberts, E. H., Hamster, W., Jurgens, P., Schumacher, H., Fondalinski, G., Reinhard, U., and Schomerus, H.: Effect of branched chain amino acids on latent portal-systemic encephalopathy In Walser, M., Williamson, J. R. [Eds.]: Metabolism and Clinical Implications of Branched Chain Amino and Ketoacids. New York, Elsevier/North-Holland, 1981, pp. 453-63.

Eriksson, L. S., Persson, A., and Wahren, J.: Branched chain amino acids in the treatment of chronic hepatic encephalopathy. Gut 23:801–806, 1982.

Fischer, J. E., and Baldesarini, R. J.: False neurotransmitters and hepatic failure. Lancet 2:75–80, 1971.

Fischer, J. E., Rosen, H. M., Ebeid, A. M., James, J. H., Keane, J. M., and Soeters, P. B.: The effect of normalization of plasma amino acids on hepatic encephalopathy. Surgery 80:77–91, 1976.

Fleming, L. W., Stewart, W. K., Fell, G. S., and Halls, D. J.: The effect of oral aluminum therapy on plasma aluminum levels in patients with chronic renal failure in an area with low water aluminum. Clin Nephrol 17:222–227, 1982.

Goldstein, D. A., Kleinman, K. S., and Swenson, R. D.: Current status of vitamin D metabolites in the treatment of renal osteodystrophy. Medicine, in press.

Greenberger, N. J., Carley, J., Schenker, S., Bettinger, I., Stamnes, C., and Beyer, P.: Effect of vegetable and animal protein diets in chronic hepatic encephalopathy. Am J Dig Dis 22:845–855, 1977.

Gretz, N., Meisinger, E., Gretz, T., Korb, E., and Strauch, M.: Low protein diet supplemented by keto-acids (KA) in chronic renal failure (CRF): A prospective controlled study. *In* Proceedings of the Third International Congress on Nutrition and Metabolism in Renal Disease, Marseille, France, September 1–4, 1982. Kidney Int (Suppl.) 16:348, 1983.

Heidland, A., and Kult, J.: Long-term effects of essential amino acid supplementation in patients on regular dialysis treatment. Clin Nephrol 3:234–239, 1975.

Heidland, A., Kult, J., Rockel, A., and Heidbreder, E.: Evaluation of essential amino acids and keto acids in uremic patients on low protein diet. Am J Clin Nutr 31:1784–1792, 1978.

Henderson, J. M., Millikan, W. J., and Warren, W. D.: Manipulation of the amino acid profile in cirrhosis with Hepatic-aid or F080 fails to reverse encephalopathy. Hepatology 2:706, 1982.

Herlong, H. F., Maddrey, W. C., and Walser, M.: The use of ornithine salts of branched-chain ketoacids in portal-systemic encephalopathy. Ann Int Med 93:545–550, 1980.

Holliday, M. A., and Chantler, C.: Metabolic and nutritional factors in children with renal insufficiency. Kidney Int 14:306–312, 1978.

Horst, D., Grace, N., Conn, H. O., Schiff, E., Schenker, S., Viteri, A., Law, D., and Atterbury, C. E.: A double-blind randomized comparison of dietary protein and an oral branched chain amino acid (BCAA) supplement in cirrhotic patients with chronic portal-systemic encephalopathy. Hepatology 1:518, 1981.

James, J. H., Ziparo, V., Jeppson, B., and Fischer, J. E.: Hyperammonaemia, plasma amino acid imbalance and blood-brain amino acid transport: A unified theory of portal-systemic encephalopathy. Lancet 2:772–775, 1979.

Kopple, J. D.: Nutritional therapy in kidney failure. Nutr Rev 39:193–206, 1981.

Maschio, G., Oldrizzi, L., Tessitore, N., D'Angelo, A., Valvo, E., *et al.*: Effects of dietary protein and phosphorus restriction on the progression of early renal failure. Kidney Int 22:371–376, 1982.

Moxley, R. T., III, Pozefsky, T., and Lockwood, D. H.: Protein nutrition and liver disease after jejunoileal bypass for morbid obesity. N Engl J Med 290:921–926, 1974.

Reiss, C., and Ahlberg, M.: Schwedendiat [Sweden diet]. Erlangen, Federal Republic of Germany, J. Pfrimmer Co., 1977.

Rossi-Fanelli, F., Riggio, O., Canhiano, C., Cascino, A., De Conciliis, D., Merli, M., Stortoni, M., and Giunchi, G.: Branched-chain amino acids vs. lactulose in the treatment of hepatic coma: A controlled study. Dig Dis Sci 27:929–935, 1982.

Slatopolsky, E., and Bricker, N. S.: The role of phosphorus restriction in the prevention of secondary hyperparathyroidism in chronic renal disease. Kidney Int 4:141–145, 1973.

Sofio, C., and Nicora, R.: High caloric essential amino acid parenteral therapy in acute renal failure. Acta Chir Scand (Suppl) 466:98–99, 1976.

Trowell, H. C., Davies, J. N. P., and Dean, R. F. A. (Eds.): Kwashiorkor. New York, Academic Press, 1982.

Vetter, K., Frohling, P.T., Kaschube, I., Gotz, K.-H., and Schmicker, R.: Influence of ketoacid-treatment on residual renal function in chronic renal insufficiency. *In* Proceedings of the Third International Congress on Nutrition and Metabolism in Renal Disease, Marseille, France, September 1–4, 1982. Kidney Int (Suppl.) 16:350, 1983.

Wahren, J., Denis, J., Desurmont, P., Eriksson, S., Escoffier, J. M., Gauthier, A. P., Hagenfeldt, L., Michel, H., Opolon, P., Paris, J. C., and Veyrac, M.: Is intravenous administration of branched chain amino acids effective in the treatment of hepatic encephalopathy? A multicenter study. Hepatology 3:475–480, 1983.

Walser, M.: Calcium carbonate–induced effects on serum Ca $\times$ P product and serum creatinine in renal failure: A retrospective study. *In* Massry, S. G., Ritz, E., and John, H. (Eds.): Phosphate and Minerals in Health and Disease. New York, Plenum Publishing Corporation, 1980, pp. 281–288.

Walser, M.: Nutritional support in renal failure: Future directions. Lancet, 1:340-342, 1983.

Walser, M.: Nutrition in renal failure. Ann Rev Nutr, 3:125-54, 1983.

Walser, M.: Therapeutic aspects of branched chain amino and keto acids. Clin Sci, 66:1-15, 1984.

Watanabe, A., Higashi, T., and Nagashima, H.: An approach to nutritional therapy of hepatic encephalopathy by normalization of deranged amino acid patterns in serum. Acta Med Okayama 32:427–440, 1978.

Weber, F. L., and Reiser, B. J.: Relationship of plasma amino acids to nitrogen balance and portal-systemic encephalopathy in alcoholic liver disease. Dig Dis Sci 27:103–110, 1982.

9
MINERAL MODIFICATIONS

Sodium Restriction

Mackenzie Walser, M.D., and
Gloria Elfert, M.S., R.D.

INTRODUCTION

Restriction of sodium intake is one of the most widely practiced and useful dietary modifications, but it is important that it be done judiciously.

The purpose of dietary sodium restriction is either to prevent or correct excess total body sodium or to maintain a moderately subnormal body sodium content in the treatment of hypertension.

RATIONALE FOR TREATMENT

Prevention or Correction of Edema

Retention of sodium and water is characteristic of congestive heart failure, hypoalbuminemic states such as the nephrotic syndrome and cirrhosis, chronic renal failure, and a number of other disorders. This problem must be differentiated from mechanical causes of edema for which dietary therapy is inappropriate. Apart from treatment of the underlying disease, the mainstay of therapy for edema is the use of diuretics, but the efficacy of diuretics is reduced unless accompanied by dietary sodium restriction. The degree of sodium restriction and the type of diuretic therapy are determined by weighing the feasibility and palatability of sodium-restricted diets against the risks and expense of long-term diuretic therapy. The efficacy of diuretics may be limited in states of severe sodium-retention; in these instances, sodium restriction becomes especially important.

212

Maintenance of a Moderately Subnormal Body Sodium Content

In hypertensive patients, a modest reduction in total body sodium content may cause a significant fall in blood pressure. Some hypertensive patients may, in fact, have a mild degree of sodium retention in the absence of edema.

DIETARY PRINCIPLES

The sodium intake of normal individuals varies according to individual preferences, cultural patterns, and cooking practices. Not only the choice of foods and manner of cooking but also the quantity of salt added at the table influences sodium intake greatly; many seasonings, such as monosodium glutamate, are high in sodium or contain NaCl. In addition, substantial quantities of sodium may be ingested in the form of bicarbonate of soda, proprietary antacids, and other medicinal products. Sodium intake can be mildly reduced to about 87 mEq/day (2000 mg) by eliminating both the use of these products and the ingestion of foods with a very high sodium content, by omitting the addition of salt or high-sodium seasonings to food, and by not using salt in cooking. An intermediate degree of sodium restriction to 43 mEq/day (1000 mg) requires, in addition, the omission of foods only moderately high in sodium content. Severe restriction to 22 mEq/day (500 mg) requires adherence to a very limited diet.

In the absence of abnormal rates of sodium loss, depletion of total body sodium content rarely results from dietary restriction alone. The kidney can decrease urinary sodium excretion to less than 1 mEq/day (23 mg); fecal excretion is negligible except in abnormal circumstances. However, when overzealous salt restriction is coupled with excessive diuretic therapy, dangerous sodium depletion can result. This may be manifested by hyponatremia, if plasma volume has been maintained by antidiuretic hormone, or by hypovolemia with its attendant signs and symptoms.

Although salt substitutes are often employed to improve the palatability of low-salt diets, most of these have a rather unsatisfactory taste, and some, especially those based on potassium, are dangerous. The ability to excrete potassium via the kidneys is critically dependent on sodium excretion. Those individuals with low rates of urinary sodium excretion are most likely to seek a salt substitute; they cannot excrete potassium readily and are therefore at risk for developing hyperkalemia when using such substitutes.

PATIENT SELECTION

The mild restriction regimen (to 2000 mg/day) is used for patients with early mild hypertension, for women prone to premenstrual edema, and for patients with mild congestive heart failure. It may also prevent hypertension in susceptible individuals, although this remains an unproven hypothesis. More severe restriction (to 1000 mg/day) is used for management of edematous states. Strict reduction of sodium intake to about 22 mEq/day (or 500 mg/day) is used only for refractory edema, as the palatability of this diet is poor.

MAJOR DIETARY MODIFICATIONS

Three levels of dietary sodium restriction are presented (Table 9–1). All of these diets require the elimination of:

1. Foods high in sodium content (see Table 9–2)
2. Medications containing substantial quantities of sodium
3. Salt- or sodium-containing seasonings added in cooking or at the table

Mild restriction can be achieved by these measures alone, provided that moderately high–sodium foods are not ingested in excess (group II foods—see Table 9–2). It should be noted that the outmoded practice of ordering a "no-added-salt" diet is to be deplored. Unless all the measures listed above are followed, adequate restriction of sodium intake cannot be achieved.

Moderate sodium restriction requires, in addition, ingestion of only group I meats and fats. However, some group II breads, cereals, vegetables, and milk are permitted.

Severe sodium restriction permits ingestion, almost exclusively, of group I foods. However, fruits, juices, and sweets are also permitted.

In Table 9–2, foods are listed in ascending order of sodium content. Foods are also arranged into exchange groups to facilitate planning of low-sodium diets at any prescribed level of sodium intake. Table 9–3 provides the average sodium content of each group. These averages may be helpful in planning a meal pattern for a low-sodium diet. Sample meal patterns are given in Table 9–4.

Text continues on page 224

TABLE 9–1.   THREE LEVELS OF DIETARY SODIUM RESTRICTION

Diet	Sodium Content		
	mEq Na/day	mg Na/day	mg NaCl/day
Mild restriction	87	2000	5000
Moderate restriction	43	1000	2500
Severe restriction	22	500	1250

TABLE 9–2. SODIUM CONTENT OF FOODS (IN ASCENDING ORDER)

Food Group	Measure	Weight (g)	Sodium (mg)
MEATS, FISH, POULTRY, NUTS, AND CHEESES			
Group I (Avg 30 mg sodium)			
Peanuts, walnuts, etc. (unsalted)	1 oz	28	1
Peanut butter, low-sodium	2 tbs	28	2
Colby cheese, low-sodium (Cellu)	1 oz	28	5
Cheddar cheese, low-sodium (Cellu)	1 oz	28	10
Tuna, canned, low-sodium	1 oz	28	12
Liver, chicken, cooked without salt	1 oz	28	18
Pork, lean, cooked without salt	1 oz	28	18
Lamb, lean, cooked without salt	1 oz	28	19
Veal, lean, cooked without salt	1 oz	28	19
Chicken, light meat, cooked without salt	1 oz	28	20
Salmon, cooked, low-sodium	1 oz	28	20
Beef, lean, cooked without salt	1 oz	28	21
Oysters, raw	1 oz	28	21
Turkey, light meat, cooked without salt	1 oz	28	23
Chicken, dark meat, cooked without salt	1 oz	28	26
Bluefish, fresh cooked without salt	1 oz	28	29
Turkey, dark meat, cooked without salt	1 oz	28	30
Cod, fresh cooked without salt	1 oz	28	31
Salmon, fresh cooked without salt	1 oz	28	33
Clams, soft, raw	2	28	34
Liver, calf, cooked without salt	1 oz	28	35
Sweetbreads, beef, cooked without salt	1 oz	28	35
Halibut, fresh cooked without salt	1 oz	28	38
Ocean perch, fresh cooked without salt	1 oz	28	50
Shrimp, fresh cooked without salt	1 oz	28	53
Liver, beef, cooked without salt	1 oz	28	55
Lobster, fresh cooked without salt	1 oz	28	59
Eggs, cooked without salt	1 medium	28	61
Clams, hard, raw	1 oz	28	62
Flounder, fresh cooked without salt	1 oz	28	67
Group II (Avg 90 mg sodium)			
Group I foods with ½ tsp salt/lb in cooking	1 oz	28	90
Kidneys, cooked without salt	1 oz	28	71
Scallops, fresh cooked without salt	1 oz	28	74
Bacon	1 slice	7	76
Group III (High-sodium)			
Salmon, pink, canned	1 oz	28	108
Cottage cheese	¼ cup	57	129
Crab, steamed	1 oz	28	137
Tuna, canned	1 oz	28	174
Peanut butter	2 tbs	28	194
Cheese, cheddar, natural	1 oz	28	198
Cheese, Swiss, natural	1 oz	28	201
Cheese, Parmesan	1 oz	28	208
Sardines	1 oz	28	233
Sausage	1 oz	28	259
Ham	1 oz	28	272
Crab, canned	1 oz	28	280
Cheese, American, processed	1 oz	28	322
Cheese, Swiss, processed	1 oz	28	331
Bologna	1 slice	28	369

Table continues on following page

TABLE 9–2.   SODIUM CONTENT OF FOODS (IN ASCENDING ORDER) (Continued)

Food Group	Measure		Weight (g)	Sodium (mg)
VEGETABLES				
Group I (Avg 6 mg sodium)				
Corn, fresh or frozen, cooked without salt	5″	ear	140	tr
Corn, fresh, cooked without salt	½	cup	83	tr
Asparagus, fresh or frozen, cooked without salt	4	spears	60	1
Beans, lima, fresh, cooked without salt	½	cup	85	1
Eggplant, fresh, cooked without salt	½	cup	100	1
Potato, fresh, peeled, cooked without salt	½	cup	77	1
Peas, fresh, cooked without salt	½	cup	80	1
Squash (composite), fresh or frozen, cooked without salt	½	cup	100	1
Beans, green or wax, frozen, cooked without salt	½	cup	68	2
Bean sprouts, fresh, cooked without salt	½	cup	63	2
Beans, green or wax, low-sodium, canned	½	cup	65	2
Okra, fresh or frozen, cooked without salt	½	cup	80	2
Parsley, raw, chopped	1	tbs	3	2
Chicory, fresh, cooked without salt	½	cup	45	3
Peas, low-sodium, canned	½	cup	128	3
Asparagus, low-sodium, canned	4	spears	118	4
Beans, lima, low-sodium, canned	½	cup	85	4
Corn, low-sodium, canned	½	cup	70	4
Cucumbers, fresh, peeled	½	cup	70	4
Rutabagas, fresh, cooked without salt	½	cup	85	4
Tomato, low-sodium, canned	½	cup	120	4
Tomato, fresh	1	medium	135	4
Kohlrabi, fresh, cooked without salt	½	cup	83	5
Lettuce, iceberg	1	cup	55	5
Mushrooms, sliced, fresh	½	cup	35	5
Tomato, fresh, cooked without salt	½	cup	121	5
Beans, navy, cooked without salt	½	cup	95	6
Cauliflower, fresh, raw or cooked without salt	½	cup	56	6
Parsnips, fresh, cooked without salt	½	cup	78	6
Pepper, green, fresh, cooked without salt	½	cup	67	6
Potato, baked with skin	1	medium	202	6
Endive, fresh	1	cup	50	7
Escarole, fresh	1	cup	50	7
Broccoli, fresh, raw or cooked without salt	½	cup	78	8
Brussels sprouts, fresh, cooked without salt	½	cup	78	8
Mustard greens, frozen, cooked without salt	½	cup	75	8
Onions, fresh, raw or cooked without salt	½	cup	95	8
Radishes, fresh	10	medium	50	8
Cabbage, fresh, shredded	½	cup	45	9
Cauliflower, frozen, cooked without salt	½	cup	90	9
Chinese cabbage, fresh	½	cup	38	9
Watercress, fresh	½	cup	18	9
Cabbage, fresh, cooked without salt	½	cup	72	10
Pepper, green, fresh, raw	½	cup	75	10
Brussels sprouts, frozen, cooked without salt	½	cup	78	11
Cabbage, red, fresh, raw	½	cup	45	12
Mustard greens, fresh, cooked without salt	½	cup	70	13
Peas, dried, split, cooked without salt	½	cup	100	13
Broccoli, frozen, cooked without salt	½	cup	93	14
Collards, frozen, cooked without salt	½	cup	65	14
Kale, frozen, cooked without salt	½	cup	65	14
Turnip greens, frozen, cooked without salt	½	cup	82	14
Collards, fresh, cooked without salt	½	cup	73	18

Table continues on following page

TABLE 9–2.   SODIUM CONTENT OF FOODS (IN ASCENDING ORDER) (Continued)

Food Group	Measure	Weight (g)	Sodium (mg)
Group II (Avg 40 mg sodium)			
Carrots, fresh, cooked without salt	½ cup	78	26
Turnips, fresh, cooked without salt	½ cup	78	26
Carrots, fresh, raw	½ cup	50	28
Artichokes, fresh, cooked without salt	1 cup	250	30
Carrots, low-sodium, canned	½ cup	78	30
Turnips, fresh, raw	½ cup	65	32
Black-eye peas, frozen, cooked without salt	½ cup	85	33
Succotash, frozen, cooked without salt	½ cup	85	33
Beets, fresh, cooked without salt	½ cup	85	37
Beets, low-sodium, canned	½ cup	85	39
Spinach, fresh, raw	1 cup	55	39
Spinach, low-sodium, canned	½ cup	116	40
Dandelion greens, fresh, cooked without salt	½ cup	100	44
Spinach, fresh or frozen, cooked without salt	½ cup	100	45
Sweet potato, canned	½ cup	100	48
Vegetables, mixed, frozen, cooked without salt	½ cup	91	48
Beet greens, fresh, cooked without salt	½ cup	73	55
Celery, fresh, cooked without salt	½ cup	75	63
Swiss chard, fresh, cooked without salt	½ cup	73	63
Peas and carrots, frozen, cooked without salt	½ cup	80	67
Celery, fresh, chopped	½ cup	60	75
Group III (High-sodium)			
Peas, frozen, cooked without salt	½ cup	80	92
Lima beans, frozen, cooked without salt	½ cup	90	116
Tomatoes, canned	½ cup	120	157
Beans, green, wax, canned	½ cup	68	160
Carrots, canned	½ cup	78	183
Corn, canned	½ cup	83	195
Lima beans, canned	½ cup	85	201
Peas, canned	½ cup	85	201
Beets, canned	½ cup	85	201
Dill pickle	1	135	1928

BREADS AND CEREALS

Group I (Avg 2 mg sodium)

Matzo	1 piece	30	tr
Popcorn, unsalted	1 cup	10	tr
Cereals, cooked without salt	½ cup	122	tr–1
Rice, regular or instant, cooked without salt	½ cup	102	tr–1
Puffed rice or puffed wheat cereal	1 cup	15	1
Macaroni, pastas, cooked without salt	½ cup	70	1
Noodles, cooked without salt	½ cup	80	5
Shredded wheat, biscuits	1	25	1
Corn flakes, low-sodium	1 cup	28	2
Crackers, low-sodium (Cellu)	4	20	2
Farina, instant	½ cup	122	5
Melba toast	2 pieces	8	6
Bread, low-sodium	1 slice	25	6

Table continues on following page

TABLE 9–2.   SODIUM CONTENT OF FOODS (IN ASCENDING ORDER) (Continued)

Food Group	Measure	Weight (g)	Sodium (mg)
Group II (Avg 125 mg sodium)			
Sugar Smacks, (Kellogg's)	1 cup	28	34
Sugar Pops, (Kellogg's)	1 cup	28	63
Raisin bread	1 slice	25	91
Graham crackers (5″ × 2½″)	1	14	95
Crackers (Nabisco), unsalted	1	11	95
Yeast doughnut	1	42	99
Hamburger bun	½	20	101
Hot dog bun	½	20	101
English muffin, (Thomas')	½	28	102
Pancake (4″)	1	27	115
Bread, white	1 slice	25	127
Dinner roll (2″ diameter)	1	28	127
Bread, cracked or whole wheat	1 slice	25	132
Bread, rye	1 slice	25	139
Cocoa Krispies	¾ cup	21	142
Cap'n Crunch, (Quaker Oats)	¾ cup	21	143
French bread	1 slice	25	144
Corn Chex, (Ralston)	¾ cup	20	147
Raisin Bran, (Kellogg's)	½ cup	25	147
Special K, (Kellogg's)	1 cup	20	154
Bran Flakes, 40%, (Kellogg's)	¾ cup	26	155
Saltine crackers	5	14	156
Kaiser roll	½	25	157
Rice Chex, (Ralston)	¾ cup	19	158
Biscuit	1	28	175
Plain muffin	1	40	176
Group III (High sodium)			
Corn Krispies	1 cup	28	189
Corn muffin	1	40	192
Cheerios	¾ cup	18	207
Cake doughnut	1	42	210
Waffle (4″ × 4″)	1	34	219
Sugar Frosted Flakes, (Kellogg's)	1 cup	37	242
Rice Krispies, (Kellogg's)	1 cup	28	251
Blueberry muffin	1	40	253
Corn Flakes, (Kellogg's)	1 cup	22	255
All-Bran, (Kellogg's)	½ cup	28	284
FRUITS AND JUICES			
Group I (Avg 2 mg sodium)			
Apples, fresh	1	115	1
Apricots, fresh	3	114	1
Banana, fresh	1	175	1
Berries, fresh (composite)	1 cup	145	1
Berries, frozen (composite)	½ cup	100	1
Cherries, sweet, canned	½ cup	135	1
Cherries, sweet, fresh	10	75	1
Dates, pitted	½ cup	89	1
Figs, fresh	1	50	1

Table continues on following page

TABLE 9–2.   SODIUM CONTENT OF FOODS (IN ASCENDING ORDER) (Continued)

Food Group	Measure	Weight (g)	Sodium (mg)
Grapefruit, sections	½ cup	100	1
Orange, sections	½ cup	90	1
Peaches, fresh or frozen	½ cup	115	1
Pineapple, fresh	½ cup	78	1
Watermelon	½ cup	80	1
Apricots, canned	½ cup	129	2
Berries, canned (composite)	½ cup	128	2
Cherries, sour, canned	½ cup	122	2
Cranberries, whole, fresh	1 cup	95	2
Cranberry sauce	½ cup	129	2
Figs, canned	3	80	2
Grapes, Concord, fresh	20	80	2
Grapes, Thompson, fresh	10	50	2
Orange section, mandarin	½ cup	98	2
Papaya, fresh	½ cup	70	2
Pears, canned	½ cup	128	2
Pineapple, canned	½ cup	128	2
Tangerine, fresh	1	116	2
Plums, canned	½ cup	136	2
Avocado, fresh	½ cup	75	3
Applesauce, canned	½ cup	128	3
Peaches, canned	½ cup	128	3
Fruit cocktail	½ cup	128	6
Nectarine, fresh	1	150	8
Cantaloupe, fresh	½ cup	80	10
Melon balls, frozen	½ cup	115	11

JUICES

Apricot nectar	½ cup	120	tr
Lemon juice	1 tbs	15	tr
Apple juice	½ cup	120	1
Blackberry juice	½ cup	120	1
Grapefruit juice	½ cup	120	1
Grapefruit-orange juice	½ cup	120	1
Lemonade, frozen, diluted	½ cup	120	1
Peach nectar	½ cup	120	1
Orange juice	½ cup	120	1
Cranberry juice	½ cup	120	2
Grape juice	½ cup	120	2
Pineapple juice	½ cup	120	2
Pear nectar	½ cup	120	2
Prune juice	½ cup	120	3
Tomato juice, unsalted	½ cup	120	4
Vegetable juice (V-8), unsalted	½ cup	120	4

Group III (High-sodium)

Tomato juice, salted	½ cup	120	250
Vegetable juice (V-8)	½ cup	120	250

DESSERTS*

Group I (Avg 50 mg sodium)

Water ice	½ cup	97	tr
D-Zerta gelatin	½ cup	120	8

*Desserts made from special low-sodium recipes average 2 mg sodium/serving portion.

Table continues on following page

TABLE 9–2.   SODIUM CONTENT OF FOODS (IN ASCENDING ORDER) (Continued)

Food Group	Measure	Weight (g)	Sodium (mg)
Sherbet	½ cup	97	10
Ice cream	½ cup	67	42
Vanilla wafers	4	16	50
Pound cake (homemade)	1 slice	30	52
Sugar wafers	4	28	52
Gelatin dessert	½ cup	120	55
Chocolate pudding (homemade)	½ cup	130	73
Animal crackers	10	26	79
Vanilla pudding (homemade)	½ cup	128	83
Oatmeal-raisin cookies	4	52	84
Group II (Avg 140 mg sodium)			
Cupcake, plain	1	33	99
Boiled custard	½ cup	132	104
Sponge cake	1 slice	66	110
Chocolate chip cookies	4	29	117
Boston cream pie	1 piece	69	128
Gingersnap cookies	4	28	160
Angel food cake	1 piece	60	170
Chocolate cake with icing	1 piece	75	176
White cake with icing	1 piece	78	183
FATS			
Group I (Avg 5 mg sodium)			
Vegetable oils	1 tsp	5	0
Butter, unsalted	1 tsp	5	tr
Margarine, low-sodium	1 tsp	5	1
Poly Perx	1 tsp	5	1
Coffee-Mate	1 tsp	2	4
Mayonnaise, low-sodium	1 tsp	5	6
Heavy cream (37%)	2 tbs	30	10
Light cream (31%)	2 tbs	30	11
Table cream (21%)	2 tbs	30	12
Sour cream	2 tbs	24	12
Group II (Avg 50 mg sodium)			
Cream cheese	1 tbs	14	42
Butter	1 tsp	5	46
Margarine	1 tsp	5	46
Mayonnaise or mayonnaise-type salad dressing	2 tsp	10	56
MILK PRODUCTS			
Group I (Avg 12 mg sodium)			
Low-sodium milk	1 cup	240	12
Group II (Avg 120 mg sodium)			
Chocolate milk	1 cup	250	118
Whole milk	1 cup	244	122
Milk (2%)	1 cup	246	122
Yogurt, partially skim	1 cup	245	125
Skim milk	1 cup	245	127

Table continues on next page

TABLE 9–2. SODIUM CONTENT OF FOODS (IN ASCENDING ORDER) (Concluded)

Food Group	Measure	Weight (g)	Sodium (mg)
Group III (High-sodium)			
Evaporated milk	½ cup	126	149
Buttermilk	1 cup	244	319
Condensed sweetened milk	1 cup	306	343
SUGARS AND SWEETS			
Confectioner's sugar	1 tbs	8	tr
Granulated sugar	1 tbs	12	tr
Popsicle, twin	1	130	tr
Honey	1 tbs	21	1
Syrup, maple	1 tbs	20	2
Jams and preserves	1 tbs	20	2
Jelly	1 tbs	18	3
Molasses, light	1 tbs	20	3
Brown sugar	1 tbs	14	3
Syrup, table	1 tbs	21	14
CANDY			
Jelly beans	1 oz	28	3
Hard candy	1 oz	28	9
Gumdrops	1 oz	28	10
Marshmallows	1 oz	28	11
Chocolate, milk with almonds	1 oz	28	23
Chocolate, milk	1 oz	28	27
Mints, butter	10 pieces	18	37
Fudge	1 oz	28	54
Caramels	1 oz	28	64

TABLE 9–3. AVERAGE SODIUM CONTENT OF VARIOUS FOOD GROUPS

Food Group	Sodium Content (mg)	Food Group	Sodium Content (mg)	Food Group	Sodium Content (mg)
MEAT, FISH, POULTRY, EGGS, NUTS, AND CHEESE		BREADS/CEREALS		FATS	
		Group I	2	Group I	5
Group I	30	Group II	125	Group II	50
Group II	90	Group III	>190		
Group III	>100			MILK	
VEGETABLES		FRUITS/JUICES		Group I	12
				Group II	120
Group I	6	Group I	2	Group III	>125
Group II	40	Group III	250		
Group III	165			SUGARS, SWEETS, LOW-SODIUM DESSERTS	2
		DESSERTS			
		Group I	50		
		Group II	140		

TABLE 9–4.   SAMPLE MEAL PATTERNS FOR LOW-SODIUM DIETS

Foods	500 mg Sodium		1000 mg Sodium	
	SERVINGS	SODIUM CONTENT (MG)	SERVINGS	SODIUM CONTENT (MG)
BREAKFAST				
Fruit/Juice	As desired	2	As desired	2
Bread/Cereal	2 from group I	4	2 (1 from group I, 1 from group II)	2 / 125
Meat	1 from group I	30	1 from group I	30
Fat	2 from group I	10	2 from group I	10
Milk	1 from group II	120	1 from group II	120
Sweets	As desired from group I		As desired from group I	
Breakfast Totals		166		289
LUNCH				
Meat	2 from group I	60	2 from group I	60
Vegetables	2 from group I	12	2 (1 from group I, 1 from group II)	6 / 40
Bread/Cereal	2 from group I	4	2 from group II	250
Fat	2 from group I	10	2 from group I	10
Fruit/Special Lo-Na Dessert*	As desired	2	As desired	2
Desserts	—		—	
Sweets	As desired from group I		As desired from group I	
Lunch Totals		88		368
DINNER				
Meat	3 from group I	90	3 from group I	90
Vegetables	2 from group I	12	2 (1 from group I, 1 from group II)	6 / 40
Bread/Cereal	2 from group I	4	2 from group II	4
Fat	3 from group I	15	3 from group I	15
Fruit/Special Lo-Na Desserts*	As desired	2	As desired	2
Desserts	—		1 from group I	70
Milk	1 from group 2	120	1 from group II	120
Sweets	As desired from group I		As desired from group I	
Dinner Totals		243		347
GRAND TOTALS		497		1004

*Low-sodium desserts that contain 2 mg or less sodium per serving.

1500 mg Sodium		2000 mg Sodium	
SERVINGS	SODIUM CONTENT (MG)	SERVINGS	SODIUM CONTENT (MG)
As desired	2	As desired	2
2 (1 from group I,			
1 from group II)	125	2 from group II	250
1 from group I	30	1 from group I	30
2 from group II	100	2 from group II	100
1 from group II	120	1 from group II	120
As desired from		As desired from	
group I		group I	
	377		502
2 from group I	60	2 from group I	60
2 from group I or II	80	2 from group I or II	80
2 from group II	250	2 from group II	250
2 from group II	100	2 from group II	100
As desired	2	As desired	2
—		1 from group I	70
As desired from		As desired from	
group I		group I	
	492		562
3 from group I	90	3 from group I	90
2 from group I or II	80	2 (1 from group I or II,	
		1 from group II or III)	205
2 (1 from group I,	2		
1 from group II)	125	2 from group II	250
3 from group II	150	3 from group II	150
As desired	2	As desired	2
1 from group I	70	1 from group I or II	140
1 from group II	120	1 from group II	120
As desired from		As desired from	
group I		group I	
	639		957
	1508		2021

Potassium

Mackenzie Walser, M.D.

INTRODUCTION

A relatively small group of patients will benefit from dietary potassium restriction. This group includes those whose conditions cause potassium retention, hyperkalemia, or both.

GOAL AND RATIONALE OF TREATMENT

Several measures can be used in the long-term management of patients who are prone to potassium retention. High-potassium foods should be avoided by all such patients. Potassium-binding resins, such as Kayexalate, or diuretics that augment the renal excretion of potassium can also be used. In selecting a method of treatment, the inconvenience and poor palatability of a low-potassium diet and the likelihood of poor patient compliance must be weighed against the possible side effects and expense associated with the use of resins or diuretics. Whenever hyperkalemia becomes pronounced (more than 7 mEq/l), the risk of sudden cardiac arrest necessitates immediate institution of measures to lower the serum potassium level very rapidly. (Dietary restriction is not effective in lowering the serum potassium promptly.)

PATIENT SELECTION

Conditions that may result in potassium retention or hyperkalemia or both include acute or chronic renal failure, adrenocortical insufficiency, and metabolic acidosis. The latter two disorders are managed by treatment of the underlying disease, but renal failure is often treated by restriction of dietary potassium.

DIETARY PRINCIPLES

The potassium intake of normal individuals is usually between 60 and 100 mEq/day (2346 to 3910 mg/day) and is less variable than sodium intake. When potassium restriction is indicated, dietary limitation to 40 mEq/day (1564 mg/day) is reasonable. More severe potassium restriction is not generally employed, because it entails simultaneous restriction of protein intake to possibly inadequate levels. Patients on low-potassium diets should avoid salt substitutes containing potassium chloride.

Potassium depletion is a theoretical hazard when potassium-restricted diets are used. However, potassium depletion is rarely a clinical problem in the absence of specific transport abnormalities in the kidney or intestine; the renal capability for potassium conservation is comparable to that of sodium.

MAJOR DIETARY MODIFICATIONS

Sample meal patterns for various potassium-restricted diets are given in Tables 8–3 and 8–4. The renal exchange lists in Chapter 8, Tables 8–5 and 8–6, give the actual potassium content of many foods and may be used in planning a specific dietary pattern. Commonly ingested foods with a relatively high potassium content include tomatoes, bananas, citrus fruits, and potatoes.

Calcium
Mackenzie Walser, M.D.

INTRODUCTION

Calcium-restricted diets are seldom employed; avoidance of a high calcium intake is recommended in some patients who form urinary calculi. Calcium supplementation, on the other hand, is widely recommended by some authorities.

GOALS AND RATIONALE OF TREATMENT

The goals of calcium restriction treatment include the control of serum calcium levels in patients prone to hypercalcemia and the reduction of urinary excretion of calcium in subjects with recurrent calcific nephrolithiasis. In calcific nephrolithiasis, severe restriction of calcium intake is usually ineffective in preventing recurrences. On the other hand, a high calcium intake could theoretically increase the risk of recurrence. Similarly, while other measures are generally more effective in patients prone to develop hypercalcemia, a high intake of calcium is obviously undesirable. There is some evidence that an increase in calcium intake in older persons, especially women, may reduce the likelihood of developing osteoporosis.

DIETARY PRINCIPLES AND MAJOR DIETARY MODIFICATIONS

Patients with calcific nephrolithiasis should limit calcium intake to 1 g/day and avoid medications containing calcium, such as calcium carbonate. In an attempt to prevent osteoporosis in older individuals, intake of high-calcium foods

TABLE 9–5.   FOODS TO BE AVOIDED ON A LOW-CALCIUM DIET

Food	Amount	Weight or Volume	Calcium (mg)
Milk (avg)	1 cup	240 ml	290
Ice cream	¾ cup	100 g	145
Cheddar cheese	1 ounce	28 g	213
Cottage cheese	½ cup	120 g	116
Cream, half and half	½ cup	121 g	131

such as milk and milk products may be increased. In subjects who dislike or cannot tolerate milk, a dose of a calcium salt, such as calcium carbonate, 0.5 g/day, can be used instead.

The foods listed in Table 9–5 should be avoided or severely restricted in patients on a low-calcium diet. The calcium content of various foods is given in the renal exchange lists in Chapter 8, Table 8–6. These values may be used in planning a restricted calcium diet.

Phosphorus

Mackenzie Walser, M.D., and Elizabeth C. Chandler, B. Sc., R.D.

INTRODUCTION

Dietary restriction of phosphorus has been employed with increasing frequency in recent years, as the danger of hyperphosphatemia and the problems associated with the use of basic aluminum salts to reduce phosphate absorption have become more generally recognized.

GOAL AND RATIONALE OF TREATMENT

The goal of dietary phosphorus restriction is to minimize phosphorus accumulation in individuals prone to develop hyperphosphatemia, a problem seen primarily in patients with hypoparathyroidism or renal failure. In patients with hypoparathyroidism, drugs are more effective than dietary means for controlling serum calcium and phosphorus, and there is little evidence that hyperphosphatemia is, in itself, harmful. This is probably because the product of serum calcium × phosphorus concentrations—a product that is directly related to the tendency for soft-tissue calcification to occur—is not significantly elevated in hypoparathyroidism. In contrast, in renal failure, the product is usually increased despite the presence of hypocalcemia. This pattern is deleterious in two ways:

1. Hypocalcemia, caused in part by hyperphosphatemia, leads to secondary hyperparathyroidism, which is believed to cause many of the signs and symptoms of uremic toxicity, as well as some forms of renal osteodystrophy.

2. Renal deposition of calcium and phosphate may play a role in the progression of chronic renal failure and in the pathogenesis of acute renal failure. Such deposition is clearly promoted by a high calcium-phosphorus product as well as by high levels of parathyroid hormone.

PATIENT SELECTION

Patients with hypoparathyroidism or renal failure who have hyperphosphatemia are appropriate candidates for a low-phosphorus diet. According to some, phosphorus restriction may be useful even when serum phosphate levels are normal.

DIETARY PRINCIPLES

The oral administration of basic aluminum salts has been the therapeutic mainstay for management of the hyperphosphatemia of chronic renal failure. However, the efficacy of this treatment is substantially improved when high-phosphorus foods are avoided.

The normal phosphorus intake in the United States is about 1.5 g/day. A practical goal for restriction of phosphorus is 700 to 800 mg/day; this entails simultaneous protein restriction to the RDA—about 50 g/day. More severe restriction of phosphorus intake can be achieved only when purified amino acids replace some dietary protein.

There are some dangers associated with phosphorus restriction. Negative phosphorus balance is not readily induced in normal subjects by dietary restriction alone, as the normal kidney can conserve phosphorus very efficiently. However, clinically significant hypophosphatemia (less than 2 mg/dl) can occur in the absence of abnormal external losses when nitrogen balance is positive or when carbohydrate is infused parenterally in large amounts; under both of these circumstances, phosphate shifts into cells. Patients with chronic renal failure who are following low-phosphorus diets and using aluminum-containing preparations may develop hypophosphatemia. A possible additional hazard of phosphorus depletion in most patients is the aggravation of renal osteodystrophy.

MAJOR DIETARY MODIFICATIONS

Since phosphate restriction usually entails simultaneous protein restriction, the limiting factor in reducing dietary phosphate is the phosphorus content of

TABLE 9–6.　AVERAGE PHOSPHORUS CONTENT OF FOODS PER GRAM OF PROTEIN

Protein Source	Phosphorus (mg/g protein)
Milk, cream, ice cream, nuts	30
Cheeses (other than cottage)	20
Egg, meat, fish, bread (other than whole grain), potato, rice, pastas, vegetables	15
Cottage cheese	10
Fruit	3

foods per gram of protein. Table 9–6 lists the average phosphorus content of five major food categories in relation to their protein content. It is also important to avoid phosphate-containing medications, such as Neutra-Phos, Fleet's Phospho-Soda, K-Phos, and instant beverages sold as powders, many of which contain substantial amounts of phosphate.

Table 9–7 shows a sample diet in which phosphorus intake is restricted to 700 to 800 mg/day; this diet entails simultaneous restriction of protein to 50 g/day. In addition, sample meal patterns for diets with phosphorus contents rang-

TABLE 9–7.　PHOSPHORUS-CONTROLLED DIET (50 G PROTEIN, 700–800 MG PHOSPHORUS)*

Food Groups	Servings Daily	Foods Included	Foods Excluded
Milk	0	Specified nondairy cream products.	Milk, yogurt, ice cream.
Meat, fish, poultry, cottage cheese	3 oz	All varieties.	All in excess of allowed amounts. Cheeses other than cottage, cream, pot.
Egg	1		
Bread, cereal, potato, or alternate	7		Whole-grain cereals or breads. Quick breads— e.g., cornbread, pancakes, any products containing bran.
Vegetables	4		Dried beans, peas.
Fruit	6	All.	None.
Fats	As desired	All.	None.
Sweets, desserts	As desired	Jelly, sugars, hard candy, Italian or water-ice popsicles.	Any made with milk.
Beverages		Coffee, tea, carbonated beverages other than cola drinks.	Any made with milk, cola beverages, powdered fruit beverage mixes.
Soups	None		
Miscellaneous		All spices and herbs, vinegar, flavoring extracts.	

*If dietary protein is reduced further, phosphorus intake will also be decreased. For example, a 40-g protein diet decreases phosphorus intake to 500–650 mg.

ing from 350 to 1070 mg are given in Chapter 8, Table 8–4. The renal exchange lists in Chapter 8, Tables 8–6 and 8–7, give the phosphorus content of many foods and may be used to plan diets requiring phosphorus restriction.

Iron

Mackenzie Walser, M.D.

INTRODUCTION

Iron is an essential mineral chiefly because it is a constituent of the heme molecule, which plays a central role in oxygen and electron transport. Total body iron, about 50 mg/kg in men and 35 mg/kg in women, is mostly contained in hemoglobin, myoglobin, cytochromes, and various enzymes. The amount of nonheme, or storage iron, ranges from 10 to 35 per cent of the total body iron but may be less in women.

Body stores of iron are efficiently conserved under normal circumstances. At least 40 mg of iron per day are utilized in synthesis of hemoglobin and other heme-containing proteins, but most of the iron so utilized is derived from the breakdown of these same proteins. In adult men, iron excretion amounts to only about 1 mg/day. Menstrual losses of iron vary widely, ranging from 10 to 60 mg/month (0.3 to 2.0 mg/day). This route of iron loss is reduced in women using oral contraceptives but is increased by intrauterine contraceptive devices.

IRON REQUIREMENTS

From these data, it is evident that the iron requirement is about 1 mg/day in normal adult males and nonmenstruating females and 2 or 3 mg/day in menstruating females (Table 9–8). Additional iron is required during pregnancy (see

TABLE 9–8.   IRON REQUIREMENTS

Group	Absorbed Iron (mg/day)
Adult males and nonmenstruating females	1
Menstruating females	2–3
Pregnancy	2–4
Growing boys	1–2
Growing girls	1–2
Infants	1.0–1.5

Chapter 1, section on nutrition in pregnancy) and for growth in children. The requirement of infants is from 1.0 to 1.5 mg/day. (All of these values refer to absorbed iron, which constitutes only a fraction of the dietary iron.)

IRON DEFICIENCY

The prevalence of iron deficiency is alarming. For example, a substantial proportion of healthy young women in the United States has been found to be iron-deficient. Premature infants are invariably iron-deficient unless they receive supplementation. In developing countries, especially those where hookworm infestation is common, a large majority of the population may be iron-deficient.

In the absence of anemia, there is no conclusive proof that iron deficiency causes any disability, although it may cause fatigue. However, anemia is extremely common in iron-deficient subjects; the diagnosis is often overlooked because the hypochromic microcytic erythrocytes of full-blown iron-deficiency anemia are not usually seen in mildly iron-deficient subjects. During an iron-deficiency state, the circulating concentrations of iron bound to specific proteins —namely, ferritin and transferrin—decrease. The first biochemical sign of iron-deficiency is a reduction in serum ferritin to below 12 mg/l. Later, serum iron decreases and there is an increase in iron-binding capacity, i.e., reduced saturation of transferrin (less than 16 per cent). When hemoglobin synthesis becomes impaired, erythrocyte protoporphyrin (the precursor of heme) rises, and soon anemia becomes manifest. The clinical picture of frank iron deficiency is well known and will not be considered here. Absorption of lead is increased in iron-deficient animals; hence, iron deficiency may contribute to the incidence of lead poisoning in exposed persons.

The causes of iron deficiency are numerous. Inadequate intake, impaired absorption, blood loss, and pregnancy are the most common. Impaired absorption of iron is seen in clay-eaters, various malabsorption syndromes, chronic diarrheal disorders, and after partial gastrectomy. Blood loss may result from excessive menstrual bleeding, occult gastrointestinal losses such as those secondary to anti-inflammatory drugs, repeated blood donations, or regular hemodialysis.

Treatment of iron deficiency should be directed at identification and elimination of the underlying cause and should include supplementation with iron. Dietary supplementation, such as by frequent feedings of liver, is impractical; hence, ferrous salts must be administered. About 50 mg/day of absorbed iron will provide sufficient iron for maximal hemoglobin synthesis. Since about 20 per cent of the iron content of the various medicinal ferrous salts is absorbed, a daily dose of about 250 mg/day of elemental iron is usually prescribed. All such supplements are associated with upper gastrointestinal complaints in about one-quarter of patients.

The duration of therapy required for correction of an iron deficiency obviously depends on the magnitude of the deficit but generally requires several months. No more than a 1-month supply of iron supplements should be kept in the home because of the danger of accidental poisoning. Iron deficiency is often recurrent unless special efforts are made to eliminate the cause.

Prevention of Iron Deficiency

The Committee on Nutrition of the American Academy of Pediatrics has recommended that supplemental iron from one or more sources be provided no later than 4 months of age in term infants and no later than 2 months of age in preterm infants. This is best accomplished by the use of iron-fortified formula or, in breast-fed infants, iron-fortified cereal. The dose should not exceed 1 mg/kg/day for preterm infants, up to a maximum of 15 mg/day.

It is difficult to prevent iron deficiency in menstruating women by fortifying foods, since few iron-fortified foods are consumed regularly by this entire population. Clearly, attempts must be made to increase either the amount of iron in the diet or its bioavailability. The proportion of women of childbearing age taking iron-containing preparations has steadily increased and may now exceed one-third.

Recommendations for iron supplementation of vegetarian diets are discussed in the section on the vegetarian diet in Chapter 1.

IRON EXCESS

Since there is no mechanism for excreting excesses of iron, absorption of excessive quantities of oral iron or parenteral injection of excess iron (usually secondary to multiple transfusions) can cause iron overload even in normal persons. Absorption may be excessive when iron supplements are administered continuously to individuals who are not iron deficient.

The symptoms of iron overload are indistinguishable from those of hemochromatosis, a relatively rare hereditary disorder characterized by excessive iron absorption. Debate continues in the United States concerning the relative merits and dangers of additional iron fortification of foods, owing to this potential problem. In Sweden, however, many foods have been fortified with iron, and no obvious ill effects have been noted so far.

IRON INTAKE

Average United States iron intakes with respect to age and sex, along with the iron content of various food sources, are presented in Table 9–9. These data indicate an average value of 5 to 7 mg of iron per 1000 kcal of ingested food, except in infants, who often receive supplements. The use of iron cooking utensils may increase iron intake substantially. Iron intake may be higher in countries whose populations consume significant quantities of organ meats or use foods prepared with blood.

TABLE 9–9. AVERAGE U.S. IRON INTAKE, MG/DAY, 1977*

	Milk	Eggs	Meat, Poultry, Fish	Other Sources	Total
MALES AND FEMALES					
0–1 yr	4.9	0.2	1.3	11.0	17.4
1–2 yr	0.5	0.4	1.8	5.2	7.9
3–5 yr	0.5	0.5	2.5	6.0	9.5
6–8 yr	0.6	0.3	3.1	7.1	11.1
MALES					
9–14 yr	0.6	0.5	4.4	8.8	14.3
15–18 yr	0.7	0.6	6.1	9.7	17.1
Adults	0.3	0.8	6.2	8.5	15.8
FEMALES					
9–14 yr	0.5	0.4	3.5	7.3	11.7
15–18 yr	0.4	0.4	3.7	6.6	11.1
Adults	0.3	0.4	3.9	6.1	10.7

*From USDA Nationwide Food Consumption Survey, 48 contiguous states, 1977.

REGULATION OF IRON ABSORPTION

Iron is absorbed chiefly in the ferrous form; however, iron in food is mostly ferric, with much less in the ferrous form. Ferric iron is solubilized and reduced to ferrous iron by acid gastric juice; hence, subjects with achlorhydria or who have had subtotal gastrectomy often exhibit impaired iron absorption.

Heme iron and nonheme iron are absorbed as two separate pools; absorption of heme iron is far more efficient, although a small fraction of the iron in heme compounds is liberated from nonheme iron during gastric digestion. Absorption of these two pools of iron occurs in the upper small intestine by two distinct mechanisms. Iron deficiency leads to more efficient absorption, particularly from the nonheme pool, but the amount that can be absorbed is limited.

BIOAVAILABILITY OF DIETARY IRON

On an average diet, normal subjects absorb 5 to 10 per cent of the iron consumed; iron-deficient subjects absorb more than twice as much. As indicated in Tables 9–8 and 9–9, these amounts of absorbed iron fail to meet the requirements of a substantial number of women. The maximum amount of iron absorbed from the average United States diet is about 1 to 2 mg/day in normal adults and 3 to 6 mg/day in iron-deficient subjects.

In estimating the amount of iron available for absorption while on a given diet, it is necessary to consider the composition of each meal. Attempts to calculate the quantity of absorbable iron in any given meal are fraught with difficulty. Computer programs have even been designed for this purpose. As mentioned earlier, heme iron is absorbed much more efficiently (15 to 35 per cent) than is nonheme iron (2 to 20 per cent). All of the literature on iron absorption, including the Recommended Dietary Allowances, states that heme iron accounts for approximately 40 per cent of the total iron in meat, poultry, and fish, but this is probably an underestimate. (Although milk iron is a nonheme iron, the iron of breast milk, in particular, appears to be relatively well absorbed.) From 50 to 80 per cent of the iron in muscle tissue is heme iron; storage iron is present in significant amounts only in organ meats such as liver and kidney. Since these organ meats constitute a very small fraction of the meat consumed in the United States, it appears that dietary intake of heme iron has been consistently underestimated.

Ascorbic acid is a major dietary component affecting iron absorption. Although it has little influence on ferrous (heme) iron, ascorbic acid solubilizes ferric iron and reduces it to the ferrous form, thereby enhancing absorption in a dose-dependent manner. This effect of ascorbic acid is eliminated completely by baking but only partially by boiling. The widespread use of vitamin C in large doses may have reduced the incidence of iron deficiency.

Substances that retard absorption of nonheme iron are also present in food. Tannic acid, present in tea and many vegetables, and EDTA, a common food additive, markedly reduce iron absorption. Phytates, phosphates, and soy products also reduce absorption to some extent.

BIBLIOGRAPHY

Sodium

Anon.: Lowering blood pressure without drugs. Lancet 2:459–461, 1980.
Dahl, L. K.: Salt intake and hypertension. In Genest, J., Koiw, E., and Kuchel, O. (Eds.): Hypertension, Physiopathology and Treatment. New York, McGraw-Hill, 1977, pp. 548-559.
Morgan, T. O., and Myers, J. B.: Hypertension treated by sodium restriction. Med J Austral 2:396–397, 1981.
Mudge, G. H.: Diuretics and other agents employed in the mobilization of edema fluid. In Gilman, A. G., Goodman, L. S., Gilman, A., Mayer, S.E., and Melmon, K. L. (Eds.): The Pharmacological Basis of Therapeutics (6th Ed.). New York, Macmillan PublishingCo., Inc., 1980, pp. 892-915.

Potassium

Cohen, J. J., Gennari, F. J., and Harrington, J. T.: Disorders of potassium balance. In Brenner, B. M., and Rector, F. C., Jr. (Eds.): The Kidney (2nd Ed.). Vol. I. Philadelphia, W. B. Saunders Co., 1981, pp. 908-939.

Calcium and Phosphorus

Coe, F. L., and Kavalach, A. G.: Hypercalciuria and hyperuricosuria in patients with calcium nephrolithiasis. N Engl J Med 291:1344–1350, 1974.
David, D. S. (Ed.): Calcium Metabolism in Renal Failure and Nephrolithiasis. New York, John Wiley and Sons, 1977.
Pak, C. Y. C.: A critical evaluation of treatment of calcium stones. In Massry, S. G., Ritz, E., and

Jahn, H. (Eds.): Phosphate and Minerals in Health and Disease: Proceedings of the Fourth International Workshop in Phosphate and Other Minerals. Strasbourg, France, 22–24, June 1979, New York, Plenum Press, 1980, pp. 451-465.

Walser, M.: Delay of progression of renal failure. *In* Avram, M. M. (Ed.): Prevention of Kidney Disease and Long-Term Survival. Plenum Publishing Corp., New York, 1982, pp. 23-29.

Iron

Anon.: Preventing iron deficiency. Lancet 1:1117–1118, 1980.

Beutler, E.: Iron. *In* Goodhart, R. S., and Shils, M. E. (Eds.): Modern Nutrition in Health and Disease (6th Ed.). Philadelphia, Lea and Febiger, 1980, pp. 324–354.

Committee on Nutrition: Iron supplementation for infants. Pediatrics 58:765–768, 1976.

Cook, J. D., and Monsen, E. R.: Vitamin C, the common cold, and iron absorption. Am J Clin Nutr 30:235–241, 1977.

Finch, C. A.: Drugs effective in iron-deficiency and other hypochromic anemias. *In* Gilman, A. G., Goodman, L. S., Gilman, A., Mayer, S. E., and Melmon, K. L. (Eds.): Goodman and Gilman's The Pharmacological Basis of Therapeutics. (6th Ed.). New York, Macmillan Publishing Co., Inc., 1980, pp. 1315–1330.

Hallberg, L.: Bioavailability of dietary iron in man. Ann Rev Nutr 1:123–147, 1981.

Layrisse, M., and Martinez-Torres, C.: Model for measuring dietary absorption of heme iron: Test with a complete meal. Am J Clin Nutr 25:401–411, 1972.

Martinez-Torres, C., and Layrisse, M.: Iron absorption from veal muscle. Am J Clin Nutr 24:531–540, 1971.

Mertz, W.: The new RDAs: Estimated adequate and safe intake of trace elements and calculation of available iron. J Am Diet Assoc 76:128–133, 1980.

Monsen, E. R., and Balintfy, J. L.: Calculating dietary iron bioavailability: Refinement and computerization. J Am Diet Assoc 80:307–311, 1982.

Monsen, E. R., Hallberg, L., Layrisse, M., *et al.*: Estimation of available dietary iron. Am J Clin Nutr 31:134–141, 1978.

Saarinen, U. M., Siimes, M. A., and Dallman, P. R.: Iron absorption in infants: High bioavailability of breast milk iron as indicated by the extrinsic tag method of iron absorption and by the concentration of serum ferritin. J Pediatr 91:36–39, 1977.

Schricker, B. R., Miller, D. D., and Stouffer, J. R.: Measurement and content of nonheme and total iron in muscle. J Food Sci 47:740–743, 1982.

ADDITIONAL READING

Nutritional information on modified sodium diets is available from:
The American Heart Association
National Center
7320 Greenville Avenue
Dallas, TX 75231

Contact the local Heart Association office for information on films, leaflets, and pamphlets.

Information on meal planning is available from some food companies, for example, the following:
Delicious Low Sodium Diets
Standard Brands, Inc.
625 Madison Avenue
New York, NY 10022—(1976)

Restricted Diets Come to Life with Tabasco
McIlkenny Company
Avery Island, LA 70513—(1980)

Books such as the following may be helpful:

Secrets of Salt Free Cooking
Jeanne Jones
101 Productions
834 Mission Street
San Francisco, CA 94103—(1980)

Craig Claiborne's Gourmet Diet
Craig Claiborne with Pierre Franey
Ballantine Books
New York, NY—(1980)

Gourmet Cooking Without Salt
Eleanor P. Brenner
Doubleday and Company, Inc.
Garden City
New York, NY—(1981)

Mayo Clinic Renal Diet Cookbook
J. Margie, C. Anderson, R. Nelson, and J. Hunt
Golden Press, New York, NY—(1974) or
Western Publishing Company, Inc.,
Racine, WI—(1974)

10
MODIFIED FIBER DIETS

Albert I. Mendeloff, M.D.,
Simeon Margolis, M.D., Ph.D., and
Lora B. Wilder, M.S., R.D.

INTRODUCTION

Dietary fiber consists of all ingested plant foods that cannot be digested by human intestinal enzymes or absorbed by the body. Fiber is largely derived from a wide variety of plant foods whose cell walls and storage carbohydrates are resistant to digestion. Although to date there are no definitive chemical methods available to solubilize and characterize these materials, fiber at present is thought to consist of lignin, cellulose polysaccharides, and a few noncellulose polysaccharides.

Fiber Versus Residue

Fiber and residue do not have the same meaning, even though these terms are often used interchangeably. Although often applied misleadingly to diets, residue actually means all stool solids resulting from ingestion of any given dietary regimen. Human stools are about 75 per cent water and 25 per cent solid. Thus, residue arises not only from unabsorbed food but also from colonic bacteria and the secretion or excretion of material into the intestine. In addition to fiber, it includes bacteria, exfoliated epithelial cells, mucus, variable amounts of undigested protein and fat from food and gastrointestinal secretions, and unabsorbed minerals. Even the starving human continues to excrete residue, although stools are infrequent and low in volume. A clear or full liquid diet is best for minimizing residue.

GOALS AND RATIONALE OF THERAPY

In general, residents of developed countries, such as the United States, ingest diets that are relatively low in fiber content. Several lines of investigation suggest that increased dietary fiber may be of importance in the prevention or treatment of some disease states. For example, diabetes is relatively uncommon in populations taking most of their carbohydrates from foods containing large amounts of fiber. Because they are rich in soluble fiber, such foods slow gastric emptying and, thereby, may decrease the blood glucose elevation expected after carbohydrate ingestion. Studies performed on a small number of diabetic patients show that an increase in dietary fiber decreases insulin requirements. Although the mechanisms are unclear, some have even suggested that high-fiber diets may prevent the development of adult-onset diabetes mellitus. Anderson has published a recent guide to the use of high-fiber diets in the management of diabetes (see Bibliography).

It has been postulated that a high-fiber diet may also be beneficial for other reasons:

1. It may cause a decrease in serum cholesterol levels, either secondary to a specific hypocholesterolemic effect of some soluble polysaccharides in fiber-rich foods or to the decreased ingestion of animal protein and fat.

2. A high-fiber diet including increased intake of vegetables or pectin may relieve some manifestations of postprandial hypoglycemia and the dumping syndrome, seen occasionally after surgical procedures that either destroy or bypass the pylorus, because it decreases the rate of gastric emptying.

3. The increased chewing required for fiber-rich foods may decrease the number of calories ingested and protect against dental caries.

Celluloses and pentose-containing hemicelluloses increase stool volume by binding considerable amounts of water, but bacterial proliferation may also contribute to increased stool wet weight. The net result of ingesting fiber at levels of 50 g/day is to increase the wet weight of the stool to 250 g/day, compared with the usual 80 to 150 g/day passed by urbanized Westerners. Motor function of the colon can be affected by increased ingestion of dietary fiber; heavy bran feeding to normal subjects increases the rate at which solid stool is excreted.

Recent epidemiologic evidence suggests that populations that ingest, beginning in childhood, diets with a total fiber content of at least 25 g/day may have a decreased incidence of irritable colon syndrome, diverticulosis, appendicitis, colonic polyps, and colonic cancer. The decreased prevalence of colon polyps and carcinoma is thought to result from both increased stool volume and decreased stool transit time, which together may cause decreased exposure of colonic epithelial cells to lower concentrations of dietary carcinogens. This hypothesis has never been tested, and many epidemiologists believe that the incidence of colonic cancer is more directly associated with a high intake of beef and saturated fat rather than with a low intake of dietary fiber. However, since these dietary patterns often coexist, evaluation of their relative epidemiologic significance is imprecise.

In addition to the possibly prophylactic effects of a high-fiber diet, a gradual increase in fiber intake seems to be indicated in the treatment of several conditions:

1. *Constipation.* Gradual increases of dietary fiber (to 25 or 30 g/day) may relieve all types of constipation, *except* those due to mechanical obstruction (*e.g.,* sigmoid volvulus, postoperative adhesions, anastomotic stricture, Crohn's disease).

2. *Irritable colon syndrome.* Patients with this problem can develop markedly increased colonic intraluminal pressures after stimulation. Most complain of episodic abdominal pain associated with the passage of small, hard stools. A variable number of these patients will develop either muscular hypertrophy or diverticula of the colon after being symptomatic for several years. Some studies have shown that colonic mural tension, intraluminal pressure, and resultant pain are decreased when attempts are made to increase stool size by ingesting large amounts of dietary fiber.

3. *Chronic diverticular disease of the colon.* An increase in dietary fiber may decrease intraluminal colonic pressure, increase stool size, and enhance colonic motility. It has been postulated that these effects may decrease the incidence of diverticulitis and slow the progression of diverticulosis.

When the diet contains more than 30 g/day of fiber, significant quantities of various trace elements may be bound to the fiber and excreted in the stool. Excessive zinc loss is particularly likely to occur when intake of coarsely particulate fiber is large; iron and copper are less apt to be depleted. Since trace element deficiencies occur mostly when young children or severely malnourished adults are maintained on high-fiber diets, this regimen is not recommended for these individuals. Fermentation of fiber, particularly of soluble polysaccharides by colonic bacteria, may result in excessive formation of gas (hydrogen, carbon dioxide, and methane) and other products that may increase laxation while on a high-fiber diet. This may cause some discomfort but is not a threat to health.

The physiologic effects of dietary fiber may vary considerably according to the type ingested. For example, bran seems to be quite beneficial in the treatment of symptomatic diverticular disease but has little apparent effect on serum cholesterol levels. On the other hand, pectin and guar lower serum cholesterol but increase intestinal gas formation as a result of their fermentation.

A decrease in dietary fiber may be indicated on occasion (see Chapter 2). In the presence of acute colitis, bleeding colonic lesions, aganglionosis coli, or diarrhea (acute or chronic), dietary fiber—particularly from those foods high in cellulose and lignin—may increase the amount of insoluble material in the colon enough to directly injure already-damaged mucosa and increase bleeding. Thus, in the acutely ill or actively bleeding patient with colonic disease, the fiber content of the diet is usually reduced drastically. Dietary fiber may be cautiously increased as the clinical condition of the patient improves.

IMPLEMENTATION OF DIETS

Sample Meal Plans for high- and low-fiber diets are presented in Tables 10–1 and 10–2, respectively. Table 10–3 lists the fiber content of many common foods.

TABLE 10–1.   HIGH FIBER DIET, SAMPLE MEAL PLAN

Breakfast

½ grapefruit
1 scrambled egg
2 slices whole wheat bread
1 pat margarine
1 tsp jam
1 cup low-fat milk
Coffee or tea

Lunch

3 oz meat, fish, or poultry
2 slices whole wheat bread
1 tsp mayonnaise
½ cup fresh carrot and celery sticks
1 fresh apple
1 cup low-fat milk

Dinner

3 oz meat, fish, or poultry
½ cup cooked fresh broccoli
½ cup sliced tomato with lettuce
1 tsp oil with vinegar
1 small baked potato
1 bran muffin
2 tsp margarine
¼ cantaloupe
Coffee or tea

Evening Snack

1 fresh orange
2 squares graham crackers

The approximate composition of this meal plan is:

Calories	1830	Calcium	930 mg
Protein	87 g	Iron	14 mg
Fat	76 g	Phosphorus	1530 mg
Carbohydrate	200 g	Potassium	3580 mg
Dietary fiber	28 g	Sodium	1720 mg*

*No salt or sodium products added in cooking process. The diet is adequate in all essential nutrients.

TABLE 10–2.   LOW FIBER DIET, SAMPLE MEAL PLAN

Breakfast

6 oz orange juice
1 scrambled egg
2 slices white bread
1 pat margarine
1 tsp jelly
1 cup low-fat milk
Coffee or tea

Lunch

3 oz meat, fish, or poultry
2 slices white bread
1 tsp mayonnaise
½ cup peeled cucumber slices on lettuce
   wedge with oil and vinegar
1 canned peach half
1 cup low-fat milk

Dinner

3 oz meat, fish, or poultry
½ cup stewed tomatoes
½ cup white rice
1 small white roll
2 tsp margarine
½ cup egg custard
Coffee or tea

Evening Snack

6 oz orange juice
6 saltines

The approximate composition of this meal plan is:

Calories	1875	Calcium	895 mg
Protein	88 g	Iron	16 mg
Fat	80 g	Phosphorus	1350 mg
Carbohydrate	200 g	Potassium	2700 mg
Dietary fiber	6 g	Sodium	1830 mg*

*No salt or sodium products added in cooking. The diet is adequate in all essential nutrients.

TABLE 10–3. FIBER CONTENT OF COMMON FOODS, ARRANGED IN DESCENDING ORDER OF FIBER CONTENT WITHIN FOOD GROUPS

Food	Common Measure	Weight (g)	Fiber (g)
VEGETABLES			
Peas, dried whole, raw	½ cup	100	16.7
Beans, baked in tomato sauce	½ cup	128	9.3
Parsley, raw, leaves	3½ oz	100	9.1
Plaintain, ripe fried in oil	1 small, 5″	100	5.8
Peas, split, cooked	3½ oz	100	5.1
Beans, butter boiled	½ cup	90	4.6
Peas, canned, drained solids	½ cup	66	4.2
fresh boiled whole peas, no pods	½ cup	75	3.9
Turnip greens, boiled	½ cup	100	3.9
Yam, boiled, flesh only	½ cup	100	3.9
Lentils, boiled	½ cup	100	3.7
Mustard greens, raw, leaves and stems	½ cup	100	3.7
Broccoli top, raw	scant cup	100	3.6
Beans, summer boiled	½ cup	100	3.4
boiled, French-style	½ cup	100	3.2
Broccoli top, boiled	½ cup	78	3.2
Eggplant, raw, diced	½ cup	100	2.5
Beets, boiled	2, 2″ diameter	100	2.5
Mushrooms, raw, small	10	100	2.5
Parsnips, boiled, flesh only	½ cup	100	2.5
Potatoes, white, baked, flesh only	2½″ diameter	100	2.5
Cabbage, boiled	½ cup	85	2.4
Carrots, boiled	½ cup	78	2.4
Brussels sprouts, boiled	½ cup	78	2.3
Carrots, raw	1 (⅛ × 7½)	81	2.3
Sweet potatoes, boiled, flesh only	1 small	100	2.3
Cabbage, white, raw shredded	1 cup	80	2.2
Tomatoes, raw, flesh, skin and seeds	1 medium	150	2.2
Turnips, white, boiled, flesh only	⅔ cup (diced)	100	2.2
Bean sprouts, canned	½ cup	63	1.9
Cauliflower, raw	1 cup	85	1.8
Celery, boiled	½ cup	75	1.7
Onions, boiled, flesh only	½ cup	100	1.3
raw, flesh only	2¼″ diameter	100	1.1
Cauliflower, boiled	½ cup	63	1.1
Celery, raw, chopped	½ cup	60	1.1
Potatoes, white boiled, flesh only	2¼″ diameter	100	1.0
Peppers, green raw, flesh only	1 large	100	0.9
Potatoes, white, flesh only, mashed	½ cup	100	0.9
with margarine and milk			
Tomatoes, canned, drained	½ cup	100	0.9
Asparagus, boiled	4 spears	100	0.8
Lettuce, raw		50	0.7
Cucumber, raw (sliced)	1 cup	105	0.4
Watercress, raw, leaves and stem	10 sprigs	10	0.3
FRUITS			
Prunes, stewed without sugar,	½ cup	125	10.1
fruit and juice, no stones			
Peaches, dried uncooked	¼ cup	40	5.7

Table continues on following page

TABLE 10–3.   FIBER CONTENT OF COMMON FOODS (Continued)

Food	Common Measure	Weight (g)	Fiber (g)
Blackberries (raw)	$\frac{1}{4}$ cup	72	5.3
Lemons, whole fruit, with skin, no seeds	1	100	5.2
Grapes, white, raw, flesh and skin — no seeds or stalks	12	50	5.0
Raspberries, raw, whole fruit	$\frac{1}{2}$ cup	67	5.0
Cranberries, raw, whole	1 cup	95	4.0
Apricots, dried, raw	2 whole	16	3.8
Prunes, dried raw, flesh and skin, no stones	2 large	20	3.2
Figs, dried	1 small	15	2.8
Banana (8 × $\frac{1}{2}$")	$\frac{1}{2}$	70	2.4
Damson plums, raw (weighed with stones)	6 – 1 "diam	66	2.4
Apples, eating	$2\frac{1}{2}$ " diam	115	2.3
Pears, eating, flesh only, no skin or core (3 × $2\frac{1}{2}$")	$\frac{1}{2}$ pear	100	2.3
Rhubarb, stewed with sugar, stems and juice	$\frac{3}{8}$ cup	100	2.2
Strawberries, raw, whole fruit	10 large	100	2.2
Plums, Victoria dessert, raw, flesh and skin, no stones	2 medium	100	2.1
Oranges, raw, flesh only, no peel or seeds	1 small	100	2.0
Tangarines, raw, flesh only, no peel or seeds	1 large	100	1.9
Pears, canned, fruit halves and 2 tbs syrup	2 small	100	1.7
Apricots, raw (with skin, no stone)	2	76	1.6
Apricots, canned, halves (no stone)	4	112	1.5
Mango, raw, flesh only	$\frac{1}{2}$ medium	100	1.5
Cherries, raw, large	10	83	1.4
Dates, dried (no stones)	2	16	1.4
Peaches, fresh, raw, flesh and skin, medium	1	100	1.4
Raisins, dried, flesh and skin	2 tbs	20	1.4
Figs, green (raw), approximately 9 per lb.	1	50	1.3
Nectarines, raw, flesh and skin (no stones), medium	1	50	1.2
Fruit salad, canned	$\frac{1}{2}$ cup	100	1.1
Melon, cantaloupe, raw, flesh only (5" diameter)	$\frac{1}{4}$ melon	100	1.0
Peaches, canned, fruit halves and 2 tbs syrup	2 medium	100	1.7
Melon, honeydew, raw, flesh only (5" diameter)	$\frac{1}{4}$ melon	100	0.9
Olives in brine, without stones	3 medium	20	0.9
Pineapple, canned, large fruit slice and syrup	1	100	0.9
Pineapple, fresh, flesh only, no skin or core	$\frac{1}{2}$ cup diced	67	0.8
Avocado	$\frac{1}{8}$	31	0.6
Grapefruit, fresh, flesh only, no skin or seeds	$\frac{1}{2}$	100	0

Table continues on following page

TABLE 10–3.   FIBER CONTENT OF COMMON FOODS (Continued)

Food	Common Measure	Weight (g)	Fiber (g)
Mandarin oranges, canned, with syrup		100	0.3
Grapes, black (raw, no skin or pits)	12 grapes	50	0.2
Grapefruit juice, canned	½ cup	120	0
Lemon juice	1 tbs	15	0
Orange juice, strained juice from fresh oranges	½ cup	120	0

CEREAL/CRACKERS/FLOUR

Food	Common Measure	Weight (g)	Fiber (g)
Bran wheat	⅓ cup	20	8.8
All-bran	⅓ cup	19	5.1
Crispbread or rye crackers	4	25	2.9
Shredded wheat biscuits	1	22	2.7
Bread, whole wheat	1 slice	28	2.4
Soya flour, low-fat	2½ tbs	20	2.4
Puffed wheat	1 cup	15	2.3
Barley, boiled	½ cup	100	2.2
Cornflakes	¾ cup	19	2.1
Grapenuts	¼ cup	28	2.0
Flour, whole meal	2½ tbs	20	1.5
Graham crackers	2 squares	14	1.4
Sugar puffs	¾ cup	22	1.3
Porridge	½ cup	120	1.0
Rice krispies	¾ cup	21	0.9
Special K	1 cup	16	0.9
Bread, white	1 slice	28	0.8
Matzo (6 × 6″)	1 piece	20	0.8
Rice, boiled	½ cup	102	0.8
Flour, household	2½ tbs	20	0.7

CAKES

Food	Common Measure	Weight (g)	Fiber (g)
Fruitcake	1 slice (3 × 3 × ½″)	40	1.4
Cake, iced	1 slice	50	1.2
Gingerbread	1 piece (2 × 2 × 2″)	57	0.7
Sponge cake	1 piece ($\frac{1}{10}$ cake)	50	0.5

OTHER DESSERTS

Food	Common Measure	Weight (g)	Fiber (g)
Fruit pie (9″ diameter with double crust), e.g., apple, plum, rhubarb)	$\frac{1}{6}$	160	3.5
Custard, egg, baked from mix	½ cup	150	0

NUTS

Food	Common Measure	Weight (g)	Fiber (g)
Almonds	10	25	3.6
Coconut, dried	2 tbs	15	3.5
Brazil	6–8	28	2.5
Peanut butter, smooth	2 tbs	32	2.4
Chestnuts, small	5	25	1.7
Peanuts	10	9	0.8

Table continues on following page

TABLE 10–3. FIBER CONTENT OF COMMON FOODS (Concluded)

Walnuts	3	12	0.6
Hazelnuts	6	8	0.5
MISCELLANEOUS			
Marzipan almond paste		100	6.4
Jam, fruit with edible seed, blackberry, black currant, gooseberry, raspberry	1 tbs	20	0.2
Jam, stone fruit, apricot, plum	1 tbs	20	0.2
Marmalade	1 tbs	20	0.1
French dressing		100	0
Mayonnaise	1 tbs	14	0
Sugar, white		100	0

BIBLIOGRAPHY

Anderson, J. W.: Diabetes: A Practical New Guide to Healthy Living. London, Martin Dunitz, 1981.
Barbolt, T. A., and Abraham, R.: The effect of bran on dimethylhydrazine-induced colon carcinogenesis in the rat. Proc Soc Exp Biol Med 157:656–659, 1978.
Brodribb, A. J. M.: Treatment of symptomatic diverticular disease with a high fibre diet. Lancet 1:665–666, 1977.
Burkitt, K. P., and Trowell, J. C. (Eds.): Refined Carbohydrate Foods and Disease. Some Implications of Dietary Fibre. London, Academic Press, 1975.
Diabetes and Dietary Fiber. Nutr Rev 36:273–275, 1978.
Findley, J. M., Mitchell, W. D., Smith, A. N., et al.: Effects of unprocessed bran on colon function in normal subjects and in diverticular disease. Lancet 1:146–149, 1974.
Heaton, K. W.: Dietary fibre in perspective. Hum Nutr Clin Nutr 37:151–170, 1983.
Howell, M. D.: Diet as an etiologic factor in the development of cancers of the colon and rectum. J Chron Dis 28:67–80, 1975.
Jenkins, D. J. A., Leeds, A. R., Gassull, M. A., Cochet, B., and Alberti, K. G. M. M.: Decrease in postprandial insulin and glucose concentrations by guar and pectin. Ann Int Med 86:20–23, 1977.
Kritchevsky, D.: Fiber, lipids, and atherosclerosis. Am J Clin Nutr 31 (Suppl.):65–74, 1978.
Kritchevsky, D.: Metabolic effects of dietary fiber. West J Med 130:123–127, 1979.
Manning, A. P., Heaton, K. W., Harvey, R. F., et al.: Wheat fibre and the irritable bowel syndrome. Lancet 2:417–418, 1977.
Mendeloff, A. I.: Dietary fiber and human health. N Engl J Med 297:811–814, 1977.
Mendeloff, A. I.: Dietary fiber and gastrointestinal diseases: Some facts and fancies. Med Clin North Am 62:165–171, 1978.
Miettinen, T. A., and Tarpila, S.: Effect of pectin on serum cholesterol, fecal bile acids and biliary lipids in normolipidemic and hyperlipidemic individuals. Clin Chim Acta 79:471–477, 1977.
Miranda, P. M., and Horwitz, D. L.: High-fiber diets in the treatment of diabetes mellitus. Ann Int Med 88:482–486, 1978.
Painter, N. S., and Burkitt, D. P.: Diverticular disease of the colon: A deficiency disease of western civilization. Br Med J 2:450–454, 1971.
Paul, A. A., and Southgate, D. A. T.: McCance and Widdowson's The Composition of Foods, Fourth revised and extended edition of MRC Special Report No. 297. New York, Elsevier/North-Holland Biomedical Press, 1978.
Phillips, R. L.: Role of life style and dietary habits in risk of cancer among Seventh-Day Adventists. Cancer Res 35:2513–3522, 1975.

Pomare, E. W., Heaton, K. W., Low-Beer, T. S., *et al.*: The effect of wheat bran upon bile salt metabolism and upon the lipid composition of bile in gallstone patients. Am J Dig Dis 21:521–526, 1976.

Reinhold, J. G., Faradji, B., Abadi, P., *et al.*: Decreased absorption of calcium, magnesium, zinc, and phosphorus by humans due to increased fiber and phosphorus consumption as wheat bread. J Nutr 106:493–503, 1976.

Southgate, D. A. T., Bailey, B., Collinson, E., *et al.*: A guide to calculating intakes of dietary fibre. J Human Nutr 30:303–313, 1976.

Spiller, G., and Kay, R. M. (Eds.): Medical Aspects of Dietary Fiber. New York, Plenum Press, 1980.

Story, J. A.: The role of dietary fiber in lipid metabolism. Adv Lipid Res 18:229–246, 1981.

Trowell, H.: Definition of dietary fiber and hypothesis that it is a protective factor in certain diseases. Am J Clin Nutr 29:417–427, 1976.

Vahouny, G. V., and Kritchevsky, D. (Eds.): Dietary Fiber in Health and Disease. New York, Plenum Press, 1982.

11

SPECIAL DIETS FOR GASTROINTESTINAL DISORDERS

Lactose Intolerance

Theodore M. Bayless, M.D., and
Jean Clark Wagner, R.D.

INTRODUCTION

Lactose or milk intolerance may be defined as the development of symptoms such as bloating, cramps, flatulence, or diarrhea after consuming one or two glasses of milk. These milk-induced gastrointestinal symptoms may require dietary limitation of lactose-containing products.

The milk sugar, lactose, is split by a specific enzyme, lactase, on the brush border of the small intestinal mucosa; the resulting monosaccharide components, glucose and galactose, are then absorbed readily. An individual with adequate ("normal") lactase levels can consume one or two glasses of milk without symptoms. Almost all full-term infants have adequate lactase levels. Low-birth-weight infants may have a temporarily impaired capacity to digest lactose. In many populations, intestinal lactase levels and the person's ability to digest lactose apparently decrease on a genetic basis during childhood or adolescence despite normal health. Neither children nor adults with low lactase levels are able to digest a large lactose load; they are defined as "lactose intolerant." For example, over 90 per cent of pure-blooded American Indians, most Oriental populations, and many native African groups are lactose intolerant. Lactose intolerance occurs in about 70 per cent of American blacks, 60 to 70 per cent of American Jews, and 60 per cent of Mexican-Americans. Approximately 5 to 15 per cent of American whites of Scandinavian or northern European ancestry have lactose intolerance.

Some individuals with low lactase levels may recognize the relationship between milk ingestion and symptoms, whereas others may come to medical attention because of their diarrhea, abdominal discomfort, or flatulence. Sometimes, lactose intolerance aggravates the symptoms of other conditions, such as the irritable bowel syndrome, Crohn's disease (regional enteritis), ulcerative colitis, or postgastrectomy diarrhea.

The frequency with which an otherwise healthy person will notice symptoms from ingestion of one or two glasses of milk is controversial. Some reports show that half these adults will be symptomatic after 8 oz of milk taken on an empty stomach, whereas others show that only larger amounts of milk will regularly cause symptoms. Also, there is concern about the absorption of nutrients from a glass of milk even if no symptoms are reported.

GOALS OF TREATMENT

In treating lactose-intolerant individuals, several goals should be considered. The intake of lactose-containing foods must be limited to amounts that will not cause intestinal symptoms. Total lactose avoidance is usually not necessary. Other well-tolerated sources of calcium and protein should be provided as dietary supplements (*e.g.*, fermented dairy products including hard cheeses). Lactose intolerance should be considered before dairy products are included in diets for individuals from populations with a high prevalence of lactose intolerance.

RATIONALE FOR TREATMENT

One way to treat patients with this problem is by administering a low-lactose diet. Patients with milk intolerance that is caused by inadequate lactose digestion can usually tolerate small amounts of milk in cooking, in coffee, with cereal, or as a small serving of ice cream. Most of these patients will benefit from simply avoiding glassfuls of milk or large servings of ice cream. Some have more symptoms from iced milk, especially on an empty stomach; warm milk or milk taken with a meal may be somewhat better tolerated. Some patients describe symptoms after very small (3 to 6 g) quantities of lactose, equivalent to 2 to 4 oz of milk. A list of lactose-containing foods to avoid or milk-free recipes or both may be given to the patient if desired.

Since there is considerable variability in the amount of milk needed to cause symptoms, a *lactose-free diet* may be prescribed. But complete lactose avoidance, as for galactosemia, is usually not necessary, even though some patients are apparently "extremely sensitive." The numerous food intolerances of patients with the irritable bowel syndrome may make evaluation of these patients difficult.

Lactose hydrolyzed milk is now commercially available as is enzyme (LACT-AID) that can be added to milk to markedly reduce the lactose content: the resultant milk is sweetened but is quite palatable.

PATIENT SELECTION

The following conditions necessitate dietary control of lactose:

CONGENITAL LACTASE DEFICIENCY. This is a *very rare* genetic trait and requires lactose restriction in the newborn.

ACQUIRED LACTASE DEFICIENCY SECONDARY TO SMALL INTESTINAL MUCOSAL INJURY. This problem occurs commonly after severe gastroenteritis in infants and children, and it may require temporary use of carbohydrates other than lactose. When the mucosal injury is very severe, malabsorption of even the monosaccharides glucose and galactose may necessitate treatment with parenteral nutrition.

Mucosal injury associated with celiac disease may cause lactose intolerance that is potentially reversible if the patient adheres strictly to a gluten-free diet. Thus, milk restriction may be necessary initially, but the patient may be able to resume the intake of milk eventually.

DIARRHEA AFTER SURGERY FOR PEPTIC ULCER DISEASE. The surgical treatment of peptic ulcer disease frequently results in bypass of the pylorus or in destruction of its competence. Consequently, there may be rapid transit of foods into the small intestine, with resultant diarrhea. Thus, the ingestion of milk may cause troublesome symptoms in patients who consumed milk regularly before their peptic ulcer surgery.

MILK-INTOLERANT OLDER CHILDREN OR ADOLESCENTS. These individuals may not recognize the relationship between milk consumption and abdominal bloating or pain. Others simply may reject milk when it is offered as a beverage as part of a nutritional program. Anecdotal reports suggest that chocolate milk is accepted more readily even by lactose-intolerant school children.

MILK-INTOLERANT ADULTS. When there is some question whether individuals with gastrointestinal symptoms are milk intolerant, they can be asked to test themselves by abstaining from milk for 3 to 5 days and then consuming 1 or 2 glasses of skim milk without other food. If there is still uncertainty about the diagnosis, a lactose-tolerance test can be performed, utilizing 50 g of lactose (equivalent to 1 qt of milk), or a breath hydrogen test.

PATIENTS RECEIVING MILK AS PART OF A NUTRITIONAL PROGRAM. The nutritionist should at least consider the possibility of milk intolerance when suggesting milk for pregnant women, peptic ulcer patients, patients with diarrhea, or as a constituent of tube feedings. This is especially true of populations with a high prevalence of lactose intolerance. A family history of milk intolerance may also draw attention to this problem. Failure of a patient to consume dairy products served on a hospital or institutional tray should also cause the nutritionist to raise this question.

DIETARY MANAGEMENT

Methods for progressive limitation of dietary lactose from liberal quantities to less than 3 g/day include the following:

1. *Minimal restriction* (9 to 22 g lactose). Milk or ice cream should be restricted to 1 to 2 cups per day. A lactose enzyme product such as LACT-AID may enhance milk tolerance. Milk should be taken in combination with solid foods and in small amounts frequently throughout the day. Some patients tolerate warmed milk, chocolate milk, buttermilk, or yogurt better than they do plain

TABLE 11–1. EXAMPLES OF
LACTOSE CONTENT OF DAIRY
PRODUCTS

Product	Lactose Content (g)
Milk (1 cup)	11
Ice cream (1 cup)	9
Cheese	
Cheddar (1 oz)	0.5
American (1 oz)	0.5
Cream (1 oz)	0.8
Cottage (1 cup)	5–6
Butter (2 tsp)	0.1

milk, although these all differ little in lactose content. Yogurt contains autodigestory lactose.

2. *Modest restriction* (5 to 6 g lactose). Milk should be limited to $^1/_2$ cup per day in cooking or on cereal. One-half cup ice cream may be substituted for the milk if taken with a meal.

3. *Omit* all milk and ice cream. Cheeses (except cottage cheese) and other dairy products are not restricted.

4. *Severe restriction* (3 g lactose or less). In this regimen, foods made with milk, milk solids, or lactose added in processing are severely limited. The lactose content of dairy products is variable. Some examples are listed in Table 11–1.

These diets can all be planned to meet all the nutritional recommendations of the National Research Council. However, as the quantity of milk and dairy products is reduced, special attention must be given to the inclusion of calcium-rich foods or a calcium supplement.

Food selections and a sample meal plan for a severely lactose-restricted diet are given in Tables 11–2 and 11–3, respectively.

TABLE 11–2. FOOD SELECTIONS FOR A SEVERELY LACTOSE-RESTRICTED DIET (3 G OR LESS)

Milk and Nondairy Substitutes: Include lactose-free infant formulas and adult total liquid feedings and supplements (see Chapters 1 and 3). Nondairy creamers and nondairy whipped toppings may be used.
   OMIT all milks — whole, low-fat, skim, buttermilk, chocolate, and malted milk.

Dairy Products: Limit cheese to 1 oz/day. Sour cream, light cream, half-and-half, and whipping cream may substitute for cheese (1 tbs = 1 oz cheese). Pure yogurt may be well tolerated.
   OMIT cottage cheese, ice cream, ice milk, and sherbet.

Bread and Baked Products: All breads are allowed. Any homemade baked goods containing less than $\frac{1}{4}$ cup milk/serving — *i.e.*, biscuits, muffins, cakes, cookies — may be used but limited to 1 serving/day.

Fats: Limit butter to 2 tsp/day. Margarine is permitted as desired.

   Unless prepared with milk, milk solids, or lactose, or excessive amounts of butter, cream, or cheese, all foods not listed above are permitted.

TABLE 11–3. 3-GRAM LACTOSE DIET—SAMPLE MEAL PLAN

Breakfast

2 servings fruit
1 egg
2 slices bread or equivalent
2 tsp margarine or equivalent
Coffee, sugar, nondairy creamer

Noon Meal

3 oz meat or equivalent
1 cup vegetable
2 slices bread or equivalent
2 tsp margarine, mayonnaise, or equivalent
2 servings fruit
Coffee, sugar, nondairy creamer

Evening Meal

3 oz meat or equivalent
1 cup vegetable (green leafy)
1 cup starchy vegetable or equivalent
1 slice bread
2 tsp margarine, mayonnaise, or equivalent
2 servings fruit
Coffee, sugar, nondairy creamer

Evening Snack

1 oz cheese
2 slices bread or equivalent
2 servings fruit

An approximate composition of this diet is:

Calories	1990	Calcium	813	mg
Protein	82 g	Iron	20.6	mg
Fat	80 g	Phosphorus	1026	mg
Carbohydrate	235 g	Potassium	4373	mg
		Sodium	1632	mg

Gluten Sensitivity

Theodore M. Bayless, M.D., and
Jean Clark Wagner, R.D.

INTRODUCTION

Individuals with celiac disease (also called sprue, gluten-induced enteropathy, or celiac-sprue) incur intestinal mucosal injury when they consume foods containing buckwheat, barley, wheat, rye, or oats. Gliadin, the protein fraction of the glycoprotein gluten, damages intestinal mucosal cells in these individuals and may cause generalized malabsorption. Affected patients respond rapidly and often dramatically to a gluten-free diet. Refeeding of gluten or the return to a regular diet usually causes a gradual recurrence of symptoms.

Intestinal damage from diarrheal or malabsorptive states other than celiac disease (chronic infantile diarrhea, infantile cow's milk allergy, or tropical sprue) can also cause temporary gluten intolerance. But a long-term gluten-free diet should be limited to those patients whose celiac disease has been confirmed by biopsy, even though a temporary, nonspecific improvement may result from gluten restriction in these other conditions as well.

GOALS OF TREATMENT

The goal of treating persons who poorly tolerate gluten is complete avoidance of wheat, rye, barley, buckwheat, and oats. Ideally, this should be a lifelong restriction, but some patients are able to titrate the amount of gluten they can consume without severe symptoms or frank malabsorption. Pleasant and acceptable dietary alternatives should be provided to supply sufficient calories for weight maintenance or weight gain and for correction of nutritional inadequacies if present. The patient must receive complete and current information on the gluten content of commercial foods. Lactose intolerance (which may be slowly reversible as mucosal injury decreases) should also be taken into consideration.

RATIONALE FOR TREATMENT

Small amounts of gluten acutely injure the mucosal absorptive cells in the small intestine of affected patients. With gluten withdrawal these cells improve in 3 to 7 days and the patient notes rapid resolution of symptoms. With prolonged, strict adherence to a gluten-free diet, mucosal structure and absorptive capacity can be kept normal. When patients do not adhere to the diet, they may notice bloating, flatulence, floating malodorous stools, or inability to maintain a desirable body weight. Patients with celiac disease should be given complete and up-to-date lists of foods they can eat and foods they must avoid (see Table 11–4). Information on commercial products is very helpful when available.

TABLE 11–4. FOOD CHOICES FOR A GLUTEN-FREE DIET

Food Group	Foods Allowed	Foods Excluded
MEAT	Beef, lamb, pork, veal, fish, or poultry, prepared with allowed foods. All-meat luncheon meats, sausage, and frankfurters (ingredients must be checked).	Prepared meats such as scrapple, sausage, frankfurters, bologna, luncheon meats, commercial hamburger products which may contain cereal or filler. Meat loaf made with prohibited products, croquettes, canned meat mixtures. Canned, packaged, or frozen meat entrees with gravies or cream sauces of unknown composition.
CHEESE	All natural cheese and cheese products unless made with gluten flours.	Processed cheese with gluten products.
EGGS	All prepared plain or with allowed foods.	None except as noted.
MILK	Avoid milk for 2 weeks after diagnosis is made; then limit to ½ cup per day and increase as tolerated.	Malted milk, commercial chocolate milk that contains cereal or additives. Milk flavoring syrups that contain malt, wheat products or of unknown content.
FRUIT AND JUICE	All.	None.
VEGETABLES	All plain vegetables and those prepared with allowed products.	Any prepared with sauces containing prohibited flours, bread crumbs, or croutons. Frozen vegetable combinations with prohibited products or of unknown composition.
SOUPS	Any clear broth or consommé, other homemade soups prepared with allowed foods. Chowders or cream soups thickened with cream, allowed starch, or flours.	Commercial, canned, or dehydrated soups unless company analysis indicates the products are gluten free.
BREADS, GRAINS, CEREALS	Products made from cornmeal; corn, rice, arrowroot, soybean, and potato flours; rice cakes, rice wafers, gluten-free bread, low-protein porridge and pastas; tapioca, cornstarch; corn and rice; cereals made from corn and rice, such as cornflakes, Corn Kix, Corn Chex, Sugar Corn Pops, Cocoa Krispies, Rice Krispies, Puffed Rice, Rice Chex, cream of rice, grits, rice flakes; Kellogg's Corn Flake Crumbs.	Whole-wheat graham, gluten, oat, rye, and white flours; barley and malt. Buckwheat and low-gluten wheat starch flour (unless tolerated); wheat germ, bran, and bran cereals; all wheat, rye, oat, and barley cereals (i.e., cream of wheat, farina, grapenuts, oatmeal, shredded or puffed wheat, Ralston, wheatena or other cereals derived from prohibited grains); zweiback, rusk, Rye Krisps, or any of the following (unless made with allowed flours): bread, biscuits, rolls, muf-

Table continues on following page

TABLE 11–4.   FOOD CHOICES FOR A GLUTEN-FREE DIET (Continued)

Food Group	Foods Allowed	Foods Excluded
		fins, waffles, pancakes, crackers, doughnuts, dumplings, bread crumbs, breaded foods, pretzels, macaroni, spaghetti, noodles and other pasta, sesame seeds, millet.
FATS	Butter, margarine, cream, sour cream, all oils, meat or poultry fat, pure mayonnaise, and salad dressings without prohibited flours; olives, nuts, and peanut butter.	Commercial salad dressings with flour or gluten stabilizers; gravies and cream sauces, unless thickened with allowed products.
DESSERTS	Cornstarch, tapioca and rice puddings; custard junket, gelatin Bavarian cream; homemade or natural ice cream; commercial ice cream, ice milk, fruit ice or sherbet without prohibited flours or stabilizers; pies, cookies, and cakes made with allowed flours, meringues; fruit.	Sherbet, ice milk, and commercial ice cream with cereal additives, commercial cakes, pastries, cookies, pies, and prepared mixes; ice cream cones; commercial puddings with gluten products.
SWEETS	All sugars, syrups, honey, molasses, sorghum, jelly, jams, preserves, marmalade; candy made with allowed products; marshmallows.	Candy containing cereal additives.
SEASONINGS	Herbs, condiment spices, pure flavoring, catsup, mustard, relish, vinegar, pure cocoa, and chocolate.	Any with malt.
BEVERAGES	Cocoa, tea, pure coffee (regular and instant); fruit juice; carbonated beverages (see also section under milk).	Coffee with cereal additives, Postum, Ovaltine, or other cereal beverages; ale, beer.
MISCELLANEOUS	Coconut, pickles, popcorn, potato chips.	Chewing gum; fried snack foods with cereal additives or prohibited flours.

PATIENT SELECTION

As stated earlier, a complete and prolonged response to a gluten-free diet can be expected only in patients with celiac disease that has been confirmed by intestinal biopsy. It is not good medical practice to use a long-term gluten-free diet in patients with vague gastrointestinal symptoms or malabsorption, without a proven diagnosis of celiac disease. Rather, the physician should make a specific diagnosis of the cause of malabsorption and limit the long-term use of a gluten-free diet to those with evidence of gluten-induced enteropathy. In infancy, the differential diagnosis between cow's milk allergy and celiac disease may be difficult, but by the age of 1 or 2 years this distinction can usually be made by assessing patient response to withdrawal of milk for a few days. Gluten refeeding and repeat biopsy may be necessary in children diagnosed as having celiac disease in infancy or early childhood.

DESCRIPTION OF THE GLUTEN-FREE DIET

The diet for the management of celiac disease eliminates all foods that contain gluten:

Omit all foods containing wheat, rye, oats, barley, and malt. [*Note*: Malt *flavoring* (as in cereals) is permitted. Although made from barley and corn, malt flavoring contains only minute quantities of water-soluble protein.] Since starch, emulsifiers, stabilizers, cereals, fillers, and hydrolyzed vegetable protein are commonly made from grains not allowed on this diet, products containing these ingredients should not be used unless the source of the ingredient is known.

Buckwheat and low-gluten wheat starch flours contain some gluten and should be used only if tolerated.

Products made from cornmeal, cornstarch, corn flour, rice, rice flour, tapioca, soybean flour, potato starch flour, and arrowroot may be used.

DIETARY MANAGEMENT

1. Advise the patient of common food sources of gluten and of alternate foods available.

2. Provide a list of gluten-free commercial products and recipe books. Advise the patient to read all labels carefully and to avoid products known to contain gluten or with questionable ingredients.

3. Individualize the diet to the needs of each patient. Give particular attention to weight gain or maintenance and correction of any nutritional inadequacies.

4. Initially, consider elimination or restriction of milk and high-lactose foods until improvement in symptoms is noted.

5. A properly selected gluten-free diet can meet nutritional requirements at levels recommended by the National Research Council. A sample meal plan for a gluten-free diet is presented in Table 11–5.

GLUTEN-FREE RECIPE SOURCES

The following publications provide the patient with gluten-free recipes:

American Dietetic Association: Allergy Recipes. 620 North Michigan Avenue, Chicago, Illinois 60611.

French, A. B.: Low-Gluten Diet with Tested Recipes. Clinical Research Unit, University Hospital, 1405 E. Ann Street, Ann Arbor, Michigan.

Wood, M. N.: Gourmet Food on a Wheat Free Diet. Springfield, Ill., Charles C Thomas Publisher, 1967.

Celiac Disease Recipes for Parents and Patients. Available from Hospital for Sick Children, 555 University, Toronto 5, Ontario, Canada.

Wood M. N.: Coping with the Gluten Free Diet. Springfield, Illinois, Charles C Thomas Publisher, 1982.

Garst, P. M.: Celiac Sprue and the Gluten Free Diet. M. Stevens Agency, P.O. Box 3004, Frankfort, Kentucky 40603, 1981.

TABLE 11–5.   GLUTEN-FREE DIET—SAMPLE MEAL PLAN

Breakfast

2 servings fruit
1 egg
2 slices gluten-free bread, or equivalent cereal or grain
   product
2 tsp margarine
1 cup milk
Coffee, sugar

Noon Meal

3 oz meat or equivalent
1 cup vegetables
2 slices gluten-free bread or equivalent cereal or grain
   product
2 tsp margarine or mayonnaise
2 servings fruit
1 cup milk

Evening Meal

3 oz meat or equivalent
1 cup vegetable
1 cup starchy vegetable or equivalent
2 tsp margarine
2 servings fruit or a dessert
Coffee, sugar

Evening Snack

2 servings fruit
2 slices gluten-free bread, or equivalent cereal or grain
   product

An approximate composition of this diet is:

Calories	2097	Calcium	1033 mg
Protein	89 g	Iron	18 mg
Fat	85 g	Phosphorus	1256 mg
Carbohydrate	244 g	Potassium	4521 mg
		Sodium	1651 mg

Gastroesophageal Reflux

Theodore M. Bayless, M.D.

INTRODUCTION

Dietary manipulation may be important in the management of gastroesophageal reflux. Many patients have an associated sliding hiatus hernia, but reflux can certainly occur in the absence of such a hernia.

GOALS OF TREATMENT

The goals of dietary treatment include avoidance of foods and eating habits that increase reflux, restriction of foods that increase gastric acidity or markedly delay gastric emptying, and buffering gastric acidity. Weight reduction in overweight patients is often an additional management goal. Intensive therapy for 8 to 10 weeks may decrease the sensitivity of the esophagus to acid or bile and the therapeutic regimen can then be somewhat less rigid.

RATIONALE OF TREATMENT

Since gastroesophageal reflux is increased by the consumption of large meals, patients are advised to eat small meals and to avoid multicourse meals. Carbonated beverages cause eructation, which carries gastric juice up into the already irritated or acid-sensitive esophagus. Since reflux is also favored by the prone position, patients are advised not to eat 90 to 120 minutes before bedtime and not to lie down for 1 to 1$^{1}/_{2}$ hours after meals. It may be necessary to restrict temporarily foods that delay gastric emptying and may increase reflux, such as fatty foods.

Excess weight puts more pressure on the stomach and increases gastroesophageal reflux. Often patients complain of heartburn initially after a weight gain of 10 to 20 lbs. Thus, weight reduction may be a key part of successful management.

In many patients with gastroesophageal reflux, acid is the irritating material. In some, however, especially those with a history of previous gastric or gallbladder surgery, bile reflux is the problem. Dietary therapy should include avoidance of substances such as coffee that increase gastric acidity. (It has been suggested recently that decaffeinated coffee can also cause gastric acid secretion.) Caffeine, chocolate, and peppermint, which decrease lower esophageal sphincter tone, should also be avoided. Frequent, small meals may help to control symptoms both by eliminating the pressure of a large meal and by buffering gastric acidity. Although bland diets were very popular in the past, especially for peptic ulcer disease, there is no evidence that ingestion of a regular diet stimulates any more acid production or delays improvement in esophagitis or healing of peptic ulceration.

Medications may also help to control symptoms of esophageal reflux or improve esophagitis. Liquid antacids, taken in 30- to 60-ml quantities between meals or at bedtime, may help to control gastric acidity. Alternatively, cimetidine decreases acid production significantly in many patients when 3000 mg is taken with meals and at bedtime. Metoclopramide increases lower esophageal sphincter tone and facilitates gastric emptying; both of these effects may be very helpful in the management of gastroesophageal reflux or its complications.

DESCRIPTION OF DIET FOR GASTROESOPHAGEAL REFLUX

The purpose of this diet is to maintain or reduce body weight in the overweight patient, while modifying foods to decrease gastroesophageal reflux and reduce gastric acid production. The following measures may be helpful:

1. Small meals, five to six per day, are recommended.
2. Avoid coffee, tea, carbonated beverages, and aspirin.
3. Avoid foods known to cause symptoms.
4. Avoid alcoholic beverages unless known to be tolerated.
5. Avoid reclining for $1^1/_2$ hours after food intake.
6. Restrict fat to low or moderate levels.
7. Avoid peppermint, chocolate, or medications—such as anticholinergics —that decrease lower esophageal sphincter pressure.
8. Weight loss may be helpful in overweight patients.

Partial Obstruction

Theodore M. Bayless, M.D., and
Helen D. Mullan, B.S., R.D.

INTRODUCTION

Partial obstruction can occur in the esophagus, stomach, small intestine, or distal colon. When available, objective radiologic evidence of partial obstruction is quite helpful in deciding whether dietary manipulation is a rational therapy. Inappropriate use of soft, low-residue, and low-roughage diets is common.

Dietary management of partial obstruction usually involves shifting the diet to materials that are more likely to pass through the compromised segment. Liquids or blended foods may be needed for esophageal obstruction. Dietary management of obstructive lesions of the stomach and upper small intestine requires small feedings that do not overload the diminished gastric capacity or the delayed emptying. With partial obstruction of the lower small intestine, one should presumably avoid high-bulk foods or those with high fiber or residue content that tend to increase the consistency of the ileal contents.

GOALS OF TREATMENT

The goal of management is to provide adequate oral nutrition in a form that will pass through the obstructed area more easily than will a regular diet. This goal includes maintenance or improvement of nutritional status while minimizing symptoms that are related to obstruction. The dietary therapy may be short term, in preparation for surgical treatment or during institution of medical therapy, or it may be chronic when the obstruction is not correctable.

RATIONALE FOR TREATMENT

Dietary therapy of partial obstruction of the gastrointestinal tract is based on identifying the specific site of dysfunction, understanding the altered physiology related to that specific lesion, and changing the diet to a smaller, more liquid, or less bulky form that can be propelled past the compromised area in adequate quantities to meet the individual's nutritional needs.

Esophageal Obstruction

Obstructing lesions, such as tumors or benign stricture after severe reflux esophagitis, cause swallowing difficulty (dysphagia). Regurgitation of food, perhaps with pulmonary aspiration and chronic pneumonia, may also be a problem, especially with motility disturbances such as achalasia. However, such disorders are usually treated by mechanical or surgical relief of the obstructed area. Intermittent esophageal spasm may cause temporary but recurrent dysphagia with solid or very elastic foods or iced beverages.

The degree and nature of the obstruction determines the dietary changes needed. For example, mere avoidance of large pieces of meat or of elastic foods, such as marshmallows or dinner rolls, may suffice for patients with esophageal spasm or stricture. However, liquid nutrition or blenderized foods may be needed for those with advanced unresectable carcinoma of the esophagus. Patients prone to regurgitate and aspirate esophageal contents should avoid evening feedings before retiring.

Gastric Obstruction

Large neoplasms that constrict and obstruct the stomach may lead to early satiety. Patients with such tumors require small frequent feedings and perhaps liquid nutrient sources. Obstruction at the pyloric or distal end of the stomach may result from active peptic ulceration and edema, scarring from healed ulceration, neoplasm, or a bezoar. Sometimes, a metabolic disorder such as diabetes may cause gastric atony and poor emptying.

Symptoms of gastric obstruction may include early satiety, weight loss, and vomiting. Dietary therapy is based on the use of small meals, usually utilizing liquid supplements. In addition, fatty foods that delay gastric emptying should be avoided. In infancy, however, pylorospasm is treated with a thicker cereal to try to overcome the altered function of the pyloric sphincter. With diabetes, metoclopramide may help decrease gastric retention.

Duodenal or Jejunal Obstruction

Partial duodenal obstruction or jejunal neoplasms or scarring may cause crampy pain, abdominal distention, or vomiting shortly after meals. This condition may require a liquid diet or even continuous parenteral infusion of nutrients.

Lower Small Intestinal Obstruction

Intestinal contents are normally a thick liquid when they reach the ileum. Partial obstruction may result from scarring or inflammation associated with regional enteritis (Crohn's disease), adhesions secondary to previous surgery, or neoplasms. Patients usually complain of cramping abdominal pain and distention 1 to 2 hours after meals. Audible peristalsis (borborygmus) may accompany the pain or be heard as the pain is relieved. Some patients may not describe a clear association of symptoms with meals but will nonetheless avoid eating to lessen their discomfort.

Before initiating dietary measures for partial obstruction, it is critical to establish its etiology. Unfortunately, the diagnosis of partial intestinal obstruction is too frequently applied inappropriately to patients with chronic abdominal distention that is often associated with chronic constipation. Many of these people have a variant of the irritable bowel syndrome and actually need a high-bulk diet rather than restriction of dietary intake.

Abdominal distention, with or without excessive flatulence, may also be incorrectly attributed to obstruction. The nutritionist may discover that the patient consumes large quantities of gas-producing foods, such as beans, cabbage, or milk (if the subject is lactose intolerant), or drinks a large quantity of carbonated beverages that aggravate the symptoms.

Dietary management of partial small bowel obstruction may require avoidance of foods with fibrous residues, such as celery, apple skins, or orange pulp. Some patients have also experienced complete obstruction after ingesting large amounts of corn, nuts, raw cauliflower, or squash. Patients with continent ileostomies (Kock pouch) may also need to avoid foods that cannot pass through the drainage catheter used to empty the pouch. Standard ileostomy patients usually do not have this problem. Low-residue nutritional supplements, as well as other liquid nutrient solutions, have proved very helpful in treating some patients with partial ileal obstruction.

Colonic Obstruction

Partial obstruction of the colon is either functional or the result of fibrous stricture from diverticulitis or granulomatous colitis. Since the contents of the colon are liquid until they reach the left or descending colon, obstruction will only occur with very advanced scarring or tumors unless the lesion is in the lower left colon. More irrational dietary restrictions are probably placed on patients with presumed colonic emptying problems or motor disorders than in any other area of gastroenterology. A liquid diet or elemental diet may be needed for high-grade distal colon obstruction.

Peptic Ulcer Disease

Theodore M. Bayless, M.D., and
Helen D. Mullan, B.S., R.D.

INTRODUCTION

Dietary manipulation and restriction have been grossly overemphasized in the management of peptic ulcer disease. Since the rate of ulcer healing is not impaired by a regular diet, there is no need for a bland, soft diet in the treatment of peptic ulceration. Instead, diet therapy is combined with an antacid or with gastric acid–suppressing medications in order to buffer gastric acidity. An effort is made to keep gastric pH above 3.5 so that pepsin, the protein-digesting enzyme in gastric juice, is not activated. The dietary approach is to keep something in the stomach as an acid buffer throughout as much of the day as possible. If effective acid blocking medications are used, less dietary manipulation will be needed.

GOALS OF TREATMENT

The goals of dietary treatment of peptic ulcer patients include the following:

1. To provide a buffering capacity to offset gastric acidity after meals, utilizing a regular diet with 3 to 6 feedings, including a night-time snack
2. To avoid delayed gastric emptying in patients with gastric ulcers
3. To avoid prolonged fasting
4. To consider dietary management of gastroesophageal reflux if symptoms suggest this disorder
5. To avoid traditional use of milk, if lactose intolerance is present
6. To avoid coffee, tea, and gastric irritants such as alcohol and spicy foods

DIETARY TREATMENT

It is not necessary to order a bland, soft diet for ulcer patients. There is no evidence that such diets enhance healing. Rather, the diet should consist of 3 to 6 feedings of a regular diet while avoiding known gastric secretory stimulants, such as coffee or caffeine-containing sodas. It may be helpful to avoid alcohol, aspirin, and specific foods poorly tolerated by the individual patient.

The usual therapeutic program would include 3 to 6 feedings and liquid antacids 1 to 3 hours after the 3 main meals and before retiring. Cimetidine, 300 mg with meals and at bedtime, may be used instead of antacids. Therapy should continue for at least 8 to 10 weeks to produce ulcer healing. In a patient with recurrent ulcer disease, diet and pharmacologic therapy are sometimes continued indefinitely.

Milk has no special healing properties; in fact, its protein content may stimulate acid production. Also, in some individuals lactose intolerance may produce flatulence, bloating, cramps, or diarrhea.

Dumping Syndrome

Francis D. Milligan, M.D.

INTRODUCTION

The clinical manifestations of the dumping syndrome result from the rapid introduction of hyperosmolar solutions into the proximal small bowel. Dumping may follow any operation that bypasses or destroys the pylorus. It is more frequent after partial gastric resection and gastrojejunostomy but also occurs after a lesser procedure such as vagotomy and pyloroplasty, since competence of the pyloric sphincter has been destroyed. As many as 20 to 30 per cent of patients suffer from some mild dumping symptoms after an operation, but symptoms usually decrease with time. Permanent disability due to dumping occurs in 5 to 10 per cent of patients.

The dumping syndrome is separated into early and late phases. The early phase, lasting 30 to 60 minutes, appears to be secondary to jejunal distention and the release of vasoactive hormones into the circulation. During this phase, blood glucose rises, peripheral hematocrit increases, and circulating blood volume, serum potassium, and phosphorus levels fall. Although a decreased blood volume is a characteristic finding, vasomotor symptoms do not depend on changes in plasma volume and may be experienced even when the blood volume is maintained at a normal level by infusion. Gastrointestinal symptoms include epigastric fullness, abdominal cramping, and occasional vomiting and diarrhea. Vasomotor manifestations include palpitations, weakness and fainting, drowsiness, dyspnea, and sweating.

The late phase of dumping is associated with symptoms of hypoglycemia. Early hyperglycemia, together with the release of intestinal glucagon, leads to excessive insulin secretion. The resultant hypoglycemia reaches a peak about 2 hours after carbohydrate ingestion. Faintness, sweating, palpitations, fatigue, and headache are common symptoms.

GOALS AND RATIONALE OF TREATMENT

Patients with this syndrome should ingest multiple small feedings, to decrease jejunal distention secondary to the rapid emptying of a large meal. The patient should avoid carbohyrates, especially simple sugars, to minimize the development of early hyperglycemia and resultant reactive hypoglycemia (see Chapter 6). Restriction of fluids at mealtime is necessary to retard gastric emptying.

DIETARY MANAGEMENT

Dietary Considerations

1. A diet high in protein, moderately high in fat, and low in carbohydrates —especially simple sugars—is divided into six small feedings. Meals should be eaten slowly.

2. No fluids of any kind are ingested during meals. Instead, fluids are taken 45 to 60 minutes before or after meals. Any fluids containing carbohydrate must be calculated into the dietary pattern.

3. Avoid concentrated sweets such as sugar, honey, and molasses. Sugar substitutes may be used.

4. Calories must be adjusted according to the patient's tolerance and needs.

5. Additional dietary modifications may be necessary for individuals with lactose intolerance.

Dietary Planning

Exchange lists (see Table A–13 in Appendix) are used to calculate the dietary pattern and to make the patient aware of food compositions. The food portions given in Lists 5 and 6 are minimal amounts; the patient may ingest greater quantities of these foods if they are tolerated well. Increased amounts of carbohydrates, starting with complex carbohydrates and graduating to the more simple forms, may be given once the patient is stabilized and can judge his tolerance of these foods.

This diet is adequate in all essential nutrients if the suggested pattern is followed. A sample meal plan is provided in Table 11–6.

TABLE 11–6.   DUMPING SYNDROME—SAMPLE MEAL PATTERN

Morning Meal

2 meat exchanges
3 fat exchanges
1 bread exchange
1 fruit exchange

Mid-Morning Meal

$\frac{1}{2}$ bread exchange
1 meat exchange
1 fat exchange
$\frac{1}{2}$ milk exchange (delay 45–60 minutes)

Noon Meal

2 meat exchanges
1 bread exchange
2 fat exchanges
1 fruit exchange

Mid-Afternoon Meal

1 meat exchange
$\frac{1}{2}$ bread exchange
1 fat exchange
$\frac{1}{2}$ milk exchange (delay 45–60 minutes)

Evening Meal

3 meat exchanges
1 vegetable exchange
1 bread exchange
3 fat exchanges
$\frac{1}{2}$ fruit exchange (may substitute extra vegetable)

Bedtime

2 meat exchanges
1 bread exchange
2 fat exchanges
$\frac{1}{2}$ milk exchange (delay 45–60 minutes)

An approximate composition of this diet is:

Calories	2066	Calcium	1140 mg
Protein	101 g	Iron	16 mg
Fat	130 g	Phosphorus	1734 mg
Carbohydrate	123 g	Potassium	2907 mg
		Sodium	2572 mg *

*Sodium content of diet without added salt.

Diet for Cystic Fibrosis

Beryl J. Rosenstein, M.D. and
Sylvia V. McAdoo, M.S., R.D.

INTRODUCTION

Cystic fibrosis is an autosomal recessive disease characterized by exocrine gland dysfunction and by altered function of mucous glands. It is manifested clinically by pancreatic insufficiency in 80 to 90 per cent of patients and by severe, diffuse obstructive pulmonary disease and infection in almost all patients. Disturbances in the secretions of the eccrine sweat glands and salivary glands are almost always present. There is great variation in the severity of the disease, allowing about one-half of the patients to survive into adulthood. In most instances, death is related to respiratory failure.

GOALS AND RATIONALE OF TREATMENT

The objectives of dietary treatment are

1. To provide an adequate diet for normal growth. Increased caloric, protein, and vitamin intakes are needed to offset nutrient losses secondary to pancreatic insufficiency and malabsorption. In general, in cystic fibrosis patients, caloric requirements are increased by 50 per cent and protein requirements by 100 per cent.
2. To relieve symptoms of abnormal stools, foul-smelling flatus, rectal prolapse, and abdominal distention or cramps.
3. To prevent, if possible, certain complications of pancreatic insufficiency such as meconium ileus equivalent, intussusception, and rectal prolapse.

The management of the maldigestive disturbances in cystic fibrosis should be individualized, since there is great variability in the degree of pancreatic enzyme insufficiency and, particularly, in tolerance to ingested fat. In contrast to fats and proteins, carbohydrates are usually well tolerated. With the use of pancreatic enzymes, most patients with cystic fibrosis are able to tolerate diets similar to those of healthy individuals of the same age.

DIETARY MANAGEMENT

Traditional methods of dietary management include supplementation with pancreatic enzymes, vitamins, calories, and protein, along with variable reductions in dietary fat.

TABLE 11–7. FOOD CHOICES FOR DIETS FOR ADOLESCENTS WITH CYSTIC FIBROSIS

	Foods Allowed	Foods to Be Avoided
MEAT, FISH, POULTRY	Lean beef, veal, lamb, chicken, turkey, liver, shrimp, crab, oysters, water-packed tuna, fresh fish, well-trimmed ham, or lean pork. Do not fry or cook in gravy.	Bacon, sausage, goose, duck, frankfurter, fish sticks, mackerel, bologna, and luncheon meats. Fried foods and gravy.
CHEESE	Dry cottage cheese or cheese made with skim milk (if tolerated).	All other cheeses.
EGGS	One whole egg allowed daily. (Egg yolks are high in fat, but egg white may be eaten as desired.) Fried and scrambled eggs allowed if cooked in Teflon skillet (with part of allowed fat).	More than one egg yolk daily.
VEGETABLES	Any vegetable except avocado.	Avocado, vegetables cooked with fat meats.
POTATOES OR SUBSTITUTES	Mashed potatoes made with skim milk and margarine, rice, plain spaghetti, grits, or plain noodles. Tomato gravy made without grease can be used on spaghetti and noodles if tolerated.	Potato chips, fried potatoes, corn chips, or frozen potatoes.
FRUITS	All fruits and juices.	None.
BREADS	Saltine crackers and sliced bread.	Cornbread and biscuits, unless tolerated. (These have a high fat content.)
CEREALS	Any cereal.	
FATS	As planned for individual.	Peanut butter, chocolate, bacon fat, saltpork, butterfat, salad oils, mayonnaise, salad dressings, fried foods, or gravies.
BEVERAGES	Low-fat or skim milk, at least 24 oz daily. Cocoa, not chocolate, may be used once a day, if tolerated.	Whole milk or cream.
SOUPS	Any soup made with skim milk or meats trimmed of excess fat.	Creamed soups made with whole milk; fatty meat broth.
DESSERTS	Gelatin desserts, fruit pudding, pudding and custard made with skim milk, sherbet, ice milk, and angel food cake.	High-fat desserts such as pie, pastry, cake, ice cream, doughnuts, and cookies made with chocolate or nuts.
SWEETS	Marshmallows, sugar, honey, jelly, jam, preserves, syrup, sugar candy, peppermint, or popsicles.	Chocolate, caramel, or nut candy.
MISCELLANEOUS	Salt, as prescribed.	Popcorn and nuts.

Tips: Sandwiches for school lunches can be made with the allowed margarine, mustard, or catsup. Tomato gravy can be made with puréed, canned, or fresh tomatoes. Celery, onions, green pepper, garlic, and parsley may be used freely, if tolerated.

Pancreatic Enzyme Supplementation

Pancreatic enzymes improve digestion of fats and proteins. The amount and type of pancreatic enzyme preparation for the cystic fibrosis patient is determined individually, by observing the patient's weight response and stool pattern. Enzymes, given immediately before meals and large snacks, may be varied in amount, depending on the size and fat content of the meal. Pancreatic enzymes are available in powder, tablet, and capsule forms and from either pork or beef sources. Selection of pancreatic enzymes varies with the physician's preference and individual patient tolerance. Preparations available commercially in this country include

(1) Pancrease (McNeil Pharmaceutical) and Cotazym S (Organon, Inc.)—these capsules contain enteric-coated microspheres of pancreatic lipase, amylase, and protease.

(2) Viokase (Viobin, Inc.)—This pancreatic enzyme concentrate of porcine origin contains lipase, protease, and amylase. It is available as a tablet or powder. Beef pancreas powder is available for those exceptional patients allergic to pork.

(3) Cotazem (Organon, Inc.)—An enzyme concentrate of porcine origin available in capsule and powder form.

Vitamin Supplementation

Fat-soluble vitamins A and D should be given in a water-miscible solution in twice the daily recommended dosage for age. Supplemental vitamin K is usually recommended for infants, patients with cirrhosis or evidence of a bleeding tendency, and those on prolonged broad-spectrum antimicrobial therapy. Vitamin E may be useful in preventing the neurologic and hematologic abnormalities that have been reported in cystic fibrosis patients with severe fat malabsorption. Vitamin B–complex supplements are recommended for patients with cirrhosis and for those on long-term broad-spectrum antimicrobial therapy or taking chloramphenicol. Multivitamin preparations should be given in twice the recommended dosage. In areas where fluoride is not added to the local water supply and where naturally occurring fluoride levels are low, a fluoride supplement should be given.

Calorie and Protein Supplementation with Dietary Fat Reduction

It is far easier to control the diet of infants than that of older children and adolescents. Fortunately, malabsorption symptoms seem to be less troublesome in older patients who learn from experience what fatty foods they can tolerate. A balance must be struck between pancreatic enzyme supplementation and the fat content of the diet.

The recommended fat intake varies with age and with total caloric intake. Although some reduction in fat may be necessary in most patients, severe fat reduction should be avoided because of high cost, sacrifice of palatability and variety of meals, and possible deficiency of essential fatty acids. A diet considered to be low in fat ranges from 30 to 50 g of fat/day. Frequent feedings may be necessary to satisfy hunger and provide adequate calories. Protein intake can be augmented by high-protein snacks and protein supplementation with milk. A product such as Polycose (Ross Labs) can be utilized to increase the caloric content of various foods.

MCT Oil

Medium-chain triglycerides (MCTs) are effective in the dietary treatment of a variety of malabsorption and other syndromes (chylothorax, pancreatitis, cystic fibrosis, tropical and nontropical sprue, biliary atresia, and postgastrectomy states).

MCT oil, obtained from coconut oil by molecular distillation, is composed predominantly of triglycerides containing caprylic (C8) and capric (C10) acids. In contrast, naturally occurring fats are long-chain triglycerides (LCTs) in which the fatty acid carbon chain is invariably greater than that of lauric acid (C12). Feeding experiments with animals and subsequently with humans indicate that MCTs and LCTs are absorbed and transported differently. MCTs, unlike LCTs, are (1) more rapidly hydrolyzed, (2) independent of bile salts for absorption, (3) not incorporated into chylomicrons, and (4) transported directly to the liver via the portal circulation. In the liver they are oxidized primarily for utilization as energy and secondarily for the synthesis of fatty acids.

Such significant differences from usual lipid metabolism allow the successful use of MCTs in the treatment of certain diseases. Although not a panacea, MCT therapy is frequently effective in the management of patients with impaired fat digestion and malabsorption problems that do not respond to other forms of treatment. For these patients, MCTs may provide a source of calories and add palatability to a diet that otherwise must be severely restricted in fat. (MCT oil is distributed commercially by Mead Johnson Company, Evansville, IL 47721).

Feeding

Feeding the cystic fibrosis patient is often difficult. At the time of diagnosis it is not unusual for the patient to be underweight and malnourished. An adjustment period is usually required for the patient to become accustomed to the recommended diet and to establish an adequate level of enzyme supplementation, as well as other forms of treatment.

NUTRITIONAL ASPECTS OF CYSTIC FIBROSIS

Dietary Recommendations

Infants

The young infant is unique because milk is the prime nutrient source of the calories and protein necessary for adequate growth and development. This is the rationale for using formulas of increased caloric energy density, exceeding the standard 20 cal/oz concentration. It may also be necessary to give more frequent feedings to younger infants. Energy requirements for infants with cystic fibrosis are in the range of 150 to 200 kcal/kg/day (50 to 100 per cent above RDAs for normal infants).

An increased protein intake is also recommended for infants with cystic fibrosis. Normal fat intake for infants is in the range of 40 to 60 g/day. Although rigid fat restriction should be avoided, some fat restriction is often necessary in those infants with pancreatic insufficiency.

FORMULAS VERSUS MILK.   Whole cow's milk has generally been an adequate base for the feeding of infants over 12 months with pancreatic insufficiency secondary to cystic fibrosis. Hypoproteinemic edema can result from feeding of formulas that are quantitatively or qualitatively low in protein content. This problem has occurred almost exclusively in children fed soy formulas or breast milk. In the first instance the problem is probably one of protein quality, whereas in the latter it is one of protein quantity.

A protein hydrolysate formula such as Pregestimil, containing 40 per cent of total fat energy as MCT oil, is usually well tolerated by infants with cystic fibrosis and pancreatic insufficiency. Its use has the advantage of reducing—but not eliminating—the need for enzyme supplements.

When stools remain excessively large and foul-smelling, it may be desirable to use Portagen (Mead Johnson) as a major source of calories. Casein is the protein source and MCT oil provides 86 per cent of the fat calories. MCT oil is known to reduce steatorrhea and to improve stool character in patients with cystic fibrosis. In addition, increased rates of gain in weight and height have been observed after introduction of diets containing MCTs.

Powdered skim milk preparations or commercially available liquid skim or low-fat milk with protein supplements can be used for infants over 12 months with cystic fibrosis. These preparations should not be used for infants under 12 months of age.

SOLID FOOD.   The infant's ability to chew is dependent on his stage of development and varies among infants of the same age. Strained foods, particularly for the young infant with respiratory difficulty, are preferred because of their soft consistency. As soon as tolerated, puréed and chopped table foods are begun. Home blenders are very helpful in preparing table foods of proper consistency. Strained and puréed foods may be needed longer for the infant with cystic fibrosis, depending on the degree of maldigestion and the stage of physical development. In some infants with pancreatic enzyme deficiency, undigested food particles may appear in the stools, and the color of the stools may vary with the color of the food ingested.

In the infant with cystic fibrosis and pancreatic enzyme insufficiency, solid foods are begun at approximately 5 to 6 months and increased as tolerated to provide additional calories and protein. Fruits and cereals are used initially, followed by vegetables, lean meat, and egg yolk. One new food is started every 2 to 3 days as tolerance is assessed. Of the fruits, applesauce, pears, apricots, and peaches are started first. Prunes and plums may have a laxative effect in some infants. Of the vegetables, carrots and squash are usually well tolerated and frequently used initially. Spinach may cause an increased number of stools in some infants.

Intolerance to starch is not present in cystic fibrosis. Cereals may be used as a means of increasing energy intake.

Mixtures of vegetables and meats and high-protein dinners should be avoided. The "high-protein dinners" are mixtures of vegetables and starches with a low meat content. Pure strained or puréed meats are better sources of protein.

SALT. In very hot weather or during febrile episodes, salt requirements may be increased and additional salt should be added to the diet. Infants may have up to $\frac{1}{4}$ tsp salt per day added to their diet.

Adolescents and Young Adults

Attention to nutritional needs is more important during the growth spurt of adolescence and young adulthood than at any other developmental period except infancy. Increased amounts of high-quality protein and other essential nutrients are needed because of rapid growth expected during this period. The adolescent or young adult with cystic fibrosis should have approximately twice the RDA for protein and 1 to $1^{1}/_{2}$ times the RDA of calories to maintain growth. The goal of adequate nutrition in the face of chronic disease and maldigestive losses makes the planning and consideration of diet particularly important in these patients.

Extra calories may be obtained from (1) high-protein snacks, (2) low-fat desserts, (3) high-protein beverages, (4) sugars and starches, and (5) MCT oil, if necessary for adequate energy intake. Amount will vary depending on the degree of malabsorption and the effectiveness of pancreatic enzymes (if used).

In planning the diet, recommendations for energy intake are based on the age, activity, and degree of weight loss of the patient. The percentages of protein, fat, and carbohydrate follow the recommendations in Chapter 1, Pediatric Nutrition. Table 11–7 lists the foods allowed and to be avoided for these patients.

BIBLIOGRAPHY

Lactose Intolerance

Barr, R. G., Levine, M. D., and Watkins, J. B.: Recurrent abdominal pain of childhood due to lactose intolerance: A prospective study. N Engl J Med 300:1499–52, 1979.

Bayless, T. M.: Recognition of lactose intolerance. Hospital Practice, 97–102, October, 1976.

Bayless, T. M. Lactose malabsorption, milk intolerance and symptom awareness in adults. In Paige, D. M., and Bayless, T. M., (Eds.): Lactose Digestion: Clinical and Nutritional Implications. Baltimore, Johns Hopkins University Press., 1981, pp. 117–123.

Bayless, T. M., and Paige, D. M.: Disaccharide intolerance in feeding programs. Reprint from Proceedings Western Hemisphere Nutrition Congress III. New York, Future Publishing Co., Inc.

Calloway, D. H., and Chenoweth, W. L.: Utilization of nutrients in milk and wheat-based diets by men with adequate and reduced abilities to absorb lactose, energy and nitrogen. Am J Clin Nutr 26:939–951, 1973.

Kolars, J. C., Levitt, M. D., Aouji, M., and Savaiano, D. A.: Yogurt—an autodigesting source of lactose. N Engl J Med 310:1–3, 1984.

Newcomer, A. D., and McGill, D. B.: Clinical importance of lactase deficiency. N Engl J Med 310:42–43, 1984.

Rosensweig, N. S.: Lactose feeding and lactase deficiency. Am J Clin Nutr 26:1166–1167, 1973.

Welsh, J. D.: Diet therapy in adult lactose malabsorption: Present practices. Am J Clin Nutr 31:592–596, 1978.

Gluten Sensitivity

Baker, A. L., and Rosenberg, I. N.: Refractory sprue: Recovery after removal of nongluten dietary products. Ann Intern Med 89:505–508, 1978.
Bayless, T. M., Yardley, J. H., and Hendrix, T. R.: Adult celiac disease: Treatment with a gluten free diet. Arch Int Med 111:83–92, 1963.
Falchuk, Z. M.: Update on gluten-sensitive enteropathy. Am J Med 67:1085–1096, 1979.

Gastroesophageal Reflux

Hendrix, T.R.: Medical treatment of reflux symptoms. *In* Skinner, D. B., Belsey, R. H. R., Hendrix, T. R., Zuidema, G. D., Gastroesophageal Reflux and Hiatal Hernia. Boston, Little, Brown, and Co., 1972, pp. 129–131.
Johnson, L. F., and Peura, D. A.: Esophageal reflux: medical management. *In* Bayless, T. M. (Ed): Current Therapy in Gastroenterology and Liver Disease, Toronto, B. C. Decker, 1984, pp. 1–5.

Peptic Ulcer Disease

Babouris, N., Fletcher, J., and Lennard-Jones, J.: Effect of different foods on the acidity of the gastric contents in patients with duodenal ulcer: Effect of varying the size and frequency of meals. Gut 6:118–120, 1965.
Buchman, E., Kaung, D. T., Dolan, K., and Knepp, R. N.: Unrestricted diet in the treatment of duodenal ulcer. Gastroenterology 56:1016–1020, 1969.
Hollander, D.: Duodenal ulcer. *In* Bayless, T. M., (Ed.): Current Therapy in Gastroenterology and Liver Disease. Toronto, B. C. Decker, 1984, pp. 53–59.
Ippoliti, A. F., Maxwell, V. A., and Isenberg, J. I.: The effect of various forms of milk on gastric acid secretion. Studies in patients with duodenal ulcer and normal subjects. Ann Intern Med 84:286–289, 1976.

Dumping Syndrome

Alexander-Williams, Jr., and Hoare, A. M.: Partial gastric resection. Clin Gastroenterol 8:321–353, 1979.
Bayless, T. M.: Current Therapy in Gastroenterology and Liver Disease Toronto, B. C. Decker, 1984.
Floch, M. H.: Nutrition and Diet Therapy in Gastrointestinal Disease. New York, Plenum Publishing Corp., 1981.

Cystic Fibrosis

Beckerman, R. C., and Taussig, L. M.: Hypoelectrolytemia and metabolic acidosis in infants with cystic fibrosis. Pediatrics 63:580–583, 1979.
Chase, H. P., Long, M. A., and Lavin, M. H.: Cystic fibrosis and malnutrition. J Pediatr. 95:337–347, 1979.
Committee on Dietary Allowances, Food and Nutrition Board: Recommended Dietary Allowances. Washington, D.C., National Academy of Sciences, 1980.
Crozier, D. N.: Cystic fibrosis. A not-so-fatal disease. Pediatr Clin North Am 21:935–950, 1974.
Farrell, P. M., Bieri, J. G., Fratantoni, J. F., Wood, R. E., and di Santi'Agnese, P. A.: The occurrence and effects of human vitamin E deficiency. J Clin Invest 60:233–241, 1977.
Fleisher, D. S., Di George, A. M., Barness, L. A., and Cornfeld, D.: Hypoproteinemia and edema in infants with cystic fibrosis of the pancreas. J Pediatr 64:341–348, 1964. (See also J Pediatr 64:349–356, 1964.)
Fomon, S. J.: Nutritional disorders of children, prevention, screening and follow-up. U.S. Dept. HEW, Public Health Service, Pub. No. (HSA) 77-51-4.
Gurwitz, D., Corey, M., Francis, P. W. J., Crozier, D., and Levison, H.: Perspectives in cystic fibrosis. Pediatr Clin North Am 26:603–615, 1979.
Hamill, P. V. V., Drizd, T. A., Johnson, C. L., Reed, R. B., and Roche, A. F.: NCHS growth charts, 1976. Vital and Health Statistics—Series II. Rockville, MD, Health Resources Administration, DHEW, 1976.
Hubbard, V. S., Barbero, G., and Chase, H. P.: Selenium and cystic fibrosis. J Pediatr 96:421–422, 1980.

Lee, P. A., Roloff, D. W., and Howatt, W. F.: Hypoproteinemia and anemia in infants with cystic fibrosis. JAMA 228:585–588, 1974.

Lloyd-Still, J. D., Johnson, S. B., and Holman, R. T.: Essential fatty acid status in cystic fibrosis and the effects of safflower oil supplementation. Am J Clin Nutr 34:1–7, 1981.

Mason, M., Wenberg, B. G., and Welsch, P. K.: The Dynamics of Clinical Dietetics. New York, John Wiley and Sons, 1977.

Muller, D. P. R., Lloyd, J. K., and Wolff, O. H.: Vitamin E and neurological function. Lancet 1:225–228, 1983.

Waring, W. W.: Current management of cystic fibrosis. Pediatrics 23:401–438, 1976.

12
KETOGENIC DIETS FOR TREATMENT OF CHILDHOOD EPILEPSY

Ernest Barbosa, M.D., John Freeman, M.D., and
Gloria Elfert, M.S., R.D.

INTRODUCTION

The beneficial effects of starvation and dehydration on epilepsy have been known for centuries. In an attempt to stimulate the metabolic effects of starvation, Wilder in 1921 introduced the ketogenic diet. He speculated that the anticonvulsant effect of fasting may be related to the level of ketosis or acidosis or both that is produced.

The standard ketogenic diet employs a high ratio of fat to carbohydrate plus protein. The initial clinical reports demonstrating the anticonvulsant value of the ketogenic diet in epilepsy were presented by Peterman in 1925 and Helmholz in 1927. In a later series of 1001 patients treated with the ketogenic diet, Livingston reported that seizures were controlled in 52 per cent, markedly reduced in 27 per cent, and unresponsive in the remainder. The beneficial effects persisted so long as the diet was maintained.

A more recent ketogenic dietary program, introduced in 1971 by Huttenlocker, employs medium-chain triglycerides (MCTs) as the primary source of lipid calories. Since MCTs appear to be more ketogenic than other dietary fats, the diet can include a greater proportion of foods containing carbohydrates and protein while maintaining adequate levels of ketosis. The reported results utilizing this dietary regimen, however, suggest that it is less effective in achieving seizure control than is the standard ketogenic diet. Ketogenic diets are now used less frequently than they were before the introduction of effective anticonvulsant medication for minor motor seizures and other types of seizure disorders.

GOAL OF TREATMENT

The goal of treatment is to control seizures with the use of little or no medication. All or most anticonvulsant medications can be discontinued while the patient is following the dietary regimen. If the patient has remained virtually free of seizures for about 3 years on the diet, additional medications are usually unnecessary once the diet has been discontinued. However, for children with intractable seizures the ketogenic diet may provide seizure control without the major side effects of multiple medications.

RATIONALE OF TREATMENT

Wilder introduced the terms *ketogenic potential (K)* and *antiketogenic potential (AK)*. These terms reflect the degree to which various foodstuffs produce ketosis following digestion and metabolism. Fat has a high ketogenic potential, protein a mixed potential, and glucose negates the ketosis effect (*i.e.,* it is antiketogenic). The K/AK ratio of 1.5:1 is needed to produce ketosis, and seizure control is greatest when a diet yields K/AK values greater than 3:1 (this is referred to as a 3-to-1 diet). All diet plans need to fulfill the minimal protein requirement for growth, approximately 1 g/kg body weight/day. The total caloric intake is initially set at 75 kcal/kg of body weight/day to minimize weight gain and maximize ketonemia.

MCTs contain medium-chain fatty acids with carbon chain lengths of between 6 and 12, mainly octanoic and decanoic acids. MCTs are more ketogenic than other dietary fats because of their more rapid absorption, transport, and oxidation.

The mechanism of action of the ketogenic diet is unclear. Its anticonvulsant effect may result from ketosis, acidosis, dehydration, electrolyte alterations in the brain, or some combination of all these effects. It does appear certain that some degree of ketosis is needed. Cases have been reported in which a seizure began just 45 minutes after a glucose infusion was started. Animal studies have shown a decrease in maximal electroshock resistance $3^{1}/_{2}$ hours after a glucose (antiketogenic) load.

The anticonvulsant effects of acidosis and dehydration are less clear. Dehydration alone has been helpful, but its effect diminishes over a week's time. Acidosis develops with the initiation of starvation and the ketogenic diet, but within 1 to 2 weeks the body has compensated and the plasma pH remains normal through the remaining period of dietary treatment. The correction of the early acidosis with sodium bicarbonate does not diminish the effectiveness of the diet. Water content and electrolyte concentration in the brain are not significantly altered. Although these factors individually may not contribute to seizure control, stress of the acid-base homeostatic mechanisms may be important. Other possible mechanisms, such as alteration of the energy potentials of the brain or of putative transmitter substances, remain to be studied.

PATIENT SELECTION

The diet is most effective in controlling childhood myoclonic epilepsy; however, it may also be helpful in some patients with major motor (grand mal) seizures. The ketogenic diet is ineffective therapy for petit mal and psychomotor seizures. Patients whose electroencephalograms show abnormalities other than the classic spike-and-wave complex of petit mal epilepsy are more apt to respond to the ketogenic diet.

The diet is usually considered only after other forms of therapy have failed and is rarely used during the first year of life because of problems in achieving and maintaining ketosis. It is also often difficult to utilize the diet in older nonretarded children because of problems with compliance. The diet can achieve seizure control in children over the age of one year when dietary supervision can be maintained and parents are cooperative.

Circumstances within the home are central in deciding whether to institute the ketogenic diet. It should be attempted only when parents can accept it, cooperate fully, and ensure the cooperation of the patient. *The diet is effective only when followed rigidly.* Ketogenic diets should not be considered when feeding problems are anticipated or the home situation makes compliance unlikely.

DIETARY MANAGEMENT

Although there are different approaches to institution and maintenance of the ketogenic diet, we have found one particular regimen to be effective, and this is described subsequently.

We hospitalize the child for initiation of the ketogenic dietary regimen Fasting blood sugar, blood urea nitrogen (BUN), serum electrolytes, cholesterol and uric acid are obtained on admission and are followed closely thereafter The patient is weighed daily at approximately the same hour every day.

The ketogenic regimen is begun with a period of starvation and dehydration. During this phase, the patient receives no food but continues his previous anticonvulsant medications. About 800 ml of water is permitted daily, except when unusual environmental conditions dictate a greater allowance. Starvation is continued until 10 per cent of the patient's body weight has been lost and urinary ketones—usually highest in the late afternoon—are strongly positive This part of the regimen usually requires 2 to 5 days. Potential problems during the starvation phase include marked acidosis, hypoglycemia, and vomiting. In travenous fluids (normal saline) may be administered or starvation discontinued and the ketogenic diet instituted immediately to counter those effects.

The ketogenic diet causes a mild hypoglycemia that persists throughout the period of treatment. Blood glucose should be monitored at least twice a day o whenever symptoms of hypoglycemia occur. Starvation must be discontinued and glucose given if the patient demonstrates *both* clinical and laboratory evi dence of hypoglycemia. Although unusual, intractable vomiting during the starvation period may necessitate cessation of the regimen, a brief interruption of the starvation, or administration of small amounts of orange juice with glucose.

Initiation of the Ketogenic Diet

After the initial starvation period, the ketogenic diet is started, usually at the 4:1 ratio. It is best to offer the child one-third of the total calculated daily intake on the first day, two-thirds on the second day, and the full allowance on the third. By doing this it is often possible to avoid the intestinal upset that may develop following a period of fasting. Once the diet has been started, water (or a calorie-free beverage) is permitted, to satisfy thirst, but total fluid intake is still restricted. After several weeks, patients can usually tolerate the sense of hunger often present between meals. Caloric intake should not be increased unless the patient continues to lose weight or becomes totally uncooperative. When absolutely necessary, intake is usually liberalized in increments of 200 kcal/day.

The patient remains hospitalized for about 5 days after the full diet has been instituted, to be certain that dietary tolerance is maintained. During this period, parents or guardians must be given complete instructions on implementation of the diet at home, and the need for rigid compliance must be emphasized.

The anticonvulsant effect of the diet may not be apparent immediately. Clinical results may be seen in a few days, but periods of a week or more are commonly required for maximal control. If the diet is not effective within 3 months, it usually will not work at all. However, if the diet has been instituted at a K/AK ratio of 4:1, this ratio may now be increased to 4.5:1 or 5:1. Once seizure control is established, the diet usually will be effective for years.

All anticonvulsant medications except barbiturates may gradually be withdrawn during the first 3 months of the regimen, as tolerated. Barbiturates are usually continued at the same level for the first 3 months and then gradually decreased over the next year of treatment. Barbiturate levels should be closely monitored, especially during the initiation period of the ketogenic diet; in a large number of patients treated with the ketogenic diet, barbiturate levels have risen considerably without a corresponding change in dosage.

Complications

All measured plasma lipid levels (cholesterol, phospholipids, triglycerides, and fatty acids) are elevated 2 to 3 times normal. The lipidemia reaches a steady state after 2 to 3 weeks of therapy. No significant long-term side effects have been noted in children after discontinuation of the diet.

The diet is rich in vitamins A and D. *The diet must be supplemented with vitamins B, C, and calcium, using preparations that contain no calories.* Usually, supplementation consists of 1 g twice daily of oral calcium gluconate or 1.5 tsp daily of tribasic calcium phosphate, and 1 chewable multivitamin per day.

The most common cause for reduced ketosis or for the recurrence of seizures in a well-controlled patient are ingestion of additional food, defective scales used in food preparation, improper food preparation, or ingestion of medications/supplements containing carbohydrates. If ketonuria becomes negative or slight, the child should be fed nothing except for water or calorie-free beverages until urinary ketones become strongly positive (usually one or two meals). Care must be taken that all medications—mouthwashes, tooth powder, aspirin, and so on—are sugar free.

If the patient develops an intercurrent illness and refuses solid food, preplanned liquid meals that have essentially the same composition as the solids are substituted. Vomiting may occur at any time while the patient is on the diet. If vomiting does not resolve rapidly, it may be advisable to discontinue all food for a few days and give the patient only water during this time.

Children on the ketogenic diet should be checked periodically for signs of protein deficiency. On occasion, linear growth may be moderately retarded while the patient is on the diet. This disturbance is temporary and accelerated growth occurs when the program is discontinued. There is no evidence that patients treated with a ketogenic diet are ultimately shorter than they would have been had the diet not been used.

Discontinuation of the Diet

The ratio of fat to carbohydrate plus protein is gradually reduced over a 1-year period, to lessen the likelihood of inducing status epilepticus or of developing recurrent seizures. The K/AK ratio is changed to 3:1 for 6 months and then to 2:1 for the next 6 months. The protein allowance may be increased to 1.5 g/kg/day at the 2:1 ratio. After the patient has been on the 2:1 ratio for 6 months, a regular diet is started. As the K/AK ratio is being decreased, ketonuria will also gradually decrease. Urine testing may be discontinued when ketosis is no longer present.

CALCULATION OF THE DIET

The child must receive sufficient calories for maintenance of growth, yet the caloric allowance must be distributed according to the prescribed ratio. The 2- to 5-year-old child requires from 60 to 80 kcal/kg/day. Caloric intake should be planned according to the nutritional status, appetite, and activity of the patient.

The diet is tailored, as much as possible, to the patient's needs and preferences. It is essential that parents and patient discuss with the dietitian food habits, likes and dislikes, and normal patterns of eating. Using this information, the dietitian can provide meal plans that fit the family's meal structure and also satisfy the dietary prescription. The prescription can be translated into meal patterns with much more flexibility than may be apparent initially.

As long as the prescribed ratio of fat to carbohydrate plus protein remains constant, the amount of food ingested from day to day or from meal to meal may be varied without altering the ketogenic effect of the diet. By increasing or decreasing each item in the meal plan by the same proportion, the diet can be arranged to correspond with the child's appetite. However, since parents usually need help in changing meal plans to avoid altering the K/AK ratio, which would jeopardize the beneficial effect of the diet, they should work out adjustments in conjunction with the dietitian.

General Rules

DIET ORDER. The physician prescribes the K/AK ratio. The dietitian or physician determines the calorie allowance based on the child's weight, age, and activity level.

CALORIES. The calorie allowance is approximately 75 per cent of the RDA for the child's age:

Ages 1–3 75 kcal/kg
Ages 4–6 68 kcal/kg
Ages 7–10 60 kcal/kg

DIETARY UNITS

1. The diet is calculated by utilizing what is termed its *dietary unit*. For example, for the 4:1 diet, a dietary unit will consist of 4 g of fat and 1 g of carbohydrate plus protein combined.

2. The caloric value and caloric breakdown of a dietary unit varies with the K/AK ratio.

Ratio	Fat Calories	Carbohydrate Plus Protein Calories	Calories/Unit
2:1	2 g fat × 9 kcal/g = 18	1 g × 4 kcal/g = 4	22
3:1	3 g fat × 9 kcal/g = 27	4	31
4:1	4 g fat × 9 kcal/g = 36	4	40
5:1	5 g fat × 9 kcal/g = 45	4	49

3. The number of dietary units permitted per day equals

$$\frac{\text{Total calories allowed per day}}{\text{Calories per dietary unit}}$$

FATS. The grams of fat allowed per day equal the number of dietary units times grams of fat per unit.

PROTEIN. At least 1 g of protein/kg poststarvation weight/day, keeping as close to the minimal daily requirement as possible, is suggested. Higher protein intake is possible with 3:1 or 2:1 diets.

CARBOHYDRATES

1. Since each unit contains 1 g of carbohydrate plus protein combined, the grams of carbohydrate plus protein allowed per day equal the number of dietary units.

TABLE 12–1.   KETOGENIC DIET NUTRIENT ALLOWANCES

Kcal/Day	2:1 F g/day	2:1 C&P g/day	3:1 F g/day	3:1 C&P g/day	4:1 F g/day	4:1 C&P g/day	5:1 F g/day	5:1 C&P g/day
1000	91	45	97	32	100	25	102	20
1100	100	50	106	36	110	27	112	22
1200	109	55	116	39	120	30	123	25
1300	118	59	126	42	130	32	133	27
1400	128	64	135	45	140	35	143	29
1500	136	68	144	48	150	38	153	31
1600	146	73	156	52	160	40	163	33
1700	154	77	165	55	170	43	174	35
1800	164	82	174	58	180	45	184	37
1900	172	86	183	61	190	48	195	39
2000	182	91	195	65	200	50	204	41
2100	191	95	203	68	210	52	214	43
2200	200	100	213	71	220	55	225	45
2300	209	105	222	74	230	57	235	47
2400	218	109	232	77	240	60	245	50
2500	228	114	242	81	250	62	255	51

Note: F = fat, C = carbohydrate, and P = protein.

2. Deduct the protein allowance from the combined carbohydrate plus protein allowance.

FLUIDS.   Restrict fluids to 600 to 1200 ml/day, including liquids given as part of the meal. (The fluid allowance *may* require liberalization during hot weather.) Fluids should be apportioned throughout the day. Diet soda may be used to satisfy some fluid needs; however, no more than 1 calorie/day should be derived from this source. Otherwise, alteration of the ratio may compromise the effectiveness of the dietary program.

FOODS REFUSED.   All fat or cream or both *must* be taken at each meal, to maintain the ratio. Substitutions should be made for the fat and/or cream not ingested. Refusal of food is rarely a problem, since the diet is hypocaloric and all menus are individually based on food preferences.

Table 12–1 provides precalculated fat, carbohydrate, and protein allowances for various ratios and total caloric allowances.

Sample Calculation

A 3-year-old child weighing 13 kg is to be placed on a 4:1 ratio diet. Total calories will consist of the following:

$$100 \text{ kcal/kg/day} \times 0.75 = 75 \text{ cal/kg/day}$$
$$75 \text{ kcal/kg/day} \times 13 \text{ kg} = 975 \text{ cal/day}$$

Each dietary unit consists of 4 g of fat and 1 g of carbohydrate plus protein. Caloric value per dietary unit will be as follows:

$$4 \text{ g fat} \times 9 \text{ kcal/g} = 36 \text{ fat kcal/unit}$$

$$1 \text{ g carbohydrate} + \text{protein combined} \times 4 \text{ kcal/g} = 4 \text{ (carbohydrate} + \text{protein)} \text{ kcal/unit}$$

$$36 + 4 = 40 \text{ kcal/dietary unit}$$

The total number of dietary units permitted per day is shown in the following formula:

$$\frac{\text{Total kcal permitted/day}}{\text{kcalories/dietary unit}} = \text{Total number dietary units}$$

$$\frac{975 \text{ kcal/day}}{40 \text{ kcal/unit}} = 24.4 \text{ units/day}$$

The child's fat allowance would be determined by

$$24.4 \text{ units/day} \times 4 \text{ g fat/unit} = 97.6 \text{ g fat/day}$$

and protein allowance would be determined by

$$1 \text{ g protein} \times 13 \text{ kg body weight} = 13 \text{ g protein/day}$$

Although this protein intake is below the RDA, a higher protein intake, in this example, is impractical because the carbohydrate allowance would then become too low for patient acceptability.

Determination of the child's carbohydrate allowance is as follows:

$$24.4 \text{ units/day} \times 1 \text{ g of carbohydrate} + \text{protein combined/unit} = 24.4 \text{ g of carbohydrate} + \text{protein/day}$$

$$24.4 \text{ g carbohydrate} + \text{protein/day} - 13 \text{ g protein/day} = 11.4 \text{ g carbohydrate/day}$$

Thus, the child's diet order will read: 975 calories, 4:1 ratio.

Fat	97.6 g
Protein	13.0 g
Carbohydrate	11.4 g

The total nutrient allowance is divided into equal thirds. Each third represents one meal. Meal plans may then be prepared.

FORMULATION OF MEAL PLANS FOR THE KETOGENIC DIET

The following process illustrates the formulation of meal plans for the diet previously calculated. This diet order specifies that each meal contain 4.3 g protein, 32.5 g fat, and 3.8 g carbohydrate. These values constitute one-third of the calculated daily dietary prescription and maintain a 4:1 ketogenic-to-antiketogenic ratio. A sample meal plan is found in Table 12–2.

TABLE 12–2. SAMPLE MEAL PLAN

		Daily		Per Meal	
DIET ORDER	Kcal	975	Kcal	325	
	Protein	13 g	Protein	4.3 g	
	Fat	97.6 g	Fat	32.5 g	
	Carbohydrate	11.4 g	Carbohydrate	3.8 g	
	Ratio	4:1	Ratio	4:1	

Meal Plan		Composition		
		PROTEIN	FAT	CARBOHYDRATE
MENU 1				
14 g meat, fish, poultry		3.3	2.3	
26 g 10% fruit		0.3		2.6
16 g fat			16.0	
40 g 36% cream		0.8	14.4	1.2
	Total	4.4	32.7	3.8
MENU 2				
11 g cheese, American, Swiss, or cheddar		3.3	3.8	
26 g 10% fruit		0.3		2.6
15 g fat			15.0	
40 g 36% cream		0.8	14.4	1.2
	Total	4.4	33.2	3.8
MENU 3				
27 g egg		3.2	3.2	
26 g 10% fruit		0.3		2.6
15 g fat			15.0	
40 g 36% cream		0.8	14.4	1.2
	Total	4.3	32.6	3.8
MENU 4				
12 g meat, fish, poultry		2.8	2.0	
37 g group B vegetable		0.7		2.6
17 g fat			17.0	
40 g 36% cream		0.8	14.4	1.2
	Total	4.3	33.4	3.8
MENU 5				
9 g cheese, American, Swiss, or cheddar		2.7	3.1	
37 g group B vegetable		0.7		2.6
15 g fat			15.0	
40 g 36% cream		0.8	14.4	1.2
	Total	4.2	32.5	3.8
MENU 6				
23 g egg		2.8	2.8	
37 g group B vegetable		0.7		2.6
16 g fat			16.0	
40 g 36% cream		0.8	14.4	1.2
	Total	4.3	33.2	3.8

Any three sample menus may be used in a given day since they all follow the 4:1 ratio.

1. Using Table 12–3, calculate the amount of cream that will provide approximately 50 per cent of the fat in the meal. Forty grams of 36 per cent cream contains 14.4 g of fat. It is important to know the butterfat content of the cream used. As indicated in Table 12–3, there is a considerable difference in the fat content of 36 per cent and 30 per cent cream. The cream allowance also provides 0.8 g of protein and 1.2 g of carbohydrate.

2. The foods used to meet the carbohydrate allowance are planned next. The carbohydrate content of the cream should be calculated to determine the amount of carbohydrate to be supplied by other foods. In the sample, the 1.2 g of carbohydrate derived from cream is subtracted from the planned 3.8 g for the meal, leaving a balance of 2.6 g to be supplied by fruits or vegetables or both. Use Table 12–3 to determine the grams of fruits and/or vegetables needed to supply the 2.6 grams of carbohydrate. In the sample plan, 26 grams of 10 per cent fruit will provide 0.3 grams of protein and 2.6 grams of carbohydrate.

3. To determine the quantity of food necessary to satisfy the remaining protein requirement, subtract the protein content of the cream and fruits (or vegetables) from the total allotted to the meal. In the sample, 1.1 g protein is derived from cream and fruit. This is subtracted from the total allowance of 4.4 g leaving a balance of 3.3 g to be supplied from primary protein sources. Using Table 12–3, determine the amount of primary protein food source that is necessary. In the sample, 14 g of meat, fish, or poultry is needed.

4. To determine the amount of additional fat to be included, it is necessary to subtract the amount of fat supplied by the cream and protein sources from the total allowed for the meal. In the sample, cream provides 14.4 g and meat, fish, or poultry supplies 2.3 g. This 16.7 g of fat is subtracted from the allotted 32.5 g, leaving a balance of 16 g to be supplied as "free fat" (foods that are essentially 100 per cent fat, listed in Table 12–4).

The fat may be mixed with the other planned foods, such as putting butter over hot meat or using mayonnaise with the allotted chicken or tuna fish. The amount of free fat is rounded off to the nearest whole value that will still ensure a 4:1 ratio for the meal plan.

5. The amount of protein, fat, and carbohydrate should not vary more than 0.2 g from the exact amount ordered, and the prescribed ratio must be maintained for each meal.

At the time the patient is discharged from the hospital, parents are given a list of ketogenic diet exchanges (Table 12–4) to add variety to the meal patterns.

MEDIUM-CHAIN TRIGLYCERIDE KETOGENIC DIET

The MCT diet is an alternative to the standard ketogenic diet for control of refractory seizures in children. The regimen is initiated with a 2- to 5-day period of starvation and fluid restriction, as described for the standard ketogenic diet. A sample meal plan is given in Table 12–5.

1. The diet order should specify the total number of calories. The usual regimen permits calories at the RDA for age and does not restrict fluids. However, in our experience moderate caloric restriction, individualized according to age

Text continues on page 290

TABLE 12–3.   REFERENCE GUIDE TO NUTRIENT CONTENT OF FOODS ACCORDING TO WEIGHT

	Weight (g)	Protein (g)	Fat (g)	Carbohydrate (g)
36% CREAM	10	0.2	3.6	0.3
	20	0.4	7.2	0.6
	30	0.6	10.8	0.9
	40	0.8	14.4	1.2
	50	1.0	18.0	1.5
	60	1.2	21.6	1.8
	70	1.4	25.2	2.1
	80	1.6	28.8	2.4
	90	1.8	32.4	2.7
	100	2.0	36.0	3.0
30% CREAM	10	0.3	3.1	0.4
	20	0.5	6.3	0.7
	30	0.8	9.4	1.1
	40	1.0	12.5	1.4
	50	1.3	15.7	1.8
	60	1.5	18.8	2.2
	70	1.8	21.9	2.5
	80	2.0	25.0	2.9
	90	2.3	28.2	3.2
	100	2.5	31.3	3.6
PEANUT BUTTER	5	1.3	2.4	1.1
	6	1.6	2.9	1.3
	7	1.8	3.4	1.5
	8	2.1	3.8	1.7
	9	2.3	4.3	2.0
	10	2.6	4.8	2.2
10% FRUITS*	10	0.1	0.0	1.0
	11	0.1	0.0	1.1
	12	0.1	0.0	1.2
	13	0.1	0.0	1.3
	14	0.1	0.0	1.4
	15	0.1	0.0	1.5
	16	0.2	0.0	1.6
	17	0.2	0.0	1.7
	18	0.2	0.0	1.8
	19	0.2	0.0	1.9
	20	0.2	0.0	2.0
	21	0.2	0.0	2.1
	22	0.2	0.0	2.2
	23	0.2	0.0	2.3
	24	0.2	0.0	2.4
	25	0.2	0.0	2.5
	26	0.3	0.0	2.6
	27	0.3	0.0	2.7
	28	0.3	0.0	2.8
	29	0.3	0.0	2.9
	30	0.3	0.0	3.0
	31	0.3	0.0	3.1
	32	0.3	0.0	3.2

*10% fruits yield 10% available carbohydrate by weight. Fruits may be fresh, frozen, or canned. They must be packaged and prepared without the addition of other ingredients. Only the edible portion is weighed. Fruits yielding 15% carbohydrate by weight are listed with the ketogenic exchanges. The amount allowed must be $\frac{2}{3}$ the weight of the 10% fruit prescribed.

Table continues on following page

TABLE 12–3.   REFERENCE GUIDE TO NUTRIENT CONTENT OF
FOODS ACCORDING TO WEIGHT (Continued)

	Weight (g)	Protein (g)	Fat (g)	Carbohydrate (g)
10% FRUITS	33	0.3	0.0	3.3
	34	0.3	0.0	3.4
	35	0.3	0.0	3.5
	36	0.4	0.0	3.6
	37	0.4	0.0	3.7
	38	0.4	0.0	3.8
	39	0.4	0.0	3.9
	40	0.4	0.0	4.0
	41	0.4	0.0	4.1
	42	0.4	0.0	4.2
	43	0.4	0.0	4.3
	44	0.4	0.0	4.4
	45	0.4	0.0	4.5
	46	0.5	0.0	4.6
	47	0.5	0.0	4.7
	48	0.5	0.0	4.8
	49	0.5	0.0	4.9
	50	0.5	0.0	5.0
	51	0.5	0.0	5.1
	52	0.5	0.0	5.2
	53	0.5	0.0	5.3
	54	0.5	0.0	5.4
	55	0.5	0.0	5.5
	56	0.6	0.0	5.6
	57	0.6	0.0	5.7
	58	0.6	0.0	5.8
	59	0.6	0.0	5.9
	60	0.6	0.0	6.0
	61	0.6	0.0	6.1
	62	0.6	0.0	6.2
	63	0.6	0.0	6.3
	64	0.6	0.0	6.4
	65	0.6	0.0	6.5
	66	0.7	0.0	6.6
	67	0.7	0.0	6.7
	68	0.7	0.0	6.8
	69	0.7	0.0	6.9
	70	0.7	0.0	7.0
GROUP B VEGETABLES[†]	10	0.2	0.0	0.7
	11	0.2	0.0	0.8
	12	0.2	0.0	0.8
	13	0.3	0.0	0.9
	14	0.3	0.0	1.0
	15	0.3	0.0	1.0
	16	0.3	0.0	1.1
	17	0.3	0.0	1.2
	18	0.4	0.0	1.3
	19	0.4	0.0	1.3
	20	0.4	0.0	1.4
	21	0.4	0.0	1.5

[†]Group B vegetables yield approximately 7% carbohydrate by weight. Vegetables containing less than 7% carbohydrate are listed under group A in the ketogenic exchange lists. Since group A vegetables yield approximately half the carbohydrate of group B vegetables, it is necessary to use double the amount.

Table continues on following page

TABLE 12–3.   REFERENCE GUIDE TO NUTRIENT CONTENT OF
FOODS ACCORDING TO WEIGHT (Continued)

	Weight (g)	Protein (g)	Fat (g)	Carbohydrate (g)
GROUP B VEGETABLES	22	0.4	0.0	1.5
	23	0.5	0.0	1.6
	24	0.5	0.0	1.7
	25	0.5	0.0	1.7
	26	0.5	0.0	1.8
	27	0.5	0.0	1.9
	28	0.6	0.0	2.0
	29	0.6	0.0	2.0
	30	0.6	0.0	2.1
	31	0.6	0.0	2.2
	32	0.6	0.0	2.2
	33	0.7	0.0	2.3
	34	0.7	0.0	2.4
	35	0.7	0.0	2.4
	36	0.7	0.0	2.5
	37	0.7	0.0	2.6
	38	0.8	0.0	2.7
	39	0.8	0.0	2.7
	40	0.8	0.0	2.8
	41	0.8	0.0	2.9
	42	0.8	0.0	2.9
	43	0.9	0.0	3.0
	44	0.9	0.0	3.1
	45	0.9	0.0	3.1
	46	0.9	0.0	3.2
	47	0.9	0.0	3.3
	48	1.0	0.0	3.4
	49	1.0	0.0	3.4
	50	1.0	0.0	3.5
	51	1.0	0.0	3.6
	52	1.0	0.0	3.6
	53	1.0	0.0	3.7
	54	1.1	0.0	3.8
	55	1.1	0.0	3.9
	56	1.1	0.0	3.9
	57	1.1	0.0	4.0
	58	1.2	0.0	4.0
	59	1.2	0.0	4.1
	60	1.2	0.0	4.2
	61	1.2	0.0	4.3
	62	1.2	0.0	4.3
	63	1.3	0.0	4.4
	64	1.3	0.0	4.5
	65	1.3	0.0	4.5
	66	1.3	0.0	4.6
	67	1.3	0.0	4.7
	68	1.4	0.0	4.8
	69	1.4	0.0	4.8
	70	1.4	0.0	4.9
	71	1.4	0.0	5.0
	72	1.4	0.0	5.0
	73	1.5	0.0	5.1
	74	1.5	0.0	5.2
	75	1.5	0.0	5.2

Table continues on following page

TABLE 12–3.   REFERENCE GUIDE TO NUTRIENT CONTENT OF
FOODS ACCORDING TO WEIGHT (Continued)

	Weight (g)	Protein (g)	Fat (g)	Carbohydrate (g)
	76	1.5	0.0	5.3
	77	1.5	0.0	5.4
	78	1.6	0.0	5.5
	79	1.6	0.0	5.5
	80	1.6	0.0	5.6
	81	1.6	0.0	5.7
	82	1.6	0.0	5.7
	83	1.7	0.0	5.8
	84	1.7	0.0	5.9
	85	1.7	0.0	6.0
	86	1.7	0.0	6.0
	87	1.7	0.0	6.1
	88	1.8	0.0	6.2
	89	1.8	0.0	6.2
	90	1.8	0.0	6.3
	91	1.8	0.0	6.4
	92	1.8	0.0	6.4
	93	1.9	0.0	6.5
	94	1.9	0.0	6.6
	95	1.9	0.0	6.6
	96	1.9	0.0	6.7
	97	1.9	0.0	6.8
	98	2.0	0.0	6.9
	99	2.0	0.0	6.9
	100	2.0	0.0	7.0
MEAT, FISH, POULTRY	5	1.2	0.8	0.0
(FRESH, FROZEN,	6	1.4	1.0	0.0
OR CANNED)	7	1.6	1.2	0.0
	8	1.9	1.3	0.0
	9	2.1	1.5	0.0
	10	2.3	1.7	0.0
	11	2.6	1.8	0.0
	12	2.8	2.0	0.0
	13	3.0	2.2	0.0
	14	3.3	2.3	0.0
	15	3.5	2.5	0.0
	16	3.7	2.7	0.0
	17	4.0	2.8	0.0
	18	4.2	3.0	0.0
	19	4.4	3.2	0.0
	20	4.7	3.3	0.0
	21	4.9	3.5	0.0
	22	5.1	3.7	0.0
	23	5.4	3.8	0.0
	24	5.6	4.0	0.0
	25	5.8	4.2	0.0
	26	6.1	4.3	0.0
	27	6.3	4.5	0.0
	28	6.5	4.7	0.0
	29	6.8	4.8	0.0
	30	7.0	5.0	0.0
	31	7.2	5.2	0.0

Table continues on following page

TABLE 12–3.   REFERENCE GUIDE TO NUTRIENT CONTENT OF
FOODS ACCORDING TO WEIGHT (Continued)

	Weight (g)	Protein (g)	Fat (g)	Carbohydrate (g)
CHEESE (AMERICAN,	5	1.5	1.7	0.0
CHEDDAR, SWISS)	6	1.8	2.1	0.0
	7	2.1	2.4	0.0
	8	2.4	2.8	0.0
	9	2.7	3.1	0.0
	10	3.0	3.5	0.0
	11	3.3	3.8	0.0
	12	3.6	4.2	0.0
	13	3.9	4.5	0.0
	14	4.2	4.9	0.0
	15	4.5	5.2	0.0
	16	4.8	5.6	0.0
	17	5.1	5.9	0.0
	18	5.4	6.3	0.0
	19	5.7	6.6	0.0
	20	6.0	7.0	0.0
	21	6.3	7.3	0.0
	22	6.6	7.7	0.0
	23	6.9	8.0	0.0
	24	7.2	8.4	0.0
	25	7.5	8.7	0.0
	26	7.8	9.1	0.0
	27	8.1	9.4	0.0
	28	8.4	9.8	0.0
	29	8.7	10.1	0.0
	30	9.0	10.5	0.0
	31	9.3	10.8	0.0
EGGS	15	1.8	1.8	0.0
	16	1.9	1.9	0.0
	17	2.0	2.0	0.0
	18	2.2	2.2	0.0
	19	2.3	2.3	0.0
	20	2.4	2.4	0.0
	21	2.5	2.5	0.0
	22	2.6	2.6	0.0
	23	2.8	2.8	0.0
	24	2.9	2.9	0.0
	25	3.0	3.0	0.0
	26	3.1	3.1	0.0
	27	3.2	3.2	0.0
	28	3.4	3.4	0.0
	29	3.5	3.5	0.0
	30	3.6	3.6	0.0
	31	3.7	3.7	0.0
	32	3.8	3.8	0.0
	33	4.0	4.0	0.0
	34	4.1	4.1	0.0
	35	4.2	4.2	0.0
	36	4.3	4.3	0.0
	37	4.4	4.4	0.0
	38	4.6	4.6	0.0
	39	4.7	4.7	0.0
	40	4.8	4.8	0.0
	41	4.9	4.9	0.0

Table continues on following page

TABLE 12–3.   REFERENCE GUIDE TO NUTRIENT CONTENT OF
FOODS ACCORDING TO WEIGHT (Continued)

	Weight (g)	Protein (g)	Fat (g)	Carbohydrate (g)
CRISP BACON	5	1.0	3.5	0.0
	6	1.2	4.2	0.0
	7	1.4	4.9	0.0
	8	1.6	5.6	0.0
	9	1.8	6.3	0.0
	10	2.0	7.0	0.0
	11	2.2	7.7	0.0
	12	2.4	8.4	0.0
	13	2.6	9.1	0.0
	14	2.8	9.8	0.0
	15	3.0	10.5	0.0
	16	3.2	11.2	0.0
	17	3.4	11.9	0.0
	18	3.6	12.6	0.0
	19	3.8	13.3	0.0
	20	4.0	14.0	0.0
	21	4.2	14.7	0.0
	22	4.4	15.4	0.0
	23	4.6	16.1	0.0
	24	4.8	16.8	0.0
	25	5.0	17.5	0.0
	26	5.2	18.2	0.0
	27	5.4	18.9	0.0
	28	5.6	19.6	0.0
	29	5.8	20.3	0.0
	30	6.0	21.0	0.0
	31	6.2	21.7	0.0
STRAINED MEAT	5	0.8	0.3	0.0
	6	0.9	0.3	0.0
	7	1.1	0.4	0.0
	8	1.3	0.4	0.0
	9	1.4	0.5	0.0
	10	1.6	0.5	0.0
	11	1.8	0.6	0.0
	12	1.9	0.6	0.0
	13	2.1	0.7	0.0
	14	2.2	0.7	0.0
	15	2.4	0.8	0.0
	16	2.6	0.8	0.0
	17	2.7	0.9	0.0
	18	2.9	0.9	0.0
	19	3.0	1.0	0.0
	20	3.2	1.0	0.0
	21	3.3	1.1	0.0
	22	3.5	1.1	0.0
	23	3.7	1.2	0.0
	24	3.8	1.3	0.0
	25	4.0	1.3	0.0
	26	4.1	1.4	0.0
	27	4.3	1.4	0.0
	28	4.5	1.5	0.0
	29	4.6	1.5	0.0
	30	4.8	1.6	0.0

Table continues on following page

TABLE 12–3.   REFERENCE GUIDE TO NUTRIENT CONTENT OF
FOODS ACCORDING TO WEIGHT (Continued)

	Weight (g)	Protein (g)	Fat (g)	Carbohydrate (g)
COTTAGE CHEESE (REGULAR)	5	0.6	0.2	0.1
	6	0.7	0.3	0.2
	7	0.9	0.3	0.2
	8	1.0	0.4	0.2
	9	1.1	0.4	0.2
	10	1.2	0.5	0.3
	11	1.4	0.5	0.3
	12	1.5	0.5	0.3
	13	1.6	0.6	0.3
	14	1.7	0.6	0.4
	15	1.9	0.7	0.4
	16	2.0	0.7	0.4
	17	2.1	0.8	0.5
	18	2.2	0.8	0.5
	19	2.4	0.9	0.5
	20	2.5	0.9	0.5
	21	2.6	0.9	0.6
	22	2.7	1.0	0.6
	23	2.9	1.0	0.6
	24	3.0	1.1	0.6
	25	3.1	1.1	0.7
	26	3.2	1.2	0.7
	27	3.4	1.2	0.7
	28	3.5	1.3	0.8
	29	3.6	1.3	0.8
	30	3.7	1.4	0.8
CREAM CHEESE	5	0.5	1.9	0.0
	6	0.6	2.3	0.0
	7	0.7	2.7	0.0
	8	0.8	3.0	0.0
	9	0.9	3.4	0.0
	10	1.0	3.8	0.0
	11	1.1	4.2	0.0
	12	1.2	4.6	0.0
	13	1.3	4.9	0.0
	14	1.4	5.3	0.0
	15	1.5	5.7	0.0
	16	1.6	6.1	0.0
	17	1.7	6.5	0.0
	18	1.8	6.8	0.0
	19	1.9	7.2	0.0
	20	2.0	7.6	0.0
	21	2.1	8.0	0.0
	22	2.2	8.4	0.0
	23	2.3	8.7	0.1
	24	2.4	9.1	0.1
	25	2.5	9.5	0.1
	26	2.6	9.9	0.1
	27	2.7	10.3	0.1
	28	2.8	10.6	0.1
	29	2.9	11.0	0.1
	30	3.0	11.4	0.1

TABLE 12–4.   KETOGENIC DIET EXCHANGES

Fruits

Drained, frozen, or canned fruits without sugar may be used. If the juice is used, it must be included in the weight. No dried fruits should be used.

10% CARBOHYDRATE

Applesauce	Papaya
Cantaloupe	Peach
Grapefruit	Strawberries
Grapes (slip skin varieties)	Tangerine
Honeydew	Watermelon
Orange	

15% CARBOHYDRATE (*Note*: Use ⅔ the amount of 10% fruit prescribed.)

Apple	Nectarine
Apricot	Pear
Blackberries	Pineapple
Blueberries	Plums (Damson)
Figs	Raspberries, black
Mango	Raspberries, red

Vegetables

Vegetables allowed may be fresh, canned, or frozen (unsweetened and without added ingredients); they may be raw or cooked, as specified (R = raw, C = cooked and drained).

Group A (*Note*: Use double the amount of group B calculated from Table 12–3.)

Asparagus—C	Radish—R
Beet greens—C	Rhubarb—R
Cabbage—C	Sauerkraut—C
Celery—R or C	Summer squash—C
Chicory—R	Swiss chard—C
Cucumbers—R	Tomato—R
Eggplant—C	Turnips—C
Endive—R	Turnip greens—C
Green pepper—R or C	Watercress—R
Poke—C	

Group B (*Note*: Use the amount calculated from Table 12–3.)

Beets—C	Kohlrabi—C
Broccoli—C	Mushrooms—R
Brussels sprouts—C	Mustard greens—C
Cabbage—R	Okra—C
Carrots—R or C	Onions—R or C
Cauliflower—C	Rutabagas—C
Collards—C	Spinach—C
Dandelion greens—C	Tomato—C
Green beans—C	Winter squash—C
Kale—C	

Meat, Fish, Poultry

All meat, fish, or poultry must be plain without breading, sauce, or gravy.

Beef	Lamb
Canned salmon (drained)	Liver (any kind)
Canned tuna (drained)	Pork
Fish (any kind)	Poultry
Frankfurters or luncheon meats	Veal
(both all-meat and without fillers)	Vienna sausage

Table continues on following page

289

TABLE 12–4.   KETOGENIC DIET EXCHANGES (Continued)

Fats

Allotted fat may be mixed with other foods, *i.e.*, mayonnaise with egg or melted margarine over vegetables or meats or both.

Bacon fat	Margarine*
Butter	Mayonnaise (real)
	Oil*

*Polyunsaturated fats (safflower, sunflower, or corn) are recommended.

Miscellaneous

Food Item	Common Measure	Protein (g)	Fat (g)	Carbohydrate (g)
Bouillon cube or powder	1 cube or 4 g	0.8	0.1	0.2
D-Zerta gelatin	1 serving	2.0	—	—
Vinegar	5 g	—	—	0.3
Lemon juice	5 g	—	—	0.4

One of the following may be given daily in addition to prescribed menus:

3 ripe olives (small)
1 English walnut
1 Brazil nut
1 butternut
2 pecans
3 filberts
1 tbs sour cream
Pepper and spices, as desired
Salt, small amount in cooking only
Lettuce, 2 leaves or ½ cup chopped
Pure vanilla or lemon extract (up to 15 drops each meal)
Artificial sweeteners without calories

and activity for each patient, and restriction of fluid to a maximum of 1000 ml results in better seizure control.

2. Caloric distribution is as follows:

MCT	60% kcal
Dietary fat	11% kcal
Carbohydrate	19% kcal
Protein	10% kcal

The caloric distribution among dietary fat, carbohydrate, and protein may be altered slightly to satisfy patient preferences, but the total should not exceed 40 per cent of the total calories permitted. Protein should meet the RDA for the child's age.

3. All of the prescribed MCT oil must be taken as planned. At lower-calorie levels, the MCT diet may not provide adequate amounts of calcium and vitamins. The diet is then supplemented with a multivitamin preparation and calcium gluconate.

4. MCT oil may be incorporated in the diet in several ways:

a. Some MCT oil may be added to the allowed vegetables or blended into allowed juices.

b. MCT oil seems best tolerated when blended in at least twice its volume of skim milk. It may then be divided into three equal portions and sipped slowly.

5. The Exchange List for Meal Planning (Appendix) is used to plan the remainder of the diet. Substitutions for food refused are not necessary.

TABLE 12–5. SAMPLE MEAL PLAN FOR 1600-CALORIE MEDIUM-CHAIN TRIGLYCERIDE KETOGENIC DIET*

MCT OIL[†]	60% total kcal = 960 kcal = 115.7 g (125 ml)
PROTEIN	10% total kcal = 160 kcal = 40 g
FAT	11% total kcal = 176 kcal = 19.5 g
CARBOHYDRATE	19% total kcal = 304 kcal = 76 g

Meal	Protein (g)	Dietary Fat (g)	Carbohydrate (g)	MCT (g)	MCT (ml)
BREAKFAST					
1 meat exchange (List 2)	7	5			
1 fruit exchange			10		
½ bread exchange	1		8		
½ cup skim milk	4		6		
39 g MCT oil	—	—	—	39	42
Total	12	5	24	39	42
LUNCH					
1 meat exchange (lean)	7	3			
free vegetable, if desired					
½ fruit exchange			5		
1 bread exchange	2		15		
½ fat exchange		2.5			
½ cup skim milk	4		6		
39 g MCT oil	—	—	—	39	42
Total	13	5.5	26	39	42
DINNER					
1 meat exchange (lean)	7	3			
2 vegetable exchanges	4		10		
1 fruit exchange			10		
1 fat exchange		5			
½ cup skim milk	4		6		
38 g MCT oil	—	—	—	38	41
Total	15	8	26	38	41
GRAND TOTALS	40	18.5	76	116	125

*This diet meets the RDA for a child age 4–6, except for the requirements for niacin and possibly for riboflavin.
[†]Medium-chain triglyceride oil: 1 g = 8.3 kcal
1 ml = 7.7 kcal

6. Uncomfortable symptoms, such as cramps, nausea, vomiting, and diarrhea, often result from ingestion of MCT oil. Equal apportionment of the oil into meals and its slow ingestion may help alleviate symptoms. When significant symptoms persist, the diet must be discontinued.

BIBLIOGRAPHY

Berman, W.: Medium-chain triglyceride diet in the treatment of intractable childhood epilepsy. Dev Med Child Neurol 20:249–250, 1978.

Davidian, N. M., Butler, T. C., and Poole, D. T.: The effect of ketosis induced by medium chain triglycerides on intracellular pH of mouse brain. Epilepsia 19:369–378, 1978.

Dodson, W. E., Prensky, A. L., DeVivo, D. C., Goldring, S., and Dodge, P. R.: Management of seizure disorders: Selected aspects. Part II. J Pediatr 89:695–703, 1976.

Gordon, N.: Medium-chain triglycerides in a ketogenic diet. Dev Med Child Neurol 19:535–538, 1977.

Helmholz, H. F.: The treatment of epilepsy in childhood. Five years of experience with the ketogenic diet. JAMA 88:2028–2032, 1927.

Huttenlocher, P. R., Wilbourn, A. J., and Signore, J. M.: Medium-chain triglycerides as a therapy for intractable childhood epilepsy. Neurology (Minn) 21:1097–1103, 1971.

Livingston, S.: Comprehensive Management of Epilepsy in Infancy, Childhood and Adolescence. Springfield, IL, Charles C Thomas Publisher, 1972.

Livingston, S.: Medical treatment of epilepsy. Parts I and II. South Med J 71:298–310, 432–447, 1978.

Millichap, J. G., Jones, J. D., and Ruchis, B. P.: Mechanism of anticonvulsive action of ketogenic diet. Am J Dis Child 107:593–604, 1964.

Nellhaus, G.: The ketogenic diet reconsidered: Correlation with EEG. Neurology (Minn) 21:424, 1971.

Peterman, M. G., The ketogenic diet in epilepsy. JAMA 84:1979–1983, 1925.

Wilder, R. M.: The effects of ketonemia on the course of epilepsy. Mayo Clin Bull 2:307–308, 1921.

Withrow, C. D.: The ketogenic diet mechanism of anticonvulsant action. In Gloser, G. H., Penry, J. K., and Woodbury, D. M. (Eds.): Antiepileptic Drugs: Mechanisms of Action: Advances in Neurology. New York, Raven Press, 1980, pp. 635–647.

13

DIETARY MANAGEMENT OF INBORN ERRORS OF METABOLISM

Introduction

David L. Valle, M.D.

Each of the disorders discussed in this section results from the abnormal function of an enzyme involved in amino acid, carbohydrate, or lipid metabolism. Some general comments are possible despite the diversity and complexity of the various disorders.

A rational approach to the dietary management of inborn errors of metabolism requires some understanding of the pathogenesis. Three pathogenetic mechanisms should be considered: (1) the accumulated substrate or its metabolites may have toxic effects, (2) the decreased synthesis of product may be deleterious, or (3) both factors may play a role. The rationale of dietary therapy depends on which of these mechanisms is thought to be important. For example, in galactosemia the goal is to reduce the accumulation of precursors (galactose and galactose-1-phosphate). In type I glycogen storage disease, the aim is to supply the deficient product (glucose), whereas in phenylketonuria both reduction of the substrate (phenylalanine) and provision of adequate amounts of the product (tyrosine) must be accomplished. A beneficial response to dietary regulation of either substrate or product may, in fact, be the best evidence regarding which mechanism is most important.

Not every inborn metabolic error can be treated by dietary manipulation. For example, nonketotic hyperglycinemia and type II hyperprolinemia do not respond clinically or biochemically to limitation of the accumulated amino acid. Since these conditions involve nonessential amino acids that are readily synthesized in the body, their accumulation cannot be regulated by restriction of dietary intake. Thus, for conditions in which substrate toxicity is the pathogenetic mechanism, a requisite for successful dietary therapy is that food be a significant source of the substrate (*e.g.,* disorders involving essential amino acids).

Similarly, if the disorder is mainly the result of product deficiency, a requisite for successful dietary control depends on the ingestibility of a biologically utilizable form of the product. For example, glucose can be supplied easily through diet for patients with type I glycogen storage disease, whereas a usable form of melanin cannot be supplied in diets of individuals with albinism.

Finally, successful dietary therapy of patients with inborn errors requires a keen appreciation of the tremendous variability among individuals and a willingness to tailor the general therapeutic approaches to the specific needs of each patient. In this chapter's discussions of inborn errors, it is assumed that all patients with a given disorder are a homogeneous group. This approach is an obvious oversimplification, since heterogeneity is the rule.

The sources of this heterogeneity are many. The function of a given gene may be impaired by any of several mutations, each with subtle differences (e.g., consider the possible mutations of the β-globin gene, each of which can affect hemoglobin function differently). Secondly, there are innumerable variations among genes other than those that are responsible for the specific disorder (e.g., the normal variability among the genes regulating amino acid transport across the gut and blood brain barrier may influence greatly both the severity and response to therapy of an amino acid disorder). Finally, each patient is influenced by a host of environmental factors (e.g., dietary customs), which may greatly affect dietary therapy.

The sections that follow discuss those disorders in which dietary therapy is most widely practiced. Table 13–1 lists less common genetic disorders in which dietary therapy has been employed.

TABLE 13–1.   SOME ADDITIONAL METABOLIC DISORDERS IN WHICH DIETARY THERAPY HAS BEEN EMPLOYED

Disorder	Enzyme Defect	Diet	Response
Abetalipoproteinemia	Inability to synthesize apoprotein B	Low-fat, with or without medium-chain triglyceride oil; large oral doses of vitamin E	Good
Beta-sitosterolemia and xanthomatosis	Unknown	Restrict plant sterols	Good
Glycogen storage disease, type III	Amylo-1,6-glucosidase	Frequent high-protein feedings	Fair
Gyrate atrophy of choroid and retina	Ornithine aminotransferase	Low-arginine	Good
Hereditary fructose intolerance	Fructose-1-phosphate aldolase	Fructose-free	Good
Hereditary tyrosinemia	Multiple	Low-tyrosine and phenylalanine	Fair
Histidinemia	Histidase	Low-histidine	Fair
Isovaleric aciduria	Isovaleryl Co-A dehydrogenase	Low-leucine	Good
Propionic acidemia and methylmalonic acidemia	Multiple	Low-protein amino acid mixture*	Fair
Refsum's disease	Phytanic acid alpha-hydrolase	Low-phytanate	Fair

*OS-IR, Milupa, Darien CT 06820.

Phenylketonuria

David L. Valle, M.D., and
Barbara Jean Cavagnaro-Wong, R.D.

INTRODUCTION

This inborn error in phenylalanine metabolism was first described in 1934 by Fölling and serves as a general model for the nutritional management of disorders involving essential amino acids. Early diagnosis by neonatal screening and institution of nutritional therapy in the first month of life has markedly improved the outlook for individuals with this disorder.

GOALS OF THERAPY

Successful dietary therapy for phenylketonuria (PKU) limits phenylalanine intake to an amount that is adequate for growth but does not lead to excessive phenylalanine accumulation. The long-term goal is that the patient achieves his or her expected intellectual potential without a severe alteration in life style.

DIETARY THERAPY

Nature of the Defect

Classic phenylketonuria is an inherited disorder in phenylalanine metabolism. It is asymptomatic in early infancy but gradually leads to severe mental retardation, diminished pigmentation, an eczematoid dermatitis, and, frequently, seizures. On a regular diet, infants with classic phenylketonuria have 20- to 60-fold elevations in plasma phenylalanine concentration and excrete large quantities of phenylalanine and certain of its metabolites in the urine.

A reduction in phenylalanine hydroxylase activity to less than 1 per cent of normal is responsible for these problems (Fig. 13–1). Phenylalanine hydroxylase catalyzes the conversion of phenylalanine to tyrosine and requires tetrahydrobiopterin as a cofactor. In normal individuals, most ingested phenylalanine undergoes this conversion. Thus, when phenylalanine intake is normal but the activity of phenylalanine hydroxylase is significantly reduced, phenylalanine accumulates. In addition, a reaction catalyzed by phenylalanine transaminase, generally of minor importance, becomes significant when plasma phenylalanine levels exceed 1 mM (16.5 mg/dl). This combination results in the production of large amounts of phenylpyruvic acid and its metabolites (phenylacetic acid,

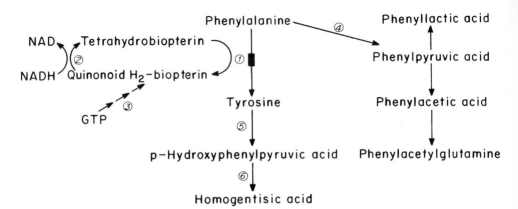

FIGURE 13–1. Metabolism of phenylalanine and tyrosine. Classical phenylketonuria results from a severe reduction in the activity of phenylalanine hydroxylase (1) which converts phenylalanine to tyrosine. Tetrahydrobiopterin is a cofactor for this reaction. Hyperphenylalaninemia may also result from partial defects in phenylalanine hydroxylase or from deficiency of dihydropteridine reductase (2) or any of a series of enzymes (3) required for the synthesis of quinonoid-dihydrobiopterin from GTP. Tyrosine transaminase (5) catalyzes the first step in tyrosine catabolism. The product is converted to homogentisic acid by p-hydroxyphenyl pyruvic acid oxidase (6). Transient deficiency of this enzyme in the newborn period causes transient tyrosinemia with elevations of plasma tyrosine and phenylalanine levels. When plasma phenylalanine levels exceed 1 mM beyond the newborn period, the reaction catalyzed by phenylalanine transaminase (4) results in the formation of phenylpyruvic acid. This compound and its further metabolites (phenylacetic acid, phenyllactic acid and phenylacetylglutamine), along with phenylalanine, are excreted in the urine.

phenyllactic acid, and phenylacetylglutamine). These compounds, along with phenylalanine, are excreted in large quantities in the urine of untreated phenylketonuric patients after the first 2 to 3 weeks of life.

The mechanism by which the block in phenylalanine metabolism leads to various clinical abnormalities is not well understood. Since the typical clinical phenotype is present in phenylketonuric individuals on a normal diet (which provides adequate amounts of tyrosine), tyrosine deficiency probably does not cause these abnormalities; rather, the high levels of phenylalanine or its metabolites or both are believed to be the responsible agents.

Classic phenylketonuria is inherited as an autosomal recessive trait and occurs in about 1 in 13,000 live births in the United States. It is seen in all ethnic groups but is less common in blacks and American Indians than in whites. Nearly all states and territories of the United States presently screen infants for hyperphenylalaninemia, utilizing the bacterial inhibition assay developed by Guthrie. Thus, typical "new" phenylketonuric patients are asymptomatic infants, usually a few weeks old, who have been detected by a screening test.

In addition to classic phenylketonuria, several other conditions are associated with elevated levels of plasma phenylalanine. The most common is hyperphenylalaninemia resulting from a less severe primary abnormality in phenylalanine hydroxylase. In this inherited condition, the residual activity of the enzyme is greater than in classic phenylketonuria but is still only a small fraction of normal. The plasma phenylalanine concentrations in individuals with this condition are significantly elevated but are less than 1 mM on a normal phenylalanine intake. Available evidence suggests that these individuals do not require therapy.

A second group of disorders that elevate plasma phenylalanine comprises inherited defects in the synthesis of the tetrahydrobiopterin cofactor required for phenylalanine hydroxylase activity. This group includes deficiencies of dihydropteridine reductase and of one or more of the enzymes in the synthetic pathway of biopterin (Fig. 13–1). The biochemical abnormalities in these individuals include hyperphenylalaninemia, abnormal concentration of biopterin metabolites, and decreased concentrations of neurotransmitters and their metabolites. The latter abnormality results from the fact that tetrahydrobiopterin is also a cofactor in reactions involved in the synthesis of serotonin and dopa. Thus, patients with abnormal biopterin metabolism require both dietary management to control hyperphenylalaninemia and pharmacologic therapy to increase central nervous system neurotransmitter levels. If therapy is not successful, these patients develop severe neurologic abnormalities despite adequate control of phenylalanine concentrations. All hyperphenylalaninemic infants should be screened for abnormalities of biopterin metabolism.

Transient tyrosinemia is a third disorder that may cause significant elevations of plasma phenylalanine during infancy. This condition is caused by a delay in the maturation of the enzymes necessary for tyrosine degradation. The resultant accumulation of tyrosine (plasma concentrations usually exceed 0.5 mM) causes a secondary modest elevation of phenylalanine. Hypertyrosinemia distinguishes this condition from all of the others causing hyperphenylalaninemia. Administration of ascorbic acid or reduction in protein intake corrects these biochemical abnormalities within a few days. Ascorbic acid prevents inhibition of p-hydroxyphenylpyruvic acid oxidase, an enzyme in the main pathway of tyrosine metabolism, by its substrate.

Hyperphenylalaninemia has a deleterious effect on the developing fetus. When women with classic phenylketonuria follow an unrestricted diet during pregnancy (plasma phenylalanine > 1.2 mM), more than 90 per cent of their offspring will be mentally retarded and microcephalic. Furthermore, available evidence suggests that women with more modest hyperphenylalaninemia (0.6 to 1.2 mM plasma phenylalanine) also have an increased risk of having mentally retarded offspring. This deleterious effect of maternal hyperphenylalaninemia on the fetus, often referred to as "maternal phenylketonuria," is thought to be the result of a direct effect of phenylalanine on the developing fetal nervous system.

These observations suggest that if a woman with significant hyperphenylalaninemia desires biologic offspring, her plasma phenylalanine should be reduced to nearly normal values by dietary means prior to conception and throughout pregnancy. The general efficacy of this form of treatment has not yet been determined.

Rationale for Dietary Therapy

In normal infants and children, the primary fate of ingested phenylalanine is either incorporation into protein (growth) or conversion to tyrosine. Since the latter pathway is blocked in phenylketonuric patients and since avoidance of extreme hyperphenylalaninemia prevents the clinical abnormalities characteristic of untreated phenylketonuria, successful therapy requires a diet that provides sufficient phenylalanine to allow the patient's growth yet prevents significant phenylalanine accumulation.

Results of Dietary Therapy

The outlook for a phenylketonuric child whose treatment is started within the first few weeks of life is remarkably improved over the outcome for an untreated phenylketonuric child. In fact, current data indicate that IQ and physical growth of well-managed phenylketonuric children at 6 years of age are indistinguishable from their normal siblings. Subtle abnormalities, such as specific learning disabilities, are probably more common in phenylketonuric children than they are in normal children. The long-term efficacy of dietary therapy is not known, since such treatment on a large scale was not started until the early 1960s.

PATIENT IDENTIFICATION AND DIAGNOSIS

Nearly all states and territories now screen newborn infants for elevated blood phenylalanine. Current evidence suggests that this procedure detects at least 95 per cent of the cases of classic phenylketonuria. An infant with a significant elevation (0.25 mM or greater) is retested to confirm hyperphenylalaninemia. Since phenylalanine hydroxylase activity is not normally present in readily accessible tissues, such as blood cells or fibroblasts, the diagnosis of phenylketonuria is made on the basis of substrate concentrations rather than by direct enzyme assay. Classic phenylketonuria is arbitrarily defined by a plasma phenylalanine concentration in excess of 1.2 mM (20 mg per cent), associated with a normal plasma tyrosine level. Abnormal phenylalanine metabolites, which result in a positive ferric chloride test on the urine, are usually not present during the first 2 to 3 weeks of life owing to the developmental characteristics of phenylalanine transaminase. All hyperphenylalaninemic infants should be screened for defects in biopterin metabolism by quantitative and qualitative measures of urinary pterins. Conditions that also may be detected by screening for elevated phenylalanine levels include:

1. Hyperphenylalaninemia caused by less severe primary defects in phenylalanine hydroxylase
2. Defects in the synthesis of the cofactor tetrahydrobiopterin
3. Transient tyrosinemia

DIETARY PRINCIPLES

Phenylalanine is an essential amino acid. Thus, the sources of phenylalanine are dietary protein and breakdown of endogenous protein. The latter is significant only in the presence of negative nitrogen balance. In a growing infant or child, it is possible, using formulas containing specially processed proteins that are low or devoid of phenylalanine, to supply an adequate amount of protein and just enough phenylalanine to meet growth requirements. Since growth rates vary greatly with age, the amount of dietary phenylalanine necessary to meet this requirement must be changed accordingly. Failure to provide sufficient phenylalanine causes cessation of growth, dermatitis, and a "paradoxic" elevation in plasma phenylalanine caused by excessive breakdown of endogenous protein. Since there is no evidence suggesting that modest hyperphenylalaninemia (to 0.5 mM) is deleterious, standard practice is to maintain plasma phenylalanine concentrations somewhat above normal in the range of 0.18 to 0.5 mM.

Tyrosine is an essential amino acid in phenylketonuric patients, since the tyrosine synthetic pathway is blocked. Thus, tyrosine intake must be adequate. In general, diets described here will provide sufficient tyrosine.

The optimal duration of therapy is not well defined in patients with phenylketonuria. This uncertainty stems from poor understanding of the pathophysiologic mechanisms in the disorder and from the limited appreciation of variability among phenylketonuric patients. In the past, many phenylketonuria centers have terminated diet control at about 6 years of age, on the basis of the assumption that by then the brain is completely matured and is no longer susceptible to the toxic effects of hyperphenylalaninemia. However, recent studies suggest that an average phenylketonuric patient exhibits a slow decline in performance on psychologic tests over the first few years following termination of the diet. Increased tremulousness and hyperactivity may also occur. On the other hand, some phenylketonuric patients have discontinued dietary treatment without the development of these problems, despite similar serum phenylalanine levels. Thus, it is not known if, when, and in whom dietary control should be terminated. Most phenylketonuria treatment centers now recommend continuation of the diet for as long as possible. Close follow-up of children who have discontinued the diet is always important.

DIETARY MANAGEMENT

Special Dietary Products. Any balanced diet containing the minimum protein requirement would introduce excessive phenylalanine into the diet of a phenylketonuric patient. Consequently, special products that are almost phenylalanine-free form the basis of the modified diet. Their composition is listed in Table 13–2.

Lofenalac is a casein hydrolysate from which most of the phenylalanine has been removed. At its usual concentration of 20 kcal/oz, Lofenalac provides 3.6 mg of phenylalanine/oz, which is not adequate for infants. When sufficient

Text continues on page 301

TABLE 13–2. NUTRITIVE COMPOSITION OF SPECIAL DIETARY PRODUCTS FOR PHENYLKETONURIA (PER 100 G OF POWDER)

Nutrient	Lofenalac*	Phenyl-Free*	PKU-Aid[†]
Calories	460	406	240
Protein (g)	15	20.3	60
Fat (g)	18	6.8	0
Carbohydrate (g)	59.6	66	0
L-AMINO ACIDS (G)			
Essential			
Histidine	0.39	0.47	1.8
Isoleucine	0.75	1.10	2.6
Leucine	1.41	1.73	6.1
Lysine	1.57	1.89	6.1
Methionine	0.45	0.63	1.5
Cystine	0.025	0.35	Nil
Phenylalanine	0.08	0	0.07
Tyrosine	0.81	0.94	6.00
Threonine	0.77	0.94	4.8
Tryptophan	0.19	0.28	0.9
Valine	1.20	1.26	4.6
Nonessential			
Arginine	0.34	0.69	3.1
Alanine	0.64	0	4.1
Aspartic Acid	1.34	5.20	8.1
Glutamic Acid	3.78	1.88	Nil
Glycine	0.35	3.35	3.1
Proline	1.13	0	3.6
Serine	1.02	0	4.8
VITAMINS			
Vitamin A (IU)	1151	2030	0
Vitamin D (IU)	288	406	0
Vitamin E (IU)	7	10	0
Vitamin C (mg)	37	53	0
Thiamine (mg)	0.36	0.6	2
Riboflavin (mg)	0.43	1	2
Vitamin B_6 (mg)	0.3	0.5	2
Vitamin B_{12} (mcg)	1.4	2.5	20
Niacin (mg)	5.8	8	25
Folic Acid (mcg)	72	102	400
Pantothenic Acid (mg)	2.2	3	20
Choline (mg)	61	86	0
Biotin (mg)	0.04	0.03	0.6
Vitamin K (mcg)	72	102	0
Inositol (mg)	22	30	0
MINERALS			
Calcium (mg)	432	609	2500
Phosphorus (mg)	324	457	1500
Magnesium (mg)	50	71	300
Iron (mg)	9	12	25
Iodine (mcg)	32	46	150
Copper (mg)	0.4	0.6	2.5
Manganese (mg)	0.7	1	3.5
Zinc (mg)	3	4	15
Sodium (mg)	216	254	1403
Potassium (mg)	468	711	2581
Chloride (mg)	324	508	2837

*Mead Johnson.
[†]Milner Scientific and Medical Research Co., Ltd., Liverpool, England. (From Pediatrics 57:785–786, 1976.)

amounts of a natural protein, such as milk, are added to furnish an adequate dietary intake of phenylalanine, the Lofenalac-based formula offers a nutritionally complete diet for most phenylketonuric infants. As the child grows, solid foods may replace the milk added to the formula.

With the decline of the child's growth rate, phenylalanine requirements decrease, and the residual phenylalanine in Lofenalac may make dietary control difficult in the child over 2 to 3 years old. Phenyl-Free is a product that has been designed to meet the needs of older patients. Its phenylalanine-free formulation allows for incorporation of a greater variety and larger amounts of natural food into the diet. The greater concentration of amino acids in Phenyl-Free allows consumption of a smaller volume of special formula. Phenyl-Free is not recommended for patients under 1 year old, because these patients have greater phenylalanine requirements.

For years, PKU-Aid has been used successfully in Europe to treat phenylketonuria. PKU-Aid contains all amino acids, both essential and nonessential, except phenylalanine. Since PKU-Aid is a very concentrated protein formula and contains no carbohydrate, protein requirements can be met with smaller quantities of formula than with Lofenalac. In addition, since it is phenylalanine-free, the patient can be permitted a larger selection of natural foods. However, care must be taken to meet the patient's caloric requirements.

DIETARY IMPLEMENTATION. Once the diagnosis of phenylketonuria has been made, plasma phenylalanine levels should be decreased as rapidly as possible. This goal is best accomplished by feeding the infant Lofenalac at its normal dilution (20 kcal/oz), without supplemental natural protein. The amount of time needed to decrease the plasma phenylalanine levels on this regimen varies but is usually about 4 days. This process should be carried out in the hospital, to permit close monitoring of the infant's weight, intake, and serum phenylalanine levels. Once the phenylalanine content of the blood has dropped to a satisfactory level (<0.5 mM), natural protein must be added to the diet to provide sufficient phenylalanine to support growth and metabolic needs.

PRESCRIPTION OF THE DIET. The diet for the patient with phenylketonuria must prescribe calorie and protein intake as well as phenylalanine content. Table 13–3 provides recommended intakes for various ages, but these are only to be used as guidelines. The patient must be followed closely. Analysis of the child's phenylalanine intake, physical growth, and serum phenylalanine levels are used to determine the allowable phenylalanine intake. The diet should contain the maximal amount of phenylalanine that will maintain phenylalanine blood levels between 0.1 and 0.5 mM while supporting growth and development. Frequent adjustments of the prescription may be needed, especially before the child reaches 6 months of age.

CALCULATION OF DIET WITH LOFENALAC. The initial step involves a determination of the amount of Lofenalac to be given, based on the total number of calories prescribed for the child. Sufficient Lofenalac, in its standard dilution of 20 kcal/oz (one packed scoop/2 oz of water) should be given to supply the child's caloric needs.

It is important that the child receive enough fluid. This is determined by the patient's age and weight and the quantity of Lofenalac being given. Infants

TABLE 13–3. RECOMMENDED PHENYLALANINE, PROTEIN, AND ENERGY
INTAKES FOR CHILDREN WITH PHENYLKETONURIA*

Age	Phenylalanine Intake	Protein Intake	Energy Intake
(MONTHS)	MG/KG/DAY	G/KG/DAY	KCAL/KG/DAY
0–3	70–90	2.5	120
4–6	60–70	2.5	115
7–9	40–50	2.5	110
10–12	30–40	2.5	105
(YEARS)		TOTAL G/DAY	KCAL/DAY
1–2	25	25.0	1300
2–3	24	25.0	1300
3–4	20	30.0	1300
4–6	18	30.0	1800
6–8	17	35.0	2000
8–10	15	40.0	2000

*Modified from Acosta, P.B., and Elsas, L.J.: Dietary Management of Inherited Metabolic Disease: Phenylketonuria,
Galactosemia, Tyrosinemia, Homocystinuria, Maple Syrup Urine Disease. Atlanta, ACELMU Publishers, 1976.

need a minimum of 150 ml of water/kg of body weight. If the fluid provided by
the formula in its standard dilution is not sufficient, additional water may be
added. The patient's parents should be cautioned to watch for signs of thirst
and to provide the patient with additional water as needed. For infants, the
Lofenalac formula should never be concentrated more than its standard 20
kcal/oz dilution owing to its high renal solute load. Older children prefer a
more concentrated formula so that they do not have to consume as large a volume. They can satisfy their increased fluid needs by drinking other liquids.

The amount of phenylalanine supplied by the formula should be calculated
next. The amount of milk or other source of natural protein to be added to the
formula to satisfy additional phenylalanine needs can then be determined. A
limited variety of solid foods can be used to provide phenylalanine for the
older child (see Table 13–4).

Finally, the total protein content of the diet is calculated. Since the protein
content of Lofenalac is high, the infant usually receives protein in excess of the
minimal daily requirement. Approximately 85 to 90 per cent of the child's protein needs should be met by the Lofenalac formula.

The caloric content of the formula is usually slightly higher than that required. When altering the prescription according to the patient's serum phenylalanine level, the quantity of natural protein given is all that is changed. Table
13–5 provides a sample prescription and calculation.

CALCULATION OF THE DIET WITH PHENYL-FREE. The daily basic ration of
Phenyl-Free (MJ Product 3229) is 98.5 g reconstituted with sufficient water to
make 16 fl oz or approximately 480 ml. This provides 25 kcal/oz or 83 kcal/100
ml. This standard portion of Phenyl-Free supplies the phenylketonuric patient
with 20 g of protein. The protein requirement of the phenylketonuric child is
met by adjusting the volume of this basic mix according to the needs of the pa-

Text continues on page 311

TABLE 13–4.   PHENYLALANINE, PROTEIN, AND CALORIC CONTENT OF VARIOUS FOODS*

Food	G/Tbs	Amount	Phenylalanine (mg)	Protein (g)	Calories (kcal)
Each serving as listed below contains approximately 15 mg phenylalanine.					
VEGETABLES — BABY FOOD (STRAINED AND JUNIOR)	14.3				
Mixed vegetables		3 tbs	16	0.5	15
Garden vegetables		2 tbs	16	0.5	8
Beets		6 tbs	15	1.1	33
Carrots		5 tbs	15	0.5	19
Creamed spinach		2 tbs	15	0.9	14
Green beans		2 tbs	15	0.3	7
Squash		3 tbs	14	0.3	13
Peas		1 tbs	17	0.5	6
FRUITS — BABY FOOD (STRAINED AND JUNIOR)	14.3				
Applesauce		11 tbs	15	0.3	127
Applesauce and apricots		10 tbs	15	0.4	124
Applesauce and cherries		18 tbs	15	0.5	239
Applesauce and pine-apple		10 tbs	15	0.4	169
Apricots and tapioca		12 tbs	14	0.7	138
Bananas and tapioca		8 tbs	15	0.8	137
Peaches		5 tbs	16	0.4	60
Pears		10 tbs	15	0.6	99
Pears and pineapple		11 tbs	15	0.6	111
Plums and tapioca		11 tbs	15	0.5	154
Prunes and tapioca		8 tbs	15	0.7	105
Bananas with pineapple and tapioca		11 tbs	15	0.6	180
Apples and pears		18 tbs	15	0.5	208
FREE FOODS (BABY)					
These foods contain little or no phenylalanine. May be used as desired.					
Applesauce and raspberries		10 tbs	4	0.1	151
Applesauce and cherries		7 tbs	6	0.2	93
Apples and cranberries		16 tbs	5	0.2	213
FRUIT JUICES (BABY)	15.0				
Apple		16 oz	14	0.5	235
Apple-apricot		16 oz	14	0.5	336
Apple-cherry		10 oz	15	0.6	135
Apple-grape		16 oz	14	0.5	312
Apple-pineapple		16 oz	14	0.5	336
Mixed fruit		6 oz	14	0.5	106
Orange		4 oz	16	0.6	60
Orange-apple		6 oz	14	0.5	97
Orange-apple-banana		4 oz	16	0.6	78
Orange-apricot		3 oz	14	0.5	55

*Modified from Acosta, P. B., and Wenz, E.: Diet Management of PKU for Infants and Preschool Children. U.S. Department of Health, Education and Welfare, Pub. No. (HSA) 77-5209, 1977. (Available from Superintendent of Documents, U.S. Government Printing Office, Washington, DC 20402.)

Table continues on following page

TABLE 13–4.   PHENYLALANINE, PROTEIN, AND CALORIC CONTENT OF VARIOUS FOODS* (Continued)

Food	G/Tbs	Amount	Phenylalanine (mg)	Protein (g)	Calories (kcal)
Orange-pineapple		4 oz	16	0.6	71
Pineapple		6 oz	14	0.5	99
Pineapple-grapefruit drink		6 oz	14	0.4	70
Prune-orange		4 oz	16	0.6	90
Apple-prune		10 oz	15	0.6	204

Each serving as listed below contains approximately 30 mg phenylalanine.

BREADS AND CEREALS—
BABY FOOD (STRAINED AND JUNIOR)

Food	G/Tbs	Amount	Phenylalanine (mg)	Protein (g)	Calories (kcal)
Dry Cereals	2.4				
Barley		2 tbs	28	0.5	18
Mixed cereal		2 tbs	28	0.6	18
Oatmeal		2 tbs	30	0.8	15
Rice cereal		4 tbs	31	0.6	36
Mixed cereal with bananas		2 tbs	29	0.6	21
Oatmeal with bananas		2 tbs	30	0.6	19
Rice cereal with strawberries		4 tbs	30	0.6	33
Barley with mixed fruit		3 tbs	31	0.6	N/A
Cereals in Jars (Strained)	14.3				
Mixed with applesauce and bananas		3 tbs	30	0.6	39
Oatmeal with applesauce and bananas		4 tbs	30	0.5	47
Rice with applesauce and bananas		15 tbs	30	0.6	148
Rice with mixed fruit		3 tbs	30	0.6	37
Cereals in Jars (Junior)					
Mixed with applesauce and bananas		3 tbs	30	0.6	39
Oatmeal with applesauce and bananas		4 tbs	30	0.5	47
VEGETABLES (STRAINED)	14.3				
Creamed corn		3 tbs	30	0.7	30
Sweet potatoes		3 tbs	29	0.6	30

Each serving as listed below contains approximately 15 mg phenylalanine.

Food	G/Tbs	Amount	Phenylalanine (mg)	Protein (g)	Calories (kcal)
VEGETABLES					
Asparagus, cooked	9	3 tbs or 1½ stalk	17	0.6	5
Beans, green, cooked	8	3 tbs	14	0.4	6

Table continues on following page

TABLE 13–4.   PHENYLALANINE, PROTEIN, AND CALORIC CONTENT OF VARIOUS FOODS* (Continued)

Food	G/Tbs	Amount	Phenylalanine (mg)	Protein (g)	Calories (kcal)
Beans, yellow, cooked	8	¼ cup	16	0.4	7
Beans, sprouts, Mung, cooked	8	1 tbs	16	0.3	3
Beets cooked	10	⅔ cup	16	1.2	34
Beet, greens, cooked	13	3 tbs	15	0.6	6
Broccoli, cooked, chopped	10	1 tbs	14	0.4	3
Brussels sprouts, cooked	—	1 medium	13	0.4	4
Cabbage, raw, shredded	6	½ cup	15	0.6	12
Cabbage, cooked	10	⅓ cup	14	0.6	11
Carrots, raw	—	½ large or 1 small	18	0.6	21
Carrots, cooked	—	⅓ cup	15	0.5	16
Cauliflower, cooked	7	3 tbs	17	0.5	5
Celery, raw	6	6 tbs or 2 stalks	15	0.3	6
Celery, cooked, diced	8	6 tbs	18	0.4	7
Chard leaves, cooked	10	3 tbs	14	0.5	5
Collards, cooked	11	1 tbs	13	0.4	4
Cucumber, pared, raw	—	1 whole	14	0.6	14
Eggplant, diced, raw	13	2 tbs	13	0.3	7
Eggplant, cooked	13	3 tbs	17	0.4	7
Kale, cooked	7	2 tbs	18	0.4	4
Lettuce	—	2 leaves	14	0.4	5
Mushroom, raw	4	3 small	17	0.8	8
Mushroom, canned	13	3 tbs	16	0.7	7
Mushroom, sautéed	17	½ large	13	0.2	10
Mustard greens, cooked	13	2 tbs	16	0.5	5
Okra, cooked	—	3 tbs	17	0.7	10
Onion, raw, chopped	10	¼ cup	15	0.6	15
Onion, cooked	13	¼ cup	16	0.6	15
Onion, young, scallion	—	2 whole	15	0.6	14
Parsley, raw, chopped	3	4 tbs	17	0.4	5
Parsnips, cooked, diced	13	3 tbs	18	0.6	26
Peppers, raw, chopped	10	3 tbs	17	0.4	7
Pickles, dill	—	1 large	16	0.7	11
Pickles, sweet	13	1 large	16	0.7	146
Pickles, sweet relish	13	8 tbs	14	0.5	144
Pumpkin, cooked	14	4 tbs	16	0.6	18
Radishes, raw	—	3 small	13	0.3	5
Sauerkraut	15	¼ cup	15	0.6	11
Spinach, cooked	11	1 tbs	15	0.3	3
Squash, summer, cooked	13	5 tbs	16	0.6	9
Squash, winter, cooked	13	¼ cup	16	0.6	20
Tomato, raw	17	½ small	14	0.6	11
Tomato, canned	17	¼ cup	17	0.7	14
Tomato juice	14	¼ cup	16	0.6	13
Tomato catsup	17	2 tbs	17	0.7	36
Tomato purée	6	6 tbs	15	0.6	14
Tomato sauce	18	3 tbs	18	0.7	52
Turnip greens, cooked	9	2 tbs	18	0.4	4
Turnips, diced, cooked	10	9 tbs	15	0.7	21

Table continues on following page

TABLE 13–4. PHENYLALANINE, PROTEIN, AND CALORIC CONTENT OF VARIOUS FOODS* (Continued)

Food	G/Tbs	Amount	Phenylalanine (mg)	Protein (g)	Calories (kcal)
Each serving as listed below contains approximately 15 mg phenylalanine.					
SOUPS (PREPARED WITH EQUAL VOLUME OF WATER)					
Asparagus (Campbell's condensed)		3 tbs	15	0.5	12
Beef broth (Campbell's condensed)		2 tbs	17	0.6	4
Celery (Campbell's condensed)		3 tbs	15	0.3	16
Minestrone (Campbell's condensed)		3 tbs	18	0.8	17
Mushroom (Campbell's condensed)		2 tbs	15	0.3	17
Onion (Campbell's condensed)		3 tbs	19	0.9	11
Tomato (Campbell's condensed)		3 tbs	17	0.4	16
Vegetarian vegetable (Campbell's condensed)		3 tbs	14	0.3	12
Vegetable and beef broth (Campbell's condensed)		4 tbs	16	0.5	15
Clam chowder and tomato (Campbell's condensed)		3 tbs	14	0.4	15
Chicken gumbo (Campbell's condensed)		2 tbs	14	0.4	7
Cream of chicken (Campbell's condensed)		2 tbs	15	0.4	12
Beef noodle (Campbell's condensed)		2 tbs	19	0.5	8
Each serving as listed below contains approximately 15 mg phenylalanine.					
FRUITS					
Apple, raw		2½ small	15	0.5	145
Applesauce	19	¾ cup	14	0.5	207
Apricots, raw		1½ medium	14	0.6	31
Apricots, canned		3 halves	14	0.6	86
Apricots, dried		2 halves	14	0.6	31
Avocado, cubed or mashed	9.5	3 tbs	14	0.6	48

Table continues on following page

TABLE 13–4.   PHENYLALANINE, PROTEIN, AND CALORIC CONTENT OF VARIOUS FOODS* (Continued)

Food	G/Tbs	Amount	Phenylalanine (mg)	Protein (g)	Calories (kcal)
Banana, raw, sliced		½ small or ⅓ cup sliced	17	0.6	43
Blackberries, canned, syrup	15.6	5 tbs	16	0.6	71
Blackberries, raw	9	6 tbs	17	0.6	31
Blueberries, raw	8.8	10 tbs	16	0.6	55
Blueberries, frozen, unsweetened	10	9 tbs	16	0.6	50
Blueberries, canned, syrup	15	10 tbs	15	0.6	151
Cantaloupe, raw, diced	15	5 tbs	16	0.5	23
Sour cherries	13	4 tbs	16	0.6	30
Sweet cherries, canned, syrup	13	5 tbs	15	0.6	53
Cranberries, raw	6	1½ cups	14	0.6	66
Cranberry sauce	20	1⅔ cups	16	0.5	780
Cranberry, sweetened, cooked	13	1½ cups	16	0.6	555
Dates	11	2 tbs	15	0.6	69
Figs, raw		1 large	15	0.6	40
Figs, canned, syrup		4 small	16	0.6	105
Figs, dried		1 small	16	0.6	41
Fruit cocktail	13	¾ cup	16	0.6	119
Grapefruit, raw	12	¾ cup or ½ large	14	0.7	59
Grapes, Thompson seedless	10	½ cup (12 grapes)	14	0.5	54
Guava, raw		1 small	16	0.6	47
Honeydew, raw, diced	13	5 tbs	16	0.5	21
Mango, raw		½ medium	18	0.7	66
Nectarines, raw		2 large	15	0.8	80
Oranges, raw		1 medium, 3″ diameter	18	1.5	74
Papaya, raw	16	⅓ medium or 6 tbs	16	0.6	39
Peaches, raw	11	1 large or ¾ cup sliced	16	0.8	50
Peaches, canned, syrup	16	4 medium halves	16	0.8	156
Peaches, dried	10	2½ tbs	16	0.8	66
Pears, raw		½ medium (3 × 2½″)	17	0.7	61
Pears, canned, syrup	16	5 small halves	15	0.5	190
Pears, dried		½ pear	12	0.4	35
Pineapple, raw	8	1 cup diced	14	0.5	67
Pineapple, canned, syrup	16	2 large slices	16	0.6	148
Plums, Damson, raw	13	2 whole	13	0.5	66
Plums, prune-type, raw	13	1½ whole	17	0.4	38
Plums, canned, syrup	14	4 whole	13	0.5	110

Table continues on following page

TABLE 13–4.   PHENYLALANINE, PROTEIN, AND CALORIC CONTENT OF VARIOUS FOODS* (Continued)

Food	G/Tbs	Amount	Phenylalanine (mg)	Protein (g)	Calories (kcal)
Prunes, dried, medium		3 whole	18	0.4	54
Raisins, dried, seedless	10	2 tbs	15	0.5	58
Raspberries, black, raw	11	¼ cup	17	0.7	32
Raspberries, red, raw	8	6 tbs	15	0.6	27
Raspberries, black, canned, syrup	13	4 tbs	15	0.6	27
Raspberries, red, canned, syrup	13	7 tbs	16	0.6	32
Rhubarb, cooked, added sugar	15	6 tbs	15	0.5	141
Strawberries, raw	9	10 large	17	0.7	37
Strawberries, frozen whole	15	15 large	15	0.6	138
Tangerine		1 small or ½ large	12	0.4	23
Watermelon balls or cubes	12.5	⅔ cup	17	0.7	36

Each serving as listed below contains approximately 30 mg phenylalanine.

BREADS AND CEREALS

Prepared Cereals

Alpha Bits		3 tbs	27	0.6	23
Apple Jacks		6 tbs	32	0.7	47
Cap'n Crunch		5 tbs	29	0.7	65
Cheerios		2 tbs	27	0.5	15
Corn Chex		½ cup	29	0.6	30
Cornflakes		¼ cup	28	0.6	31
Froot Loops		5 tbs	36	0.6	40
Kix		½ cup	28	0.6	32
Lucky Charms		3 tbs	29	0.5	23
Puffed Rice		10 tbs	31	0.6	40
Puffed Wheat		¼ cup	32	0.9	12
Cap'n Crunchberries		¼ cup	31	0.5	47
Cap'n Crunch Peanut Butter		3 tbs	32	0.6	38
Rice Chex		6 tbs	31	0.6	44
Rice Krinkles		½ cup	28	0.5	63
Rice Krispies		¼ cup	28	0.5	30
Quisp		½ cup	31	0.8	68
Shredded Wheat		¼ biscuit	29	0.6	21
Sugar Frosted Flakes		½ cup	30	0.6	62
Sugar Pops		½ cup	30	0.6	43
Sugar Smacks		7 tbs	31	0.7	55
Trix		6 tbs	30	0.7	47
Wheaties		¼ cup	31	0.7	25
Wheat Chex		7 biscuits	31	0.7	25
Cocoa Krispies		½ cup	29	0.5	48
Team Flakes		10 tbs	30	0.6	39

Table continues on following page

TABLE 13–4.   PHENYLALANINE, PROTEIN, AND CALORIC CONTENT OF VARIOUS FOODS* (Continued)

Food	G/Tbs	Amount	Phenylalanine (mg)	Protein (g)	Calories (kcal)
Quaker Life		1 tbs	30	0.6	12
King Vitamin		½ cup	32	0.6	63
Special K		2 tbs	29	0.6	11
Franken Berry		7 tbs	30	0.6	50
Count Chocula		6 tbs	28	0.6	42
Sir Grapefellow		5 tbs	27	0.5	39
Boo Berry		5 tbs	27	0.5	39
Granola		1 tbs	32	0.6	19
Grapenuts		1 tbs	27	0.6	26
Grapenut Flakes		3 tbs	29	0.7	30
Cooked Cereals					
Cornmeal		4 tbs	29	0.7	30
Cream of Rice		5 tbs	31	0.6	38
Cream of Wheat		2 tbs	28	0.6	17
Farina		3 tbs	31	0.6	19
Malt-O-Meal		2 tbs	30	0.6	20
Oatmeal		2 tbs	33	0.6	17
Pettijohns		2 tbs	32	0.7	23
Ralston		2 tbs	31	0.6	16
Rice, white		3 tbs	28	0.5	29
Rice, brown		2 tbs	28	0.5	25
Wheatena		2 tbs	31	0.6	22
Wheat Hearts		2 tbs	31	0.7	17
Crackers					
Animal Crackers		5	33	0.7	43
Arrowroot Cookies		2	30	0.6	45
Graham Crackers		1	28	0.6	21
Ritz Crackers		3	35	0.7	45
Saltines		2	27	0.5	26
Tortilla, corn (6″-diam)		¼	33	0.7	27
Wheat Thins		4	34	0.7	32
Meal Mates		1	25	0.5	24
MISCELLANEOUS					
Corn, cooked		2 tbs	29	0.5	17
Hominy grits, cooked		6 tbs	32	0.7	31
Macaroni, cooked		2 tbs	32	0.6	20
Noodles, cooked		2 tbs	32	0.7	20
Potato chips (2″-diam)		6	29	0.6	68
Potato, Irish, cooked		⅓ potato (2¼″)	29	0.6	21
Potatoes, French-fried		3 (½ × ½ × 2″)	30	0.6	41
Instant potatoes (dry) without milk		5 tbs	33	0.7	36
Popcorn, popped, plain		5 tbs	29	0.6	19
Spaghetti, cooked		2 tbs	32	0.6	20
Sweet potatoes, cooked		3 tbs	28	0.6	38
Instant sweet potatoes, dry without milk		2 tbs	29	0.6	53

Table continues on following page

TABLE 13–4.   PHENYLALANINE, PROTEIN, AND CALORIC CONTENT OF VARIOUS FOODS* (Continued)

Food	G/Tbs	Amount	Phenylalanine (mg)	Protein (g)	Calories (kcal)

Each serving as listed below contains approximately 5 mg phenylalanine.

Food	G/Tbs	Amount	Phenylalanine (mg)	Protein (g)	Calories (kcal)
FATS					
Butter		1 tbs	4	0.1	100
French Dressing, commercial		5 tbs	5	0.2	442
Margarine		1 tbs	5	0.1	108
Miracle Whip		1 tbs	5	0.1	68
Olives, green		2 tbs	5	0.2	16
Olives, ripe		2 tbs	5	0.2	18
Mayonnaise		2 tbs	5	0.1	72
DESSERTS — COMSTOCK					
Apple pie filling		¼ cup	1	‡	89
Apricot pie filling		3 tbs	6	0.3	59
Blackberry pie filling		¼ cup	1	‡	109
Blueberry pie filling		¼ cup	6	0.2	83
Boysenberry pie filling		2 tbs	6	0.2	47
Cherry pie filling		2 tbs	6	0.2	42
Peach pie filling		¼ cup	4	0.2	78
Pineapple pie filling		¼ cup	4	0.1	70
Raspberry pie filling		3 tbs	6	0.1	79
Strawberry pie filling		¼ cup	5	0.2	79
MISCELLANEOUS					
Cake flour		1 tbs	29	0.6	29
Corn starch		1 tbs	1	trace[†]	29
Tapioca, granulated		1 tbs	2	0.1	35
Wheat starch		1 tbs	1	trace	25
NONDAIRY CREAMS					
Coffee Rich		1 tbs	3	trace	23
Cool Whip		1 tbs	2	trace	14
Dzert Whip, liquid		1 tbs	9	0.2	44
Rich's Topping		1 tbs	—	—	43
Mocha Mix		1 tbs	2	trace	13
FREE FOODS					

These foods contain little or no phenylalanine. May be used as desired.

Food	G/Tbs	Amount	Phenylalanine (mg)	Protein (g)	Calories (kcal)
Apple juice		6 oz			85
Candies					
Butterscotch		1 piece			20
Cream mints		1 piece			7
Fondant, patties or mint		1 piece			40
Gumdrops		1 large			35
Hard candy		2 pieces			39
Jelly beans		10 pieces			110
Lollipops (2″-diam)		1 medium			108

[†]Less than 0.04 g protein = trace.
[‡]Less than 0.1 g protein.

TABLE 13–4.   PHENYLALANINE, PROTEIN, AND CALORIC CONTENT OF VARIOUS FOODS* (Concluded)

Food	G/Tbsp	Amount	Phenylalanine (mg)	Protein (g)	Calories (kcal)
Carbonated beverages		6 oz			78
Corn syrup		1 tbs			58
Danish dessert		½ cup			123
Fruit butter		1 tbs			37
Fruit ices		½ cup			69
Jellies		1 tbs			55
Kool Aid		4 oz			48
Lemonade		4 oz			53
Maple syrup		1 tbs			50
Molasses		1 tbs			46
Popsicle		1 twin bar			95
Shortening		1 tbs			123
Sugar, brown		1 tbs			46
Sugar, granulated		1 tbs			43
Sugar, white, powdered		1 tbs			59
Tang liquid		4 oz			59

tient. The phenylalanine requirements of the patient receiving Phenyl-Free are met by natural foods (Table 13–4).

INTRODUCTION OF SOLID FOODS.   Generally, solid foods may be added at the same age in the same order as for nonphenylketonuric children but in more limited amounts. Eventually, breads and cereals, fruits and vegetables should replace all of the natural protein added to the Lofenalac formula as a source of phenylalanine in the diet. The phenylalanine content of cereals, fruits, and vegetables ranges from 2.5 to 5 per cent of the protein content of the food. Most high-protein foods such as meat and eggs contain correspondingly large amounts of phenylalanine and should be avoided.

Serving lists have been compiled to simplify and add variety to the low-phenylalanine diet. Foods in each group can be substituted for each other, as in diabetic dietary exchanges. A variety of special low-protein products are also available (Table 13–6).

TERMINATION OF DIET.   If the decision has been made to terminate a phenylketonuria diet, a program is instituted that allows for a gradual return to a normal dietary intake. During and after this period, the child must be followed closely psychologically, medically, and nutritionally.

The diet is terminated in the following manner:

Weeks 1 and 2	Low-phenylalanine diet, but with fruits and vegetables as desired.
Weeks 3 and 4	As above, but adding breads, cereals, and starches as desired.
Weeks 5 and 6	Add meats, cheese, legumes, and dairy foods (except cow's milk).

TABLE 13–5. SAMPLE PRESCRIPTION AND CALCULATION OF LOW-PHENYLALANINE DIET UTILIZING LOFENALAC

Prescribe and calculate a diet for a 3.4-kg, 1-month-old infant recently diagnosed as having phenylketonuria.

1. Using Table 13–3, determine the phenylalanine, protein, water, and energy allowances:
   3.4 kg × 120 kcal/kg/day = 408 kcal/day
   3.4 kg × 150 ml water/kg/day = 510 ml water/day
   3.4 kg × 88 mg phenylalanine/kg/day = 299.2 mg phenylalanine/day
   3.4 kg × 2.5 g protein/kg/day = 8.5 g protein/day
2. Determine the amount of Lofenalac to be used:

$$408 \text{ kcal} \times \frac{\text{oz Lofenalac}}{20 \text{ kcal}} = 20.4 \text{ oz Lofenalac (rounded off to 20 oz)}$$

3. Determine whether the minimum fluid requirement is met, by the following formula:

$$20 \text{ oz formula} \times \frac{30 \text{ ml}}{\text{oz}} = 600 \text{ ml fluid}$$

The infant requires 510 ml, so the formula satisfies this requirement.

4. Determine the amount of phenylalanine provided by the formula, then calculate the amount of milk needed to satisfy the patient's phenylalanine requirement:
   a. 20 oz Lofenalac × 3.6 mg phenylalanine/oz Lofenalac = 72 mg phenylalanine
   b. 299 mg phenylalanine required − 72 mg phenylalanine from Lofenalac = 227 mg phenylalanine needed from additional milk
   c. $227 \text{ mg phenylalanine} \times \dfrac{1 \text{ oz milk}}{53 \text{ mg phenylalanine}} = 4.3 \text{ oz milk}$

Rounding off to the nearest half ounce gives 4.5 oz whole milk.

5. Check the protein content of the following formula:
   20 oz Lofenalac × 0.65 g protein/oz = 13 g protein
   4.5 oz whole milk × 1 g protein/oz = 4.5 g protein

Total protein given by the formula is thus 17.5 g protein, which is in excess of that required.

6. Convert the formula prescription to packed measures of Lofenalac powder and ounces of water:
   1 packed measure Lofenalac powder and 2 oz of water make 2⅛ oz of formula. 20 oz formula divided by 2⅛ oz gives approximately 9.5 packed scoops. Add 19 oz of water to this to give approximately 21.5 oz formula.
7. Check the caloric, fluid, phenylalanine, and protein content of the total formula:

	Amount	Phenylalanine (mg)	Protein (g)	Energy (kcal)
Lofenalac	9½ scoops	71.2	13.3	408
Water	19 oz	0	0	0
Whole Milk	4.5 oz	238	4.5	90
Total	26 oz (approximately)	309	17.8	498

8. Monitor infant and adjust prescription as needed.

Week 7   Switch from Lofenalac or Phenyl-Free to
                                        regular cow's milk.

BREAST FEEDING. A phenylalanine-restricted diet involving a mixture of breast feeding and Lofenalac supplementation is feasible but somewhat more complicated than the routine diet therapy. Mature human breast milk has the advantage of being low in protein (0.9 g/dl) compared with the milk of other species (3.3 g/dl for cow's milk). There is individual variation, however, and the protein content of human milk is highest in colostrum (2.3 to 2.7 g/dl) and decreases with duration of lactation.

The current procedure recommended for breast feeding the phenylketonuric infant involves feeding the infant supplements of Lofenalac at each nursing and substituting Lofenalac for one or two feedings per day. The infant should be weighed before and after each breast feeding to determine the exact intake. Close attention to plasma phenylalanine is necessary. Ernest *et al.* have published a guide to breast feeding the phenylketonuric infant in which the procedures are discussed.

PHENYLKETONURIA DIET DURING PREGNANCY

Formula. A well-balanced amino acid mixture with little or no phenylalanine is essential in the management of the pregnant female with phenylketonuria.

Implementation of the diet. If the phenylketonuria diet had been discontinued, it would be optimal to restart the low-phenylalanine diet several months prior to conception. When this is not possible, the diet should be instituted as soon as the pregnancy has been confirmed.

Prescription of the diet. There is very little practical experience on the dietary management of a pregnant woman with phenylketonuria. It has been suggested that the prescribed diet should contain sufficient phenylalanine (5 to 10 mg/kg/day) to maintain blood phenylalanine levels between 0.2 and 0.4 mM, but the optimal range is not known with certainty. The phenylalanine requirement is likely to increase substantially in the last half of the pregnancy.

The diet prescription must also take into account the Recommended Dietary Allowances for Pregnancy (see Chapter 1, section on nutrition in pregnancy). A diet using either Phenyl-Free or Lofenalac and a variety of natural foods will meet all the requirements except that additional zinc and folate may be necessary.

Planning the diet. The amount of special formula to be given to the pregnant phenylketonuric female should be adjusted according to the individual needs of the patient. The quantities of solid food incorporated into the maternal low-phenylalanine diet depend on the type of formula used, the mother's prescription for phenylalanine, the phenylalanine content of specific solid foods utilized, and the number of special low-protein products used in the diet (Tables 13–4 and 13–6).

The dietary prescription should take into account the food preferences and special food cravings of the pregnant phenylketonuric patient. Other factors to consider include the possible presence of nausea and vomiting, appropriate

TABLE 13–6. LOW-PROTEIN PRODUCTS AND THEIR SOURCES

Product	Source
Aproten Low-Protein Pasta, Rusks, Porridge Dietetic Paygel Baking Mix Dietetic Paygel Wheat Starch Low-Protein Canned Bread Prono Imitation Jello	Dietary Specialties, Inc. P.O. Box 227 Rochester, NY 14601
Cellu Wheat Starch Lo Pro Pastas Low-Protein Baking Mix and Bread	Chicago Dietetic Supply, Inc. 405 East Shawnut Avenue La Grange, IL 60525
Controlyte	D. M. Doyle Pharmaceutical Co. Highway 100 at West 23rd Street Minneapolis, MN 55416
Low-Protein Bread and Mix Potato Mix Egg Replacer	Ener-G Foods, Inc. 1526 Utah Avenue, South Seattle, WA 98134
Welplan Bread Welplan Golden Raisin Cookies Welplan Savory (Cheese) Cookies	Anglo-Dietetics LTD. 641 Lancaster Pike Frazer, PA 19355

Low-Protein Chocolate-Flavored
  Chip Cookies; Low-Protein
  Butterscotch Chip Cookies
Low-Protein Bread
Baking Mix
Wheat Starch
Anellini (Ring Macaroni)
Ditalini (Short-Ribbed Macaroni)
Rigatoni (Long-Ribbed Macaroni)
Tagliatelle (Flat Noodles)
Rusks
Prono (low-protein gelatin—lime,
  cherry, orange, and strawberry)
Cal Plus (powdered high-calorie supplement)
	Dietary Specialties, Inc.
	P.O. Box 227
	Rochester, NY 14601

Product 80056	Mead Johnson Laboratories Evansville, IN 47721

weight gain, cost of the special diet, possible altered fluid and electrolyte status, possible constipation, and psychosocial problems. The prescription of an appropriate diet should be combined with counseling of the mother on the importance of careful adherence to the diet. These factors should enhance compliance with the special dietary regimen and help make it feasible for the phenylketonuric female to bear healthy children.

Galactosemia

David L. Valle, M.D., and
Barbara Jean Cavagnaro-Wong, R.D.

INTRODUCTION

This inborn error in carbohydrate metabolism involves multiple organ systems and is effectively treated by elimination of galactose from the diet.

DIETARY THERAPY

Nature of the Defect

Galactosemia is a clinical syndrome consisting of liver failure, cataracts, and mental deficiency associated with high serum levels of galactose. This inherited disorder results from a deficiency of galactose-1-phosphate uridyltransferase, the second enzyme in the pathway by which galactose is converted to glucose (Fig. 13–2). An inherited deficiency of the first enzyme in this pathway (galactokinase) also is associated with elevated blood levels of galactose but with a milder clinical entity characterized by juvenile-onset cataracts.

Most neonates with galactosemia develop a typical clinical picture within days after they begin to ingest lactose-containing formula. These infants develop vomiting, diarrhea, failure to gain weight, jaundice, metabolic acidosis, hemolytic anemia, and excessive bleeding. Cataracts may be apparent by slit

FIGURE 13–2. Conversion of galactose to glucose-1-phosphate. Galactokinase (1) forms galactose-1-phosphate from galactose and ATP. Deficiency of this enzyme leads to galactose accumulation and cataract formation without hepatic, renal or central nervous system involvement. Classical galactosemia, which arises from a defect in galactose-1-phosphate uridyltransferase (2), results in the accumulation of both galactose and galactose-1-phosphate. UDP galactose is converted by UDP galactose-4-epimerase (3) to UDP glucose. The latter is metabolized to glucose-1-phosphate by UDP glucose pyrophosphorylase (4).

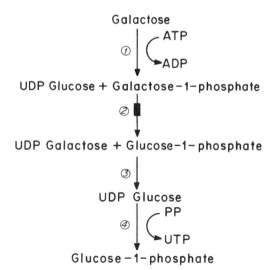

lamp examination within a few weeks after birth. Sepsis, usually due to *Escherichia coli*, occurs not uncommonly. If the infant survives, developmental milestones are delayed. Laboratory abnormalities include increased amounts of galactose in the blood and urine, deranged liver function, proteinuria, and generalized aminoaciduria.

Although this description applies to most galactosemic infants, there are some who are less severely affected. These patients may come to medical attention at a few months of age with failure to thrive, unexplained hepatomegaly, and cataracts. Occasionally, a patient—usually black—is completely asymptomatic. These infants presumably have sufficient residual enzymatic activity to prevent the onset of symptoms.

Patients with galactokinase deficiency are normal during infancy but usually develop perinuclear cataracts in the second decade of life. Although some of the reported patients have been also retarded, this has not been universal and may reflect ascertainment bias.

Symptoms are thought to develop as a result of the toxic effects of accumulated galactose metabolites. An accumulation of galactitol in the lens, from the conversion by aldose reductase within the lens of galactose to galactitol, is thought to cause cataracts. Since the lens epithelium is relatively impermeable to galactitol, large amounts of it accumulate, and, by osmosis, cause swelling and cataract formation.

The pathophysiology of the mental retardation and liver and renal diseases in galactosemia is not well understood. Since these problems are not features of galactokinase deficiency and are clearly prevented by a low-galactose diet, the major toxic agent is thought to be galactose-1-phosphate.

Rationale for Dietary Therapy

Since all of the manifestations of this disorder are believed to be secondary to impaired metabolism of galactose, a rational form of therapy involves elimination of galactose, which is derived primarily from lactose, or milk sugar.

Results of Dietary Therapy

A galactose-free diet produces a striking regression of symptoms and signs. Liver abnormalities, proteinuria, and aminoaciduria disappear; cataracts regress and vision returns to normal if treatment is initiated early. Subsequent growth is normal. The intellectual outcome of early treatment of these patients is good. Galactosemic females have a high frequency of primary or secondary ovarian failure.

PATIENT IDENTIFICATION AND DIAGNOSIS

Several states now screen for galactosemia in the neonate. Two general types of tests are used: (1) detection of increased serum levels of galactose and (2) actual measurement of erythrocyte galactose-1-phosphate uridyltransferase activity. The former screening test will also detect galactokinase deficiency.

In states that do not screen, and for those galactosemic infants who become symptomatic before the results of their screening test are available, diagnosis depends on a high degree of suspicion. The presence of non–glucose-reducing substances in the urine (negative dipstick and positive Clinitest tablet) should always suggest a disorder of galactose metabolism. Final diagnosis requires direct measurement of the activity of the appropriate enzyme in either erythrocytes or cultured skin fibroblasts.

DIETARY PRINCIPLES AND MANAGEMENT

Description and Goal of Diet

The dietary goal is the complete exclusion of galactose from the diet. Large amounts of galactose are not found in most foods; however, galactose is a component of lactose, the predominant sugar in milk. Thus, all milk and milk products must be eliminated.

Milk Substitutes

Milk substitutes that are essentially lactose-free include Nutramigen,* a casein hydrolysate, and the soybean formulas ProSobee* and Isomil.† The use of soybean milks has been challenged, since they contain galactose oligosaccharides, such as raffinose and stachyose. However, these galactose-containing sugars are not hydrolyzed by the human intestinal mucosa, and these products have been used successfully in patients with galactosemia. Table 13–7 lists the nutrient contents of Nutramigen, Isomil, and ProSobee. Coffee whiteners or nondairy creamers should not be used as replacements for milk in galactosemic children.

Nutritional Adequacy of the Diet

Infants and children with galactosemia have the same nutritional requirements as do those without the defect. It is essential that the patient receive a balanced diet containing adequate amounts of milk substitutes, fruits, vegetables, meats, breads, cereals, and fats. Additional allowed foods may be added as desired, to fulfill caloric requirements.

Foods Included or Omitted in Galactose Restriction

Table 13–8 lists the foods that may be included in or must be excluded from the galactose-free diet. Fruits and vegetables may be eaten as desired, un-

---

*Mead Johnson Laboratories, Evansville, IN.
†Ross Laboratories, Columbia, OH.

TABLE 13–7.   NUTRIENT COMPOSITION OF MILK SUBSTITUTES
(per 1000 ml)

Nutrient	Nutramigen (Mead Johnson)		Isomil (Ross Labs)		ProSobee (Mead Johnson)	
Calories	683		680		680	
Protein (g)	22	(13%)	20	(12%)	20	(12%)
Carbohydrate (g)	88	(52%)	68	(40%)	69	(40%)
Fat (g)	27	(35%)	36	(48%)	36	(48%)
VITAMINS						
Vitamin A, IU	1691		2500		2114	
Vitamin D, IU	425		400		423	
Vitamin E, IU	10.5		15		10.5	
Vitamin C (mg)	54.9		55		55	
Folic Acid (mcg)	108		100		105.7	
Thiamine (mg)	0.42		0.40		0.52	
Riboflavin (mg)	0.63		0.60		0.63	
Niacin (mg)	8.4		9		8.4	
Vitamin B_6 (mg)	0.42		0.40		0.42	
Vitamin B_{12} (mcg)	2.1		3.0		2.1	
Biotin (mcg)	52.8		150		53	
Pantothenic acid (mg)	3.1		5		3.1	
Vitamin K (mcg)	106		150		105.7	
Choline (mg)	89.8		not listed		52.8	
MINERALS						
Calcium (mg)	634		700		634.2	
Phosphorus (mg)	475.6		500		502	
Iodine (mcg)	47.5		40		68.7	
Iron (mg)	12.6		12		12.7	
Magnesium (mg)	73.9		50		74	
Copper (mg)	0.63		0.50		0.63	
Zinc (mg)	4.2		5		5.2	
Manganese (mg)	1.05		0.20		0.2	
Chloride (mg)	475.6		530		549.6	
Potassium (mg)	687		710		687	
Sodium (mg)	317		300		290.7	

TABLE 13–8.   FOOD LISTS FOR THE DIETARY TREATMENT OF GALACTOSEMIA

Food Group	Foods Included	Foods Excluded
MILK AND MILK PRODUCTS	None. Galactose-free preparations such as soybean milks, meat base formulas, or protein hydrolysates are used: Isomil, ProSobee, Nutramigen, Pregestimil, Neo-Mullsoy, Casec, Cho-Free. Cream substitutes free of milk or milk derivatives, such as Dzerta Whip, Mocha Mix, Rich's Whipped Topping.	Any milk from an animal source in any form: whole, nonfat, evaporated, condensed, chocolate dry milk solids, whey, casein, curds, lactose, yogurt, cheeses, ice milk, ice cream, sherbet, Ovaltine, malted milk, cream, butter.

Table continues on following page

TABLE 13–8. FOOD LISTS FOR THE DIETARY TREATMENT OF GALACTOSEMIA
(Continued)

Food Group	Foods Included	Foods Excluded
MEAT, FISH, AND FOWL	Plain beef, fish, poultry, pork, lamb, veal, or ham.	Liver, pancreas, brain, or any organ meats. Creamed or breaded meat, fish, or poultry; processed products such as sausage, frankfurters, or cold cuts containing milk.
EGGS	Any prepared with allowed foods.	Any prepared with milk or milk products.
FRUITS	Any fresh, canned, dried, or frozen fruits, unless processed with lactose.	Any canned or frozen processed with lactose.
VEGETABLES	Any fresh, canned, or frozen unless processed with lactose.	Any prepared with lactose or milk products.
POTATOES AND SUBSTITUTES	White potatoes, sweet potatoes, yams, macaroni noodles, spaghetti, or rice.	Any creamed, breaded, buttered, French-fried, or instant if lactose is added in processing.
BREAD AND CEREAL PRODUCTS*	Cooked and dry cereals without added milk or lactose. Bread and crackers without milk or lactose added; saltines and graham crackers; unbuttered popcorn.	Cereals, breads, crackers that contain milk, milk products, or added lactose; prepared mixes such as muffins, biscuits, waffles, and pancakes; some dry cereals such as Total, Special K, Instant Cream of Wheat.
FATS	Vegetable oils, such as soybean, corn, cottonseed, safflower, olive, peanut oils; shortening, lard, margarines, and dressings that do not contain milk or milk products; bacon; nuts and nut butters.	Margarines and dressings containing milk or milk products; butter, cream, cream cheese, peanut butter with milk-solid fillers.
SOUPS	Clear soup; vegetable soups that do not contain peas or lima beans; consommés; cream soups made with cream substitutes listed.	Cream soups, chowders, commercially prepared soups containing lactose.
DESSERTS	Water and fruit ices; gelatin, angel food cake, homemade cakes, pies, and cookies made from foods permitted; fruit-flavored corn starch puddings made with water.	Commercial cakes, cookies, and mixes; custard, puddings, ice cream made with milk; sherbet; gelatin made with carrageen; any containing milk chocolate.
SWEETS	Jelly, jam, marmalade, sugar, pure sugar candy, carob powder, marshmallows, corn syrup, molasses, honey, Karo syrup. Unsweetened cocoa, cooking chocolate, semisweet chocolate.	Any made with chocolate or cocoa; toffee, peppermints, butterscotch, caramels, commercial candy with lactose; chewing gum. Sugar substitutes that contain lactose, such as Sweet 'n Low.
SEASONINGS	Salt, pepper, cinnamon, paprika, nutmeg, mustard, catsup, vinegar, garlic, pure spices.	
BEVERAGES	Fruit juices: fresh, canned, or frozen if not processed with lactose; ground coffee, tea, carbonated beverages, some powdered soft drinks.	Milk chocolate and presweetened punch base with lactose, milk, or malted milk.

*In each geographic area, bakeries will need to be contacted and a list of acceptable products made available.

TABLE 13–9.   PRODUCTS THAT MAY CONTAIN ADDED LACTOSE

Simulated mother's milk—infant food formulas	Easter egg dyes and dye carrier
Health foods—geriatric foods	Meat products
Diabetic and dietetic preparations	Spice blends
Pie crusts and pie fillings	Buttermilk
Cakes and sweet rolls	Yogurt
Cookies and cookie sandwich filling	Modified skim milks
Sweetened condensed milk	Cottage cheese and cottage cheese dressings
Caramels, fudge, and tableted candies	Starter cultures
French-fried potatoes and corn curls	Cheese foods and spreads
Canned and frozen vegetables	Sour cream
Instant potatoes	Party dips
Canned and frozen fruits	Salad dressings
Instant coffee	Sherbets, frozen desserts, and ices
Powdered coffee cream	Dried soups
Pharmaceutical bulking agents and fillers	Monosodium glutamate extender
Tinctures	Powdered soft drinks, Sweet 'n Low
Tablets—pharmaceutical and food	Puddings
Vitamin and mineral mixtures	Cordials and liqueurs
Vitamin C and citric acid mixtures	

less lactose has been added in processing. In the meat group, galactose-storing organs such as liver, pancreas, and brain should be avoided. Frequently, milk products of some sort are added to baked goods, cereals, and other foods to improve their flavor, browning, texture, or nutritional value, so these should be avoided. Lactose is also added to many processed foods and medicines. Table 13–9 lists products that may contain added lactose.

LABELS.   Product labels should be scrutinized carefully. They must be checked not only for the presence of milk, cheese, cream, and other excluded foods but also for alternate forms of milk such as dry milk solids, casein, whey, lactose, and curds. Foods that contain lactate, lactic acid, lactalbumin, or calcium compounds need not be avoided.

Termination of Diet

Enzyme activity in galactosemia patients remains reduced throughout life, and most investigators now believe that galactose restriction is a lifelong requirement. However, there may be psychologic problems associated with adherence to a rigid galactose-free diet by the older school-age child. It has been suggested that inclusion of the small amounts of galactose found in bread, cake, sauces, and similar prepared foods should eventually be allowed, while continuing to exclude milk, cheese, and other milk products completely. Each case must be assessed individually.

Maple Syrup Urine Disease

David L. Valle, M.D., and
Barbara Jean Cavagnaro-Wong, R.D.

INTRODUCTION

The nutritional management of this inborn error in the catabolism of the branched-chain amino acids is particularly challenging because three essential amino acids are involved and because measurements of the branched-chain ketoacids are not readily available. However, early diagnosis by astute clinicians or neonatal screening tests or both and careful nutritional management have markedly improved the outcome of affected individuals.

GOAL OF THERAPY

The goal of dietary therapy of this disease is to provide enough dietary branched-chain amino acids to maintain a normal rate of growth, while restricting their intake sufficiently to prevent accumulation and the development of symptoms therefrom.

DIETARY THERAPY

Nature of the Defect

Maple syrup urine disease, or branched-chain ketoacidemia, is an inherited disorder of the second step in the degradation pathway of the three branched-chain amino acids—leucine, isoleucine, and valine. The first step in their degradation involves reversible transamination reactions catalyzed either by valine transaminase or by leucine-isoleucine transaminase (Fig. 13–3). The ketoacid products of transamination are decarboxylated in a reaction catalyzed by a thiamine-dependent, branched-chain ketoacid decarboxylase. The activity of this enzyme is deficient in individuals with maple syrup urine disease; the resulting metabolic block causes an accumulation of the branched-chain ketoacids. Branched-chain amino acids also accumulate because the transamination is reversible. The high levels of branched-chain amino acids (leucine elevation usually greatly exceeds that of valine or isoleucine) are readily detectable with an amino acid analyzer, whereas special techniques are required to demonstrate accumulations of the branched-chain ketoacids.

When isoleucine is metabolized by transamination, the resulting branched-chain ketoacid contains an asymmetric carbon atom. This asymmetric center tends to become racemized in the body by an unknown mechanism. When the ketoacid with the opposite configuration is transaminated, alloisoleucine is

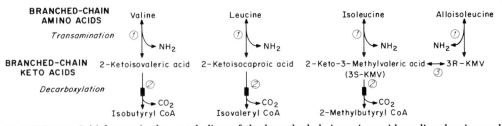

FIGURE 13-3. Initial steps in the metabolism of the branched-chain amino acids, valine, leucine and isoleucine. Transamination to ketoacids by branched-chain amino acid transaminases (1) is the first step in the catabolism of branched-chain amino acids. Maple syrup urine disease results from a defect in branched-chain ketoacid decarboxylase (2), an enzyme which acts on each of the ketoacids and requires thiamine as a cofactor. Deficiency of this enzyme leads to an accumulation of the branched-chain ketoacids and amino acids because the transaminase reactions are readily reversible. The initial ketoacid derivative of isoleucine, 2-keto-3-methylvaleric acid (3S-KMV), has a second asymmetric carbon atom and can be racemized to 3R-KMV(3) and transaminated (1) to form alloisoleucine. This amino acid is normally present in plasma in trace amounts, but accumulates in maple syrup urine disease.

formed. Since branched-chain ketoacid decarboxylation is impaired in this disease, both stereoisomers accumulate. Thus, an additional characteristic of these patients is a high plasma concentration of alloisoleucine, an amino acid that is usually present only in trace amounts.

In addition to high levels of the branched-chain amino acids and alloisoleucine, patients with maple syrup urine disease have a propensity for developing life-threatening metabolic acidosis and ketosis. Hypoglycemia may also occur during episodes of metabolic imbalance. The causal mechanisms for these additional biochemical abnormalities are not known.

Typically, an infant with maple syrup urine disease is normal at birth but develops lethargy, vomiting, and dehydration at age 3 to 7 days. If unrecognized, the illness usually progresses to seizures, coma, and death. Metabolic acidosis and ketonuria are present. The patient's urine smells like maple syrup, because of the presence of a derivative of the ketoacid of isoleucine. A plasma amino acid determination is diagnostic showing 20- to 40-fold increases in leucine, 5- to 10-fold increases in isoleucine and valine, and high levels of alloisoleucine.

Older patients with maple syrup urine disease have episodes characterized by similar clinical and biochemical abnormalities. These attacks usually occur either when excessive amounts of the branched-chain amino acids are ingested or when an intercurrent infection causes increased breakdown of tissue protein.

In some individuals, a less severe inherited deficiency of branched-chain ketoacid decarboxylase leads to a milder form of the illness. The defect may cause mildly abnormal amino acid concentrations in some patients on a regular diet; in others, the concentrations of these compounds are only abnormal during acute episodes. At least one family has been described with a deficiency of branched-chain ketoacid decarboxylase that was ameliorated by pharmacologic doses of thiamine.

Rationale for Dietary Therapy

Since leucine, isoleucine, and valine are essential amino acids, their accumulation can be prevented by reduction of dietary intake. The clinical symptoms correlate well with their serum levels (particularly that of leucine) so that the toxicity of the accumulated precursors appears to be the pathogenetic mechanism. It is also necessary to avoid overzealous restriction of these essential amino acids. Skin rash, growth failure, and neurologic problems have been reported as sequelae of a deficiency of one or more of the branched-chain amino acids.

Results of Dietary Therapy

There is meager information available regarding the long-term outcome of dietary therapy in maple syrup urine disease. It is clear that careful management can nearly or completely correct the biochemical abnormalities and allow normal growth. Many of the patients have modest to moderately severe intellectual deficits and spasticity resembling that seen with cerebral palsy. These deficits are static and presumably represent damage that occurred during the neonatal illness. Other patients—particularly those detected in the first few days of life—are physically and intellectually normal.

PATIENT IDENTIFICATION AND DIAGNOSIS

Maple syrup urine disease and other inborn errors causing acute metabolic disease should be considered in the differential diagnosis of infants with vomiting and lethargy. Plasma amino acid levels are diagnostic of maple syrup urine disease. The diagnosis can be confirmed further by assay of branched-chain ketoacid decarboxylase in cultured skin fibroblasts or leukocytes. Pharmacologic doses (10 mg/day) of thiamine should be administered during a period of defined intake to assess vitamin responsiveness.

Some states screen all neonates for hyperleucinemia by a method similar to that used to screen for phenylketonuria. A positive screening test should be confirmed by measurement of all plasma amino acids. The goal is to detect affected infants prior to the occurrence of neurologic damage.

DIETARY PRINCIPLES

The intake of leucine, isoleucine, and valine must be limited. Since the requirement for each is different and since natural proteins contain different amounts of each, it is frequently necessary to manipulate the amounts ingested individually. Failure to provide sufficient amounts of any of the three amino acids will impair growth and cause excessive breakdown of endogenous protein.

DIETARY MANAGEMENT

An amino acid mixture free of branched-chain amino acids but containing adequate calories is used for this purpose. Until recently, this was prepared by

TABLE 13–10. SPECIAL DIETARY PRODUCTS FOR MAPLE SYRUP URINE DISEASE
(per 100 g powder)

Nutrient	MSUD Diet Powder*	MSUD-Aid†	MSUD‡ 71004	Product 80056*
Calories	476	248		490
Protein equivalent (g)	8.2	64.4		0
Carbohydrate (g)	63.7	0		22.5
Fat (g)	20.1	0		71.8
VITAMINS AND MINERALS				
Vitamin A, IU	1190	0		1439
Vitamin D, IU	297	0		360
Vitamin E, IU	7	0		9
Vitamin C, mg	39	0		45
Folic Acid, mcg	74	400		90
Thiamine, mg	0.37	2		0.45
Riboflavin, mg	0.45	2.5		0.54
Niacin, mg	5.9	25		7.2
Vitamin B_6, mg	0.3	2		0.36
Vitamin B_{12}, mcg	1.5	20		1.8
Biotin, mg	0.04	0.6		0.045
Pantothenic Acid, mg	2.2	20		2.7
Vitamin K, mcg	74	0		90
Choline, mg	63	0		76
Inositol, mg	22	250		27
Calcium, mg	491	2500		540
Phosphorus, mg	268	1500		297
Iodine, mcg	33	150		41
Iron, mg	9	50		11
Magnesium, mg	52	300		63
Copper, mg	0.4	2.5		0.54
Manganese, mg	0.7	3.5		0.9
Chloride, mg	372	2600		135
Potassium, mg	335	2600		337
Sodium, mg	223	1400		72
ESSENTIAL AMINO ACIDS (G)				
Histidine	0.25	2.7	3.9	0
Leucine	0	0	0	0
Isoleucine	0	0	0	0
Lysine	0.80	7.1	7.2	0
Methionine	0.25	1.9	2.8	0
Phenylalanine	0.55	3.8	5.6	0
Threonine	0.55	3.3	6.1	0
Tryptophan	0.20	1.2	2.2	0
Valine	0	0	0	0
NONESSENTIAL AMINO ACIDS				
Arginine	0.50	5.1	5.0	0
Alanine	0.45	7.1	3.9	0
Aspartic Acid	1.14	12.1	8.9	0
Cystine	0.25	2.1	5.6	0
Glutamic Acid	2.09	13.3	25.0	0
Glycine	0.60	3.9	3.3	0
Proline	0.90	2.3	8.9	0
Serine	0.60	2.4	6.1	0
Tyrosine	0.65	3.8	5.6	0

*From Mead Johnson and Co., Product Description, Evansville, IN 47721, 1979.
†From Milner Scientific and Medical Research Co., Ltd., Liverpool, England. Available from: Institute for Developmental Research, Center for Mental Retardation Research, Children's Hospital Research Foundation, Ellard and Bethesda Avenues, Cincinnati, OH 45229.
‡From Grand Island Biological Company (GIBCO), Grand Island, NY 14072.

mixing MJ 80056 (Mead Johnson) with GIBCO amino acid mixture #71004 (Grand Island Biological Company, Grand Island, New York). The latter product, a mixture of L-amino acids from which the branched-chain amino acids have been omitted, provides all other amino acids in adequate amounts. MJ Product 80056 is a protein-free mixture of carbohydrates, fats, vitamins, and minerals. A new product, MSUD Diet Powder (Mead Johnson)—an otherwise complete infant formula that lacks only the branched-chain amino acids—is largely replacing this constructed mixture (Table 13–10).

The plasma levels of leucine, isoleucine, and valine should be monitored daily during institution of treatment. The period required for each of these amino acids to return to normal levels varies, with isoleucine becoming normal within 2 to 3 days, followed by valine, and finally by leucine at 8 to 10 days. As the plasma level of each branched-chain amino acid returns to normal, the diet is supplemented to prevent a deficiency state from developing. Once plasma levels become stable, a carefully measured quantity of natural protein (e.g., evaporated milk, whole milk, or standard infant formula may be used as a source for branched-chain amino acids. The amount of natural protein is calculated from the amount of leucine required. Additional valine or isoleucine may be required.

The diet for the patient with maple syrup urine disease must contain the recommended daily allowances for protein and energy. Since the requirements for the branched-chain amino acids are only estimates, plasma levels are used to determine the exact amounts to provide in the diet. Every effort should be made to keep plasma levels within or close to the normal range. In the young infant, the following dietary ranges may be used as guidelines for the initial formulation of the diet:

Leucine	75–150 mg/kg/day
Isoleucine	80–100 mg/kg/day
Valine	85–105 mg/kg/day

The patient should be started on the lower values within a range; adjustments are then based on plasma levels of the branched-chain amino acids and on the child's growth rate.

There are no data available on requirements from 7 months to 10 years of age. As in all patients with this disorder, the specific dietary allowance for these children is determined by plasma levels of the branched-chain amino acids and by the growth rate. As the child grows and develops, solid foods may be added to the diet at the usual times.

Two new formulas are now available for the treatment of infants with maple syrup urine disease and have generally replaced the aforementioned constructed formula. MSUD-aid (Milner) is a mixture of crystalline L-amino acids devoid of the branched-chain amino acids. The product also contains water-soluble vitamins and minerals (see Table 13–10). Fat-soluble vitamins and additional calories from carbohydrate and fat are needed to meet general nutritional requirements. Additional protein is needed as a minimal source of the branched-chain amino acids (Tables 13–11, 13–13, and 13–14). Sample prescriptions and menus are given in Table 13–12. MSUD Diet Powder (Mead John-

Text continues on page 331

TABLE 13–11. NITROGEN, PROTEIN, ENERGY, AND BRANCHED-CHAIN AMINO ACID CONTENT OF WHOLE COW'S MILK*

Component	Whole Cow's Milk (per 100 ml)
Protein (g)	3.5
Energy (kcal)	67
Isoleucine (mg)	223
Leucine (mg)	344
Valine (mg)	240

*From Acosta, P.B., and Elsas, L.J.: Dietary Management of Inherited Metabolic Disease: Phenylketonuria, Galactosemia, Tyrosinemia, Homocystinuria, Maple Syrup Urine Disease. Atlanta, ACELMU Publishers, 1976.

TABLE 13–12. SAMPLE PRESCRIPTIONS AND MENUS FOR CHILDREN, UTILIZING MSUD*

9 Months; 9 kg

PRESCRIPTION

Isoleucine: 50 mg × 9 kg = 450 mg
Leucine: 110 mg × 9 kg = 990 mg
Valine: 65 mg × 9 kg = 585 mg
Protein: 2 g × 9 kg = 18 g
Calories: 110 × 9 kg = 990 kcal
Thiamine: 100 mg

FOOD USING MSUD DIET POWDER

	Ileu (mg)	Leu (mg)	Val (mg)	Protein (g)	Energy (kcal)
MSUD Diet powder, 131 g	—	—	—	10.7	623
Mixed with:					
Milk, whole 50 ml	112	172	120	1.7	34
Water to make 900 ml					
Vegetables, 3 servings	69	90	81	2.1	45
Fruits, 3 servings	45	75	75	1.8	270
Bread/cereal, 4 servings	60	140	80	1.6	80
Total:	538	999	788	18.0	1052

FOOD USING MSUD-AID

	Ileu (mg)	Leu (mg)	Val (mg)	Protein (g)	Energy (kcal)
MSUD-Aid, 15 g				9.3	37
Mixed with:					
Milk, whole 150 ml	334	516	360	5.2	100
Vegetable oil, 1 tbs					126
Dextrimaltose, 6 tbs					162
Water to make 24 oz					
Vegetables, 4 servings	92	120	108	2.8	60
Fruits, 4 servings	60	100	100	2.4	360
Bread/cereal, 6 servings	90	210	120	2.4	120
Total	576	946	688	22.1	965

*Modified from Acosta, P.B., and Elsas, L.J.: Dietary Management of Inherited Metabolic Disease: Phenylketonuria, Galactosemia, Tyrosinemia, Homocystinuria, Maple Syrup Urine Disease. Atlanta, ACELMU Publishers, 1976.

TABLE 13–13.   AVERAGE COMPOSITION OF SERVING LISTS FOR DIETS RESTRICTED IN ISOLEUCINE, LEUCINE, AND VALINE*

List	Ileu (mg)	Leu (mg)	Val (mg)	Protein (g)	Energy (kcal)
Vegetables	23	30	27	0.7	15
Fruits	15	25	25	0.6	90
Breads/Cereals	15	35	20	0.4	20
Fats	7	10	8	0.1	70

*From Acosta, P.B., and Elsas, L.J.: Dietary Management of Inherited Metabolic Disease: Phenylketonuria, Galactosemia, Tyrosinemia, Homocystinuria, Maple Syrup Urine Disease. Atlanta, ACELMU Publishers, 1976.

TABLE 13–14.   SERVING LISTS FOR DIETS RESTRICTED IN ISOLEUCINE, LEUCINE, AND VALINE

	Ileu (mg)	Leu (mg)	Val (mg)	Protein (g)	Energy (kcal)
VEGETABLES					

This group will contain (per serving) an average of 23 mg isoleucine, 30 mg leucine, 27 mg valine, 0.7 g protein, and 15 kcal. Vegetable protein is approximately 3.5% isoleucine, 4.6% leucine, and 4% valine.

	Ileu (mg)	Leu (mg)	Val (mg)	Protein (g)	Energy (kcal)
Asparagus, raw, 1½ spears (33 g)	18	32	26	0.70	9
Asparagus, canned, green, 2 medium spears (38 g)	26	32	35	0.70	7
Beans, green raw, cooked in small amount of water, ¼ cup (31 g)	22	29	24	0.50	8
Beans, green, canned, drained solids, ¼ cup (31 g)	20	26	21	0.40	8
Beans, yellow wax, canned, drained solids, ¼ cup (50 g)	32	40	33	0.70	12
Beets, canned, drained, ½ cup (100 g)	29	28	25	0.80	31
Beet greens, cooked, 2 tbs (25 g)	18	27	21	0.20	4
Brussels sprouts, cooked, drained, 1 sprout (17 g)	29	31	31	0.70	6
Cabbage, raw, ½ cup shredded (50 g)	26	26	20	0.60	12
Cabbage, cooked in small amount of water, 5 tbs (50 g)	22	22	16	0.60	10
Carrots, raw, ½ large (50 g)	16	25	25	0.55	21
Carrots, canned, drained solids, ½ cup	24	34	30	0.64	24
Chard, frozen, cooked, 3 tbs (33 g)	26	32	23	0.80	8
Collards, frozen, cooked, 1½ tbs (18 g)	16	30	27	0.60	6

Adapted from Acosta, P.B., and Elsas, L.J.: Dietary Management of Inherited Metabolic Disease: Phenylketonuria, Galactosenina, Tyrosinenia, Homocystinuria, Maple Syrup Urine Disease. Division of Medical Genetics, Department of Pediatrics, Emory University School of Medicine, Atlanta, Georgia 30322, 1976.

Table continues on following page

TABLE 13–14.   SERVING LISTS FOR DIETS RESTRICTED IN ISOLEUCINE, LEUCINE, AND VALINE (Continued)

	Ileu (mg)	Leu (mg)	Val (mg)	Protein (g)	Energy (kcal)
Cucumber, not pared, 1 medium (100 g)	18	26	20	0.10	16
Eggplant, cooked, drained, ¼ cup (50 g)	26	31	30	0.50	10
Kale, frozen, cooked, 2 tbs (17 g)	17	32	24	0.50	5
Lettuce, raw (25 g)	12	21	18	0.30	4
Mustard greens, frozen, cooked, ¼ cup (50 g)	36	30	52	1.10	10
Okra, cooked, 2 pods (25 g)	21	31	28	0.55	10
Onion, raw, 6 tbs chopped (60 g)	18	30	40	1.20	24
Potato, boiled in skin, ⅓ medium (33 g)	31	35	37	0.70	25
Spinach, frozen, cooked, 1 tbs (12 g)	17	28	20	0.40	3
Squash, summer, cooked, drained, ½ cup (100 g)	29	41	33	0.90	14
Squash, winter, boiled, 3 tbs (50 g)	17	25	20	0.55	19
Sweet potato, baked, ¼ small (25 g)	25	30	39	0.52	35
Tomato, raw, 1 small (100 g)	32	45	31	1.10	22
Tomato, canned, 6 tbs (75 g)	22	31	21	0.75	16
Tomato juice, canned, ½ cup (100 g)	26	37	25	0.90	16
Turnip greens, cooked in small amount of water (12 g)	14	27	19	0.37	4

GERBER'S STRAINED AND JUNIOR VEGETABLES

In 7-tbs (100-g) Amounts

Beets	47	46	41	1.30	38
Carrots	26	37	33	0.70	30
Green Beans	57	75	62	1.30	29
Squash	25	36	29	0.80	27
Sweet Potatoes	67	81	105	1.40	69

In 1-tbs Amounts

Beets	6.7	6.6	5.9	0.19	5.4
Carrots	3.7	5.3	4.7	0.10	4.3
Green Beans	8.1	10.7	8.9	0.19	4.1
Squash	3.6	5.1	4.1	0.11	3.9
Sweet Potatoes	9.6	11.6	15.0	0.20	9.9

FRUITS

This group will contain (per serving) an average of 15 mg isoleucine, 25 mg leucine, 25 mg valine, 0.6 g protein, and 90 kcal. Fruit protein is approximately 2.9% isoleucine, 4.4% leucine, and 3.7% valine.

Apple, raw, 1 small, 2″ diam (100 g)	13	23	15	0.4	58
Applesauce, canned, sweetened, ⅔ cup (200 g)	13	23	15	0.4	182
Apple juice, 1½ cup	13	23	15	0.4	174
Apricot, raw, 2–3 medium (100 g)	14	23	19	0.8	51
Apricot, canned, sweetened, 4 medium halves (133 g)	14	23	19	0.8	115

Table continues on following page

TABLE 13–14.   SERVING LISTS FOR DIETS RESTRICTED IN ISOLEUCINE, LEUCINE, AND VALINE (Continued)

	Ileu (mg)	Leu (mg)	Val (mg)	Protein (g)	Energy (kcal)
Apricots, dried, 3 halves (18 g)	14	23	19	0.8	52
Avocado, 3½ tbs (33 g)	16	25	21	0.5	56
Banana, ½ small (50 g)	16	26	22	0.6	42
Dates, domestic natural, 2 medium pitted (20 g)	15	15	19	0.4	55
Figs, raw, 1 large (50 g)	18	26	23	0.6	40
Orange, raw, 1 small, 2½″ diam. (100 g)	23	22	31	0.8	49
Orange juice, canned, $\frac{2}{5}$ cup (100 g)	23	22	31	0.8	48
Peach, raw, 1 medium (100 g)	13	29	30	0.8	38
Peaches, canned, 4 medium halves, and 4 tbs syrup (200 g)	13	29	30	0.8	156
Peach nectar, canned, 1½ cup (370 g)	13	29	30	0.8	178
Pear, canned, in syrup,* 6 small halves and 6 tbs syrup (300 g)	17	26	22	0.6	226
Pear, raw,* ½ pear (100 g)	20	30	26	0.7	61
Pineapple, raw,* 1½ cup diced (200 g)	23	35	30	0.8	104
Pineapple juice,* 1 cup (240 g)	23	35	30	0.8	128
Pumpkin, canned, 3⅓ tbs (50 g)	19	26	19	0.5	17
Strawberries, fresh, 7½ large (75 g)	14	32	17	0.6	28
Strawberries, frozen and sugar, ½ cup (128 g)	14	32	17	0.6	140

GERBER'S STRAINED AND JUNIOR FRUITS

In 7-tbs (100-g) Amounts

	Ileu (mg)	Leu (mg)	Val (mg)	Protein (g)	Energy (kcal)
Applesauce	6	12	8	0.2	81
Applesauce and Apricots†	7	13	9	0.3	87
Applesauce with Pineapple†	6	10	7	0.2	77
Apricots with Tapioca‡	6	12	9	0.4	80
Bananas with Tapioca‡	14	23	19	0.5	88
Bananas with Pineapple and Tapioca†,‡	8	13	11	0.3	83
Peaches	10	22	22	0.6	82
Pears	11	17	15	0.4	69
Pears and Pineapple†	11	17	15	0.4	71
Apple Juice	3	6	4	0.1	49
Orange Juice	14	14	19	0.5	50
Orange Apple Juice	9	13	11	0.3	54
Orange Apricot Juice	14	17	19	0.6	61
Orange Pineapple Juice	14	22	19	0.5	59

In 1-tbs Amounts

	Ileu (mg)	Leu (mg)	Val (mg)	Protein (g)	Energy (kcal)
Applesauce	<1	1.7	1.1	0.003	11.6
Applesauce and Apricots	1	1.9	1.3	0.004	12.4
Applesauce with Pineapple	<1	1.4	1	0.003	11.0
Apricots with Tapioca	<1	1.7	1.3	0.060	11.4
Bananas with Pineapple and Tapioca	2	3.3	2.7	0.007	12.6
Peaches	1.4	3.1	3.1	0.009	11.7
Pears	1.6	2.4	2.1	0.006	9.9
Pears and Pineapple	1.6	2.4	2.1	0.006	10.1

*Amino acid content based on mean percentage of protein found in 10 fruits.
†Calculated on basis that product is one-half of each fruit noted.
‡Calculated on basis that fruit provides all the protein.

Table continues on following page

TABLE 13–14.   SERVING LISTS FOR DIETS RESTRICTED IN ISOLEUCINE, LEUCINE, AND VALINE (Continued)

BREAD AND CEREAL

This group will contain (per serving) an average of 15 mg isoleucine, 35 mg leucine, 20 mg valine, 0.4 g protein, and 20 kcal. Bread and cereal protein is approximately 3.8% isoleucine, 8% leucine, and 5% valine.

	Ileu (mg)	Leu (mg)	Val (mg)	Protein (g)	Energy (kcal)
Ready to Serve					
Bran, All, Kellogg's, 1 tbs (3.5 g)	13	26	19	0.4	12
Bran Flakes, 40%, 2 tbs (4.7 g)	16	32	24	0.5	17
Bran, Raisin, Kellogg's, 2 tbsp, (5 g)	15	30	22	0.4	18
Cheerios, 2 tbs (3 g)	17	33	23	0.4	13
Cornflakes, 2 tbs (3 g)	10	24	12	0.3	12
Rice Krispies, 4 tbs (¼ cup) (7 g)	18	35	24	0.4	27
Rice, Puffed, 8 tbs (½ cup) (6 g)	18	35	24	0.4	25
Cooked					
Farina, 2 tbs	23	33	21	0.5	18
Rice, brown, 2 tbs	16	30	24	0.4	17
Rice, white, 2 tbs	17	30	0.4	0.4	17
Special Low-Protein Products[§,‖]					
Aproten Macaroni Products					
Anellini, uncooked, ¾ cup (100 g)	13	26	15	0.5	340
Rigatoni, uncooked, 1½ cup (100 g)	13	26	15	0.5	340
Tagliatelle, uncooked, 1¼ cup (100 g)	13	26	15	0.5	340
Paygel Low-Protein Bread, 1 slice (32 g)				0.3	83
Aproten Rusks, 1 slice (11.5 g)	4	6	4	0.1	48
GERBER'S DRY CEREALS					
In 1-tbs (2.4-g) Amounts					
Barley	10	19	14	0.269	9
Oatmeal	14	6	20	0.359	9
Rice	6	12	10	0.159	9
GERBER'S CEREALS IN JARS					
In 1-tbs Amounts					
Mixed with applesauce	6	12	8	0.2	12
Oatmeal with applesauce-bananas	5	9	6	0.2	11
Rice with applesauce-bananas	2	4	2	<0.1	10
Rice with mixed fruit	9	18	12	<0.1	10

FATS

These contain (per serving) an average of 7 mg isoleucine, 10 mg leucine, 8 mg valine, 0.1 g protein, and 70 kcal.

Butter, 1 tbs (14 g)	6	10	7	0.1	100
Cream, whipping (40%), 1 tbs (5 g)	6	10	7	0.1	17

§Manufactured by Henkel, Special Dietary Foods, 4620 W. 77 St., Minneapolis, MN 55440.
‖ Not calculated in mean figures for amino acid content of Bread/Cereal List.

Table continues on following page

TABLE 13–14.   SERVING LISTS FOR DIETS RESTRICTED IN ISOLEUCINE, LEUCINE, AND VALINE (Concluded)

	Ileu (mg)	Leu (mg)	Val (mg)	Protein (g)	Energy (kcal)
Coffee Rich, liquid, 1 tbs (14 g)	8	11	8	0.1	24
French Dressing, 2 tbs (28 g)	6	7	7	0.2	114
Margarine, 2 tsp (10 g)	5	7	5	0.1	72
Mayonnaise, 1 tbs (14 g)	10	13	11	0.15	101
Tartar Sauce, ½ tbs (10 g)	7	9	7	0.1	47
Thousand Island Dressing, 1 tbs (14 g)	7	10	8	0.11	70

son), a complete formula for infants with maple syrup urine disease, will facilitate the treatment of this disorder. Older patients who have developed a taste for the MJ 80056–GIBCO amino acid mixture currently being used may have to be continued on the more cumbersome formula.

When solid foods are incorporated into the diet, exchange lists are utilized. Consult Table 13–13 for the average content of branched-chain amino acids in various food groups and Table 13–14 for the contents of specific foods.

When infection or fever interferes with the control of biochemical or clinical abnormalities, all branched-chain amino acids should be eliminated from the diet. At the same time, intravenous fluid therapy may be necessary to correct acidosis. Peritoneal dialysis or hemodialysis may be needed with severe episodes.

There is not enough experience now to indicate when, if ever, the special diet may be discontinued. It probably must be maintained throughout life, though it may be possible to ease stringent controls in older patients.

Congenital Hyperammonemia and Related Disorders

Mackenzie Walser, M.D.,
Mark L. Batshaw, M.D., and
Sylvia Ann Smith, M.S., R.D.

INTRODUCTION

Nutritional management is the mainstay of treatment for the deficiencies of any of the six enzymes of the urea cycle and a related disorder, lysinuric protein intolerance. It is now well established that, with proper dietary care, normal growth and development are possible in the complete inability of the patient to excrete waste nitrogen as urea.

GOAL OF THERAPY

The goal of therapy is to prevent hyperammonemia by reducing the patient's requirement for ureagenesis or by providing alternate pathways for excretion of waste nitrogen or both, without impairing the patient's growth and development.

DIETARY THERAPY

Nature of the Defect

Six enzymes are involved in the biosynthesis of urea (Fig. 13–4). The combined action of two enzymes, N-acetylglutamate synthetase and mitochondrial carbamoyl phosphate synthetase (N-acetylglutamate is a required activator of the latter enzyme), results in the production of carbamoyl phosphate from ammonium and bicarbonate. The remaining four enzymes operate in a cyclic manner, using ornithine as the regenerated substrate: (1) ornithine carbamoyltransferase (ornithine transcarbamylase) condenses carbamoyl phosphate with ornithine to produce citrulline (Fig. 13–5); (2) argininosuccinate synthetase condenses citrulline with aspartate (the source of the second nitrogen atom of urea) to produce argininosuccinate (Fig. 13–6); (3) argininosuccinate lyase (argininosuccinase) cleaves argininosuccinate to arginine and fumarate (Fig. 13–7); and (4) arginase cleaves arginine to urea and ornithine (Fig. 13–8). Congenital deficiencies of all six enzymes have been described.

N-ACETYLGLUTAMATE SYNTHETASE (NAGS) DEFICIENCY.   In the absence of N-acetylglutamate, mitochondrial carbamoyl phosphate synthetase is completely inactive *in vitro*. The first instance of an individual lacking this enzyme, a neonate, has recently been described in preliminary form. The presenting picture was that of typical neonatal hyperammonemia, as seen with carbamoyl phosphate synthetase deficiency.

Carbamoyl phosphate Synthetase Deficiency
and N–acetylglutamate Synthetase Deficiency

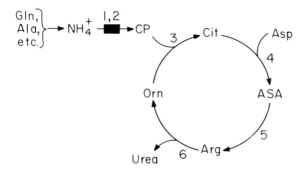

FIGURE 13–4. Steps in the biosynthesis of urea, illustrating the metabolic consequences of N-acetylglutamate synthetase deficiency or carbamoyl phosphate synthetase deficiency. The accumulated metabolites are Gln, Ala, and NH_4^+; the deficient metabolites are CP, Cit, Arg, and Urea; Orn and Asp are unchanged, and the fate of ASA is unknown. Abbreviations: Gln = Glutamine, Ala = alanine, CP = carbamoyl phosphate, Cit = citrulline, Asp = aspartate, ASA = argininosuccinic acid, Arg = arginine, Orn = ornithine.

Ornithine Carbamoyltransferase Deficiency

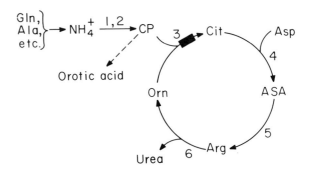

FIGURE 13–5. The metabolic consequences of ornithine carbamoyltransferase (ornithine transcarbamylase)
deficiency. The accumulated metabolites are Gln, Ala, NH_4^+, CP: The
deficient metabolites are Cit, Arg, and
Urea; Orn and Asp are unchanged,
and the fate of ASA is unknown. For
abbreviations see Figure 13–4.

Argininosuccinate Synthetase Deficiency
(Citrullinemia)

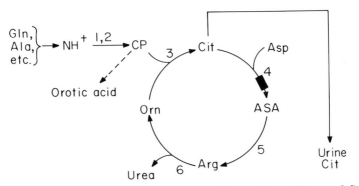

FIGURE 13–6. Metabolic consequences of argininosuccinic acid synthetase deficiency. The
accumulated metabolites are Gln, Ala, NH_4^+, CP, and Cit, which appears in the urine; the deficient
metabolites are Urea, Arg, and ASA; Orn is unchanged. Accumulated CP is diverted to orotic acid.
For abbreviations see Figure 13–4.

Argininosuccinase Deficiency
(Argininosuccinic Aciduria)

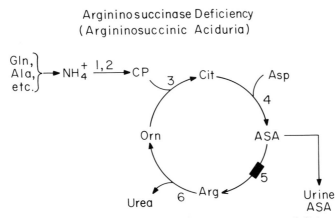

FIGURE 13–7. Metabolic consequences of argininosuccinase deficiency. The accumulated
metabolites are Gln, Ala, Cit, NH_4^+, Asp, and ASA, which appears in the urine; the deficient
metabolites are Orn, Arg, and Urea; the fate of CP is unknown. For abbreviations see Figure 13–4.

Arginase Deficiency
(Argininemia)

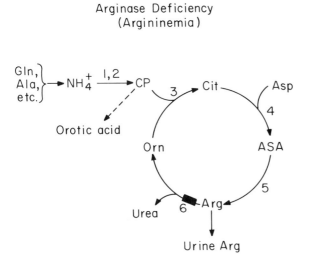

FIGURE 13–8. Metabolic consequences of arginase deficiency. The accumulated metabolite is Arg, which appears in the urine; the deficient metabolites are Orn and Urea; Gln, Ala, and NH_4^+ are unchanged, although NH_4^+ occasionally accumulates; the fate of CP and ASA is unknown; however, orotic aciduria is seen. For abbreviations see Figure 13–4.

CARBAMOYL PHOSPHATE SYNTHETASE (CPS) DEFICIENCY. At least 28 cases of this disorder have been described, of which 13 had complete or virtually complete enzyme deficiency and the remainder had a partial deficiency. The disorder is inherited as an autosomal recessive condition. The clinical picture in neonates is one of fulminant hyperammonemia with vomiting, lethargy, seizures, and coma within the first few days of life.

ORNITHINE CARBAMOYLTRANSFERASE (ORNITHINE TRANSCARBAMYLASE, OR OTC) DEFICIENCY. This sex-linked trait is the most common urea cycle enzyme defect, having been reported in at least 110 patients. Females are carriers; affected males are hemizygous and usually present with complete defects and fulminant neonatal hyperammonemia. However, a number of males have been described with onset later in the first year of life. Most females heterozygous for OTC deficiency remain clinically asymptomatic throughout life, even though subtle mental impairment or reduced tolerance to high-protein loads may be present. Some females who have adversely lyonized, inactivating their normal X chromosome, will have symptoms ranging from cyclic vomiting to pronounced hyperammonemia leading to physical and mental retardation.

ARGININOSUCCINATE SYNTHETASE (AS) DEFICIENCY (CITRULLINEMIA). This disorder occurs in three forms: (1) a neonatal form usually associated with complete or nearly complete enzyme deficiency and severe hyperammonemia, as described in some 20 cases; (2) a subacute type (approximately 8 cases) with onset in infancy or early childhood, associated with marked but incomplete enzyme deficiency; and (3) a late-onset variant (at least 22 cases) seen almost exclusively in Japan, with few or no symptoms in infancy but bizarre mental dysfunction and episodic coma described as beginning between the ages of 9 and 48 years. Enzyme measurements in this variant form usually show only partial deficiency. Citrullinemia is inherited as an autosomal recessive trait, at least in the neonatal type. The mode of inheritance of the Japanese type is not established.

ARGININOSUCCINATE LYASE (AL), OR ARGININOSUCCINASE, DEFICIENCY (ARGI-NINOSUCCINIC ACIDURIA). This disorder also occurs in two forms: (1) a neonatal variety, reported in at least 21 cases, associated with virtually complete enzyme deficiency in the liver, but occasionally with normal enzyme levels in other tissues; and (2) a subacute or delayed onset variety, reported in some 50 cases, in which hyperammonemic episodes begin during infancy or childhood and lead to psychomotor retardation. The incidence is approximately 1 in 30,000 live births in the United States. The disorder is inherited as an autosomal recessive trait.

ARGINASE (ARGL) DEFICIENCY (ARGININEMIA). This defect is quite rare. Only 15 cases have been reported, 7 of whom were of Spanish or Spanish-American origin. Since the enzyme defect does not affect the kidney, some urea is produced from citrulline synthesized in the gut and subsequently transported to the kidney. The clinical picture is distinct, being characterized by progressive spasticity beginning in infancy or childhood and mental retardation. Hyperammonemia occurs only intermittently, and either the accumulated intermediate, arginine, or its metabolites are believed to be responsible for producing the clinical disorder. Argininemia is inherited as an autosomal recessive trait.

LYSINURIC PROTEIN INTOLERANCE (LPI). This disorder is usually classified with the congenital hyperammonemias even though the urea cycle enzymes are normal. The defect involves an impairment of dibasic amino acid transport in gut and kidney, leading to defective intestinal absorption and increased renal excretion of lysine, ornithine, and arginine. For uncertain reasons, protein intolerance with episodic hyperammonemia is the presenting problem. Mental retardation is common. About 80 cases have been identified, at least two-thirds of whom are Finnish. The disorder is inherited as an autosomal recessive trait.

Rationale for Dietary Therapy

All six urea cycle disorders are characterized by protein intolerance and hyperammonemia owing to limited capacity to synthesize urea. The basic rationale for dietary therapy, therefore, is (1) to provide as little dietary nitrogen as possible without impairing growth and development and (2) to provide alternative pathways of waste nitrogen excretion. Nitrogen restriction is accomplished by a low-protein diet supplemented with essential amino acids or their nitrogen-free analogues. Alternate pathways may be exploited by administering arginine or sodium benzoate or both. Sodium phenylacetate may also be useful for this purpose.

Arginine becomes an essential amino acid in all these disorders, except in arginase deficiency. In citrullinemia and argininosuccinic aciduria, arginine supplementation also promotes urinary excretion of the accumulated intermediates, citrulline and argininosuccinate, which are alternate waste nitrogen products. Sodium benzoate conjugates with glycine in the liver to yield hippurate that is readily excreted, thereby removing 1 mol of waste nitrogen per mol of benzoate administered. Sodium phenylacetate conjugates with glutamine to form phenylacetylglutamine, removing 2 mols of waste nitrogen per mol of phenylacetate.

Substantial experience with the use of benzoate has shown it to be effective on a long-term basis. Experience with phenylacetate is as yet limited.

Carbamoyl glutamate, a substance that mimics the action of *N*-acetylglutamate, can be used to replace the latter when it is deficient, as in *N*-acetylglutamate synthetase deficiency, or possibly, to stimulate residual urea synthetic capacity in carbamoyl phosphate synthetase deficiency. Experience with this compound is very limited. A number of other therapeutic approaches have been tried with no clear benefit.

Results of Dietary Therapy

N-ACETYLGLUTAMATE SYNTHETASE DEFICIENCY. Protein restriction plus carbamoyl glutamate therapy (300 to 400 mg/kg/day) has resulted in nearly normal growth and development in the only infant so far identified with this disorder.

CARBAMOYL PHOSPHATE SYNTHETASE DEFICIENCY. Two males with complete carbamoyl phosphate synthetase deficiency were treated with a combination of protein restriction and essential amino acids supplemented with sodium benzoate (250 mg/kg/day), sodium phenylacetate (250 mg/kg/day), and arginine free base (175 mg/kg/day). Both are alive at 14 and 18 months and have exhibited normal growth and development. Two females with complete deficiencies were treated with protein restriction and nitrogen-free analogues of 5 essential amino acids and several other amino acids as such (including histidine and arginine). One remained severely retarded until her death at 5 months of age; the other developed normally until a fatal hyperammonemic crisis, unresponsive to peritoneal dialysis and sodium benzoate, occurred at 15 months of age.

ORNITHINE CARBAMOYLTRANSFERASE DEFICIENCY. Seven males with complete ornithine transcarbamoylase deficiency have been treated with protein restriction, essential amino acids plus sodium benzoate, sodium phenylacetate, and arginine for periods of 8 to 20 months. Four have died of intercurrent hyperammonemic crises. Physical and intellectual development have varied with the severity of neonatal hyperammonemic coma. An additional 5 males were treated with protein restriction plus nitrogen-free analogues. Four died in the first year of life. One survives at 6 years of age but is severely mentally retarded with cerebral palsy.

ARGININOSUCCINATE SYNTHETASE DEFICIENCY. Seven infants with complete argininosuccinate synthetase deficiency have been treated for 8 to 42 months with protein restriction supplemented with arginine (500 to 700 mg/kg/day) and sodium benzoate. Six have survived but only 1 has normal intellectual function. Three were treated with protein restriction, arginine, nitrogen-free analogues, and (in 1) sodium benzoate; none of these 3 survived past 1 year of age.

ARGININOSUCCINATE LYASE DEFICIENCY. Ten infants with argininosuccinate lyase deficiency have been treated for 7 to 50 months with protein restriction and arginine (500 to 700 mg/kg/day). All have survived, but most are mentally retarded. Whether argininosuccinic acid (or citrulline in argininosuccinate synthetase deficiency) is toxic in the brain is uncertain.

ARGINASE DEFICIENCY (ARGL).   Recently it has been established that a ow-arginine diet, achieved by adding essential amino acids to a low-protein diet, can prevent the symptoms and signs of this disease. Benzoate may also be useful.

LYSINURIC PROTEIN INTOLERANCE.   Protein restriction alone is not adequate n this disorder because it aggravates the deficiency of basic amino acids, even though the frequency of hyperammonemic episodes is reduced. Citrulline supplementation has proven successful in counteracting most, but not all, of the clinical manifestations. Since it is not a dibasic amino acid, citrulline is absorbed normally by the intestine and is converted readily to arginine and ornithine, thus correcting the deficiencies of these amino acids. Attempts to correct lysine deficiency by oral supplementation of lysine usually results in cramps and diarrhea.

PATIENT IDENTIFICATION AND DIAGNOSIS

A flow chart for the differential diagnosis of hyperammonemia caused by urea cycle defects or organic acidemias is shown in Figure 13–9.

N-ACETYLGLUTAMATE SYNTHETASE DEFICIENCY AND CARBAMOYL PHOSPHATE SYNTHETASE DEFICIENCY.   These disorders are presently indistinguishable clinically. The diagnosis should be suspected in any child with hyperammonemia with low to absent plasma citrulline levels who does not exhibit organic acidemia, argininemia, or orotic aciduria. (Orotic aciduria reflects overproduc-

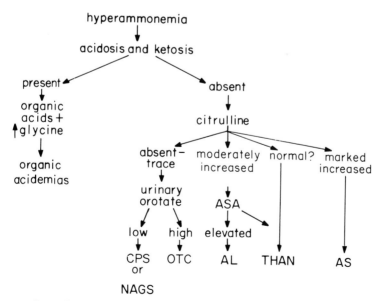

FIGURE 13–9. Flow diagram for diagnosing neonatal hyperammonemia. THAN—transient hyperammonemia of the newborn. Organic acidemias include propionic acidemia, methylmalonic acidemia, glutaric acidemia type II, isovaleric acidemia, beta-ketothiolase deficiency, and multiple carboxylase deficiency. (Modified from Brusilow et al., 1982.)

tion of orotic acid from accumulated carbamoyl phosphate.) Such cases may be presumptively diagnosed, but confirmation requires a needle biopsy of the liver (or of duodenal or rectal mucosa) for enzyme assay.

ORNITHINE CARBAMOYLTRANSFERASE DEFICIENCY. Hyperammonemia with low to absent citrulline but without argininemia or organic acidemia, accompanied by pronounced orotic aciduria, is virtually pathognomonic for this disorder. In neonates at risk the diagnosis can be made before hyperammonemia or orotic aciduria develops by the demonstration of a very low or absent peak for citrulline on plasma amino acid analysis. Needle biopsy of liver (or of rectal or duodenal mucosa) will confirm the diagnosis but is not necessary.

ARGININOSUCCINATE SYNTHETASE (AS) DEFICIENCY. Diagnosis of this deficiency should be suspected in any child with symptoms of hyperammonemia or in adults with episodes of bizarre behavior accompanied by hyperammonemia. Plasma or urine analysis for amino acids will reveal a pronounced increase in citrulline (over 0.5 mM). If confirmation of the diagnosis is desired, a variety of tissues, including liver, skin fibroblasts, and leukocytes, may be assayed for the enzyme.

ARGININOSUCCINATE LYASE (AL) DEFICIENCY. This diagnosis should be suspected in children with symptoms of hyperammonemia, and is based on the finding of large quantities of citrulline (0.2 to 0.4 mM) and argininosuccinate in blood or urine. Enzyme assay is not necessary to confirm the diagnosis.

ARGINASE DEFICIENCY. The diagnosis of this deficiency should be suspected in infants or children with unexplained spasticity and mental retardation. Arginine levels are greatly elevated (0.5 to 1.0 mM) in blood and urine. The enzyme defect is readily demonstrable in erythrocytes.

LYSINURIC PROTEIN INTOLERANCE. This diagnosis is suspected in children who have protein intolerance not otherwise diagnosed and in those who have dibasic aminoaciduria without cystinuria. A reduced response of plasma lysine or arginine to oral loads of these amino acids or to whole protein is also required to confirm that the defect involves the gut as well as the kidney.

DIETARY PRINCIPLES

Long-Term Therapy

Protein Restriction

At least the minimum daily requirement of protein should be given (see Appendix) when protein is restricted on a long-term basis, unless a supplement of essential amino acids or their analogues is provided. Such patients, as well as others on more severe protein restriction, commonly require vitamin supplementation.

Essential Amino Acids

Sufficient quantities of supplementary essential amino acids should be included so that the combined intake of each essential amino acid from dietary protein and from the supplement is adequate to meet minimum daily requirements (see Appendix). Histidine should always be included, and arginine should be included in all urea cycle disorders except argininemia. Neonates may also benefit from the inclusion of cystine, tyrosine, and taurine. Food-grade amino acids may be obtained from Tanower, Inc., San Diego, CA, or from Ajinomoto, Inc., New York, NY.

Nitrogen-Free Analogues

Keto-analogues of the essential amino acids, valine, leucine, isoleucine, and phenylalanine are available, as is the D,L-hydroxy-analogue of methionine. All are effective as dietary substitutes for the corresponding amino acids. Infants should not be given substantial doses of R,S-α-keto-β-methylvalerate (a racemic mixture of the keto-analogues of isoleucine and alloisoleucine) because it produces a profound increase in plasma alloisoleucine and a paradoxical fall in isoleucine. Instead, infants given such supplements should receive either L-isoleucine itself or S-α-keto-β-methylvalerate (the keto-analogue of isoleucine). These analogues are usually given as sodium salts; the use of calcium salts would entail an intake of calcium great enough to be harmful, at least in infants. The dosage of the branched-chain keto-acids will, in general, need to be higher than the requirements for the corresponding amino acids, because substantial oxidative decarboxylation of these compounds occurs. When these analogues are used, nitrogen intake is reduced, compared with supplements containing the corresponding amino acids. Although one might predict that nonessential nitrogen would become limiting for growth, this has not been noted, presumably because the regimen still includes some nitrogen (as protein and amino acids, especially arginine), or perhaps because "obligatory" ureagenesis ceases in complete defects. These analogues are investigational at present. They may be purchased as chemicals from Degussa Corp., Teterboro, NJ.

Arginine

Arginine as the free base is provided at a dose of 175 mg/kg/day for patients with carbamoyl phosphate synthetase (CPS) or ornithine carbamoyltransferase (OTC) deficiency. It comes as a white powder and is mixed with the daily formula, given three times a day mixed with Tang, or given as capsules to older children. Citrulline may be substituted for arginine. Arginine at a dose of 500 to 700 mg/kg/day is given to patients with AS and AL deficiencies. Arginine and citrulline may be obtained from the sources listed under Essential Amino Acids.

Sodium Benzoate

Sodium benzoate, an investigational new drug, at a dose of 250 mg/kg/day is given in CPS, OTC, and AS deficiencies and may be used in arginase deficiency. This is administered with arginine. Folate 0.5 mg/day and pyridoxine 5 mg/day are given to avert glycine depletion. Sodium benzoate can be obtained from Amend Drug and Chemical Co., Irvington, NJ.

A summary of this approach to therapy is shown in Table 13–15. Repeated measurements of plasma amino acids are important as a guide to adjusting the dosage of individual components, especially in patients receiving analogues. Plasma benzoate levels should be monitored in patients receiving this drug.

TABLE 13–15.   COMPOSITION OF LONG-TERM THERAPY (g/kg/day)[†]

Defect	Protein	Essential Amino Acids or Keto-Analogues	Arginine	Sodium Benzoate	Citrulline
CPS (or NAGS)*	0.5–0.7	0.5–0.7	0.175	0.25	—
OTC	0.5–0.7	0.5–0.7	0.175	0.25	—
AS	0.5–0.7	0.5–0.7	0.5	0.25	—
AL	1.5–2.0	—	0.5–0.7	—	—
ARGL	0.5–0.7	0.5–0.7	—	0–0.25	—
LPI	1.5	—	—	—	0.2

*Abbreviations: CPS = carbamoyl phosphate synthetase deficiency
           NAGS = N-acetylglutamate synthetase deficiency
           OTC = ornithine carbamoyltransferase deficiency
           AS = argininosuccinic acid synthetase deficiency
           AL = argininosuccinase deficiency
           ARGL = arginase deficiency
           LPI = lysinuric protein intolerance
[†]Folate 0.1 mg/day and pyridoxine 5 mg/day are also given when benzoate is used. Caloric intake is maintained between 100 and 120 kcal/day with Mead Johnson Product 80056. Citrulline 0.15 gm/kg/day may be substituted for arginine 0.175 gm/kg/day. In NAGS deficiency, carbamoyl glutamate, 375 mg/kg/d, may be employed.

Alloisoleucine accumulation appears to be of no clinical significance. Assay of plasma ketoacids is unnecessary, since these compounds are very rapidly utilized.

Amino acid imbalance may be detectable clinically as decreased growth, asymptomatic hyperammonemia or hyperglutaminemia, or frank symptoms of ammonia intoxication.

Acute Therapy

Intercurrent illnesses may also lead to symptomatic hyperammonemia and severe clinical consequences if not identified and treated early. The occurrence of lethargy, irritability, or vomiting in a patient with a urea cycle defect should lead to immediate hospitalization. After measuring plasma ammonium and amino acids, intravenous therapy is begun. Hyperammonemic patients with CPS and OTC deficiencies should receive a bolus of sodium benzoate (250 mg/kg) plus arginine hydrochloride (200 mg/kg) over 60 minutes. This should be followed by a continuous infusion of benzoate (500 mg/kg/24 hr) and arginine (200 mg/kg/24 hr). Maximal calories should be provided as 10 per cent glucose without supplemental protein. If plasma ammonium levels do not fall toward normal within 6 hours, peritoneal dialysis or hemodialysis should be started. During dialysis benzoate and arginine are continued.

Patients with AS deficiency follow the same regimen, except that for them arginine dosage is increased to a bolus of 800 mg/kg followed by 800 mg/kg/24 hr as a continuous infusion. Patients with AL deficiency generally respond to the same regimen without benzoate.

DIETARY MANAGEMENT

In infants with these disorders, food protein is provided as Similac mixed with MJ 80056, a protein-free powder containing carbohydrate, fat, vitamins and minerals (Table 13–16). Essential amino acids or ketoacids, arginine, or cit-

TABLE 13–16.   NUTRIENT COMPOSITION OF MJ
80056 POWDER*

Nutrient	Mead Johnson Product 80056 (per 100 g powder)
Calories	490
Protein, equivalent (g)	0
Carbohydrate (g)	71.8
Fat (g)	22.5
CALORIC DISTRIBUTION	
Protein (% of calories)	0
Carbohydrate (% of calories)	41
Fat (% of calories)	59
VITAMINS AND MINERALS	
Vitamin A, IU	1439
Vitamin D, IU	360
Vitamin E, IU	9
Vitamin C (mg)	45
Folic Acid (mcg)	90
Thiamine (mg)	0.45
Riboflavin (mg)	0.54
Niacin (mg)	7.2
Vitamin B_6 (mg)	0.36
Vitamin B_{12} (mcg)	1.8
Biotin (mg)	0.045
Pantothenic Acid (mg)	2.7
Vitamin K (mcg)	90
Choline (mg)	76
Inositol (mg)	27
Calcium (mg)	540
Phosphorus (mg)	297
Iodine (mcg)	41
Iron (mg)	11
Magnesium (mg)	63
Copper (mg)	0.54
Zinc (mg)	3.6
Manganese (mg)	0.9
Chloride (mg)	135
Potassium (mg)	337
Sodium (mg)	72

*From Mead Johnson and Co., Evansville, IN 47721 (1979).

rulline, and sodium benzoate are added in the amounts indicated in Table 13–15.

In children older than 9 months of age, protein provided in formula is progressively replaced by protein from foods selected from low-protein food lists (see Table 8–7 and Tables 13–4 and 13–6). Daily intake of animal protein from foods should be divided into 2 to 3 servings throughout the day to increase its utilization.

Solid foods should be introduced in the usual order for infants, starting with cereals, then fruits and vegetables. Low-protein products (Table 13–6) can

TABLE 13–17. DIETARY REGIMENS FOR UREA CYCLE DISORDERS

(1) 3-KG NEWBORN INFANT WITH ORNITHINE CARBAMOYLTRANSFERASE DEFICIENCY

	Protein Equivalent (g)	Energy (kcal)	Volume (ml)
Essential amino acids or ketoacids	2.10	8	0
Arginine or citrulline	0.52	2	0
Similac-20, 135 ml	2.10	92	135
MJ 80056, 53 g	0.00	260	315
Total	4.72	362	450

(Add sodium benzoate 0.75 g/day, folate 0.1 mg/day, and pyridoxine 5 mg/day.)

(2) 10-KG CHILD, 1 YR OLD, WITH ARGININOSUCCINASE DEFICIENCY.

	Protein Equivalent (g)	Energy (kcal)	Volume (ml)
Essential amino acids or ketoacids	5.0	20	0
Arginine or citrulline	5.0	20	0
Similac-20, 135 ml	2.1	92	135
Food	3.0	200–300	varies
MJ 80056, 130 g	0.0	637	773
Total	15.1	969–1069	varies

(Add sodium benzoate 2.5 g/day, folate 0.5 mg/day, and pyridoxine 5 mg/day.)

be used as calorie sources as the child grows older and energy needs increase. The child should be encouraged to develop a preference for these low-protein foods. Introduction of concentrated protein sources such as meat, eggs, and dairy products should be delayed. These foods provide too few calories/g of protein and displace low-protein foods from the diet.

Older children who no longer consume a minimum of 100 g MJ 80056/day do not receive adequate amounts of vitamin D, riboflavin, vitamin B$_{12}$, iron, zinc, or calcium. A multivitamin preparation that contains iron and zinc should be provided along with a calcium supplement that meets RDA requirements.

Examples of diets are given in Table 13–17.

Homocystinuria From Cystathionine - β - Synthase Deficiency

David L. Valle, M.D., and
Barbara Jean Cavagnaro-Wong, R.D.

INTRODUCTION

This inborn error of methionine metabolism involves complex pathways that not only degrade methionine but also provide the means for cysteine biosynthesis and the donation of methyl groups. The clinical consequences of this disorder reflect widespread organ involvement but develop slowly over several years. Therefore, evaluation of the efficacy of nutritional therapy is not yet complete.

GOAL OF THERAPY

The goal of dietary treatment of this disorder is to provide a diet that contains sufficient methionine and cysteine to support normal growth without causing an accumulation of methionine or homocystine.

DIETARY THERAPY

Nature of the Defect

The homocystinurias are a group of autosomal recessively inherited disorders in the metabolism of the essential amino acid methionine (Fig. 13–10). Me-

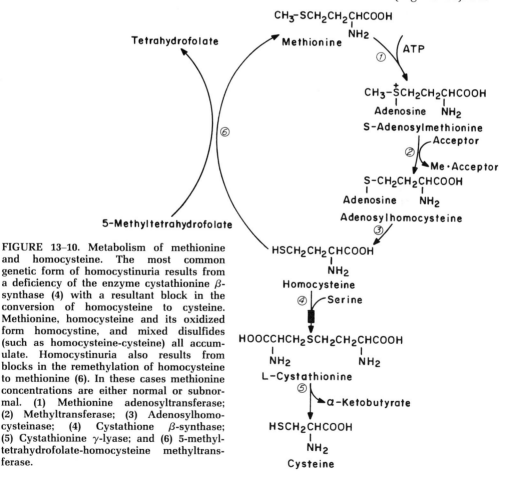

FIGURE 13–10. Metabolism of methionine and homocysteine. The most common genetic form of homocystinuria results from a deficiency of the enzyme cystathionine β-synthase (4) with a resultant block in the conversion of homocysteine to cysteine. Methionine, homocysteine and its oxidized form homocystine, and mixed disulfides (such as homocysteine-cysteine) all accumulate. Homocystinuria also results from blocks in the remethylation of homocysteine to methionine (6). In these cases methionine concentrations are either normal or subnormal. (1) Methionine adenosyltransferase; (2) Methyltransferase; (3) Adenosylhomocysteinase; (4) Cystathione β-synthase; (5) Cystathionine γ-lyase; and (6) 5-methyltetrahydrofolate-homocysteine methyltransferase.

thionine is first converted to the active methyl donor *S*-adenosylmethionine. Transfer of the methyl group to various methyl acceptors results in the formation of *S*-adenosyl homocysteine. This compound is located at an important metabolic branch point. It may be remethylated to form methionine or condensed with serine to form cystathionine and thereby cysteine. Blocks in either of these pathways result in homocysteine accumulation and homocystinuria.

The most common genetic cause of homocystinuria is a block in the conversion of homocysteine to cystine caused by a deficiency of the pyridoxine-dependent enzyme cystathionine-β-synthase. This inborn error leads to the accumulation of methionine, homocysteine, homocystine, and mixed disulfides (such as homocysteine-cysteine). Blocks in the remethylation of homocysteine to methionine, which also result in homocystine accumulation, can be differentiated from cystathionine-β-synthase deficiency because methionine levels are reduced (rather than increased). Confirmation of cystathionine-β-synthase deficiency by assaying the enzyme activity in cultured fibroblasts should be performed in each patient suspected of having the disorder.

Patients with cystathionine-β-synthase deficiency are normal at birth but eventually may develop problems in four major areas: ocular, skeletal, cardiovascular, and intellectual. The major ocular problem is an acquired dislocation of the lens (ectopia lentis) that occurs in childhood or early adulthood in almost all untreated patients. The major skeletal abnormalities are osteoporosis and arachnodactyly. The cardiovascular problems result from an increased incidence of spontaneous thromboembolic phenomena that can lead to problems such as focal neurologic deficiencies, myocardial infarction, pulmonary embolism, and/or death. The final major clinical problem is mild to moderate mental retardation in about one-half to two-thirds of the patients.

Rationale for Dietary Therapy

Since the product of the pathway, cysteine, can also be obtained from dietary protein and since patients with isolated hypermethioninemia do not manifest the symptoms of homocystinuria from cystathionine-β-synthase deficiency, the ocular, skeletal, and cardiovascular manifestations of this disorder are all thought to be secondary to the accumulation of homocysteine and homocystine.

The accumulation of methionine and homocystine can be prevented by limiting dietary methionine. The diet must supply cysteine, which becomes an essential amino acid because of the metabolic block.

Results of Dietary Therapy

Properly managed methionine-restricted diets can lead to complete correction of the biochemical abnormalities. In the few reported cases treated by this diet, growth and development have been normal and the ocular lenses have not become dislocated. Long-term follow-up of a large group of patients is required, however, to determine the ultimate success rate of this form of therapy.

PATIENT IDENTIFICATION AND DIAGNOSIS

The most commonly used screening test for cystathionine-β-synthase deficiency in the newborn is the detection of elevated levels of methionine in the same blood sample used to screen for phenylketonuria. Infants found to have hypermethioninemia by the screening test should then have a complete amino acid analysis. Those with cystathionine-β-synthase deficiency will have increased homocystine and decreased cystine levels in addition to hypermethioninemia. The homocystine is excreted in the urine, where it is detected by amino acid analysis or by the cyanide-nitroprusside test. The latter test should also be performed on all patients coming to medical attention with ectopia lentis. Final confirmation requires measurement of enzyme activity in cultured skin fibroblasts.

DIETARY PRINCIPLES AND MANAGEMENT

Objectives and Rationale

Since the homocystinuric patient is unable to metabolize the essential amino acid methionine, the objective of dietary management is to provide a nutritionally complete diet that contains only that amount of methionine required for net protein synthesis and growth. Furthermore, since the metabolic block prevents cysteine synthesis (*i.e.*, cysteine becomes an essential amino acid), care must be taken to supply adequate amounts of this amino acid in the diet.

In actual practice, the plasma amino acid values and the physical growth of the patient must be followed closely. Methionine intake needs to be sufficient to support normal growth, yet not so high as to result in methionine and homocystine accumulation. Patients who are well controlled grow normally and have plasma methionine values that range from normal to twice normal, no detectable plasma homocystine, and normal cysteine levels.

Protein Sources

In order to provide a low-methionine diet that is adequate in essential amino acids, 3 special products are currently available: Methionaid,* 3200 K,† and Low-Methionine Isomil‡ (Table 13–18).

Methionaid is a blend of beef serum protein hydrolysate, selected L-amino acids, water-soluble vitamins, and minerals. When this product is used, fat and carbohydrate must be added in amounts sufficient to meet the patient's nutrient requirements and energy needs. This goal can be achieved by mixing Methionaid with Product MJ 80056† (Table 13–16). Polycose‡ may be added as needed to fulfill carbohydrate and caloric needs. Whole milk or solid foods or both are used to supply adequate methionine in the diet.

---

*Milner Scientific and Medical Research Co., Ltd., Liverpool, England.
†Mead Johnson.
‡Ross Laboratories.

TABLE 13–18. NUTRIENT COMPOSITION OF SPECIAL DIETARY PRODUCTS FOR HOMOCYSTINURIA (per 100 g powder)

Nutrient	3200 K* (Mead Johnson)	Low-Methionine Isomil[†] (Ross Labs)	Methionaid[‡] (Milner)
Calories	518	516	250
Protein (g)	15.8	12.5	63
Carbohydrates (g)	51	57	0
Fat (g)	28	28.1	0
VITAMINS AND MINERALS			
Vitamin A, IU	1296	2200	0
Vitamin D, IU	324	340	0
Vitamin E, IU	8	12	0
Vitamin C (mg)	42	60	0
Folic Acid (mcg)	81	0.12	400
Thiamine (mg)	0.40	0.0005	2
Riboflavin (mg)	0.49	0.6	2.5
Niacin (mg)	6.5	0.009	5
Vitamin B$_6$ (mg)	0.3	0.0005	2
Vitamin B$_{12}$ (mcg)	1.6	35	20
Biotin (mg)	0.04	0.00013	0.6
Pantothenic Acid (mg)	2.4	0.007	20
Vitamin K (mcg)	81	0.12	0
Choline (mg)	69	94	0
Inositol (mg)	24	0	100
Calcium (mg)	486	650	2500
Phosphorus (mg)	324	440	1500
Iodine (mcg)	36	120	150
Iron (mg)	10	10	50
Magnesium (mg)	49	40	300
Copper (mg)	0.5	0.5	2.5
Zinc (mg)	4	4	15
Manganese (mg)	0.8	0	3.5
Chloride (mg)	324	450	2800
Potassium (mg)	445	406	2600
Sodium (mg)	202	239	1400
L-ESSENTIAL AMINO ACIDS (G)			
Histidine	0.38	0.28	2.8
Isoleucine	0.76	0.56	2.4
Leucine	1.31	1.02	3.2
Lysine	0.98	0.77	6.0
Methionine	0.18	0.14	0.2
Cystine	0.11	0.15	3.7
Phenylalanine	0.86	0	4.3
Tyrosine	0.55	0.40	4.3
Threonine	0.59	0.51	3.2
Tryptophan	0.18	0.12	0.9
Valine	0.80	0.52	3.2
NONESSENTIAL AMINO ACIDS (G)			
Arginine	1.08	0.83	4.4
Alanine	0.68	0.53	5.6
Aspartic Acid	1.94	1.29	9.5
Glutamic Acid	3.12	2.48	11.0
Glycine	0.67	0.52	4.3
Proline	0.77	0.6	1.6
Serine	0.81	0.68	1.7

*From Products for Dietary Management of Inborn Errors of Metabolism and Other Special Feeding Problems. Mead Johnson and Co., Evansville, IN 1979.
[†]From American Academy of Pediatrics, Committee on Nutrition: Special diets for infants with inborn errors of amino acid metabolism. Pediatrics 57:786, 1976.
[‡]From Management of Aminoacidopathies, Milner Scientific and Medical Research Co., Ltd., Liverpool, England.

Low-Methionine Isomil and 3200 K are soy protein formulas that are complete when reconstituted according to directions. Both formulas contain moderate amounts of methionine, and in our experience it has not been possible to restrict methionine intake sufficiently with these products.

Description of Diet

When planning the low-methionine diet, all protein, energy, vitamin, mineral, and fluid needs should be assessed. Table 13–19 gives suggested methionine, protein, and energy values to be used when initially calculating the diet. These are only general guidelines, and each individual patient must be followed closely with plasma amino acid determinations and growth measurements to make the final dietary adjustments. Plasma amino acid determinations will indicate whether a dietary formula needs to be supplemented with pure L-cystine. The L-cystine already present in the formula is probably sufficient for the needs of most patients.

Once solid foods are started, the low-methionine diet omits all forms of animal protein and continues to utilize the special formula as an alternate protein source. Exchange lists have been developed to add variety to the diet (see Tables 13–20 and 13–21). On the average, methionine makes up 0.67 to 1.42 per cent of the protein in vegetables, 0.62 per cent in fruits, 1.33 per cent in breads and cereals, and 3.0 to 3.5 per cent in meats.

Dietary Prescription and Calculation

The following procedure should be used to calculate a methionine-restricted diet (a sample dietary prescription and calculation is provided in Table 13–22):

1. Using Table 13–19, determine the patient's requirements for protein, calories, and methionine.

2. Calculate the amount of Methionaid that will supply the minimum protein requirement (including the requirement for cystine).

Text continues on page 351

TABLE 13–19. SUGGESTED METHIONINE, PROTEIN,
AND ENERGY REQUIREMENTS FOR USE IN
TREATMENT OF HOMOCYSTINURIA

Age (years)	Methionine (mg/kg)	Protein (g/kg)	Energy
0–0.5	42	2.00	120 kcal/kg
0.6–1.0	20	1.50	110 kcal/kg
1–3	10–23	1.25	1300 kcal/day
4–6	10–18	1.00	1800 kcal/day
7–10	10–13	1.00	2400 kcal/day

TABLE 13–20.   SERVING LISTS FOR METHIONINE-RESTRICTED DIET

VEGETABLES: GROUP 1*

Contains per serving an average of 10 mg methionine, 0.7 g protein, and 10 kcal.

	Methionine (mg)	Protein (g)	Energy (kcal)
Asparagus, cooked	11	0.7	7
3½ tbs (33 g)			
Beans, green, cooked	10	0.7	10
⅓ cup (42 g)			
Broccoli, cooked	9	0.6	5
2 tbs (20 g)			
Brussels Sprouts, cooked	7	0.7	6
1 sprout			
Cabbage, raw	9	0.6	12
1 cup shredded (50 g)			
Cauliflower, cooked	11	0.6	5
3½ tbs (25 g)			
Celery, raw	10	0.9	17
1 cup diced (100 g)			
Collards, cooked	11	0.9	9
3 tbs (33 g)			
Cucumber, raw	8	0.8	16
1 medium (100 g)			
Kale, cooked	10	1.1	9
¼ cup (33 g)			
Lettuce, raw	8	0.4	6
(33 g)			
Peppers, green, raw	8	0.6	11
½ large shell (50 g)			
Spinach, cooked	11	0.7	5
2 tbs (22 g)			
Squash, summer, cooked	12	0.9	14
½ cup (100 g)			

*All vegetables are fresh or frozen and cooked in small amount of water.

VEGETABLES: GROUP 2

Contains per serving an average of 10 mg methionine, 1.5 g protein, and 35 kcal.

	Methionine (mg)	Protein (g)	Energy (kcal)
Beets, cooked	8	1.8	68
⅞ cup (200 g)			
Carrots			
raw: 1 large (100 g)	14	1.2	42
cooked: 11 tbs (100 g)	7	0.9	31
Onion, cooked	11	1.2	29
½ cup (100 g)			
Potato, no skin, cooked	8	0.6	21
⅓ medium (33 g)			
Squash, winter, baked	12	0.9	32
¼ cup (50 g)			
Sweet Potato, baked	10	0.5	35
⅛ small (25 g)			
Tomatoes			
raw: 1 small (100 g)	8	1.1	22
canned: ½ cup (100 g)	7	1.0	21
juice: 1 cup (200 g)	12	1.8	38

Table continues on following page

TABLE 13–20. SERVING LISTS FOR METHIONINE-RESTRICTED DIET (Continued)

GERBER'S STRAINED AND JUNIOR VEGETABLES

In 7-tbs (100-g) amounts

	Methionine (mg)	Protein (g)	Energy (kcal)
Beets	5	1.3	38
Carrots	6	0.7	30
Green Beans	18	1.3	29
Squash	10	0.8	27
Sweet Potato	28	1.4	69

FRUITS

Contains per serving an average of 5 mg methionine, 0.8 g protein, and 75 kcal.

	Methionine (mg)	Protein (g)	Energy (kcal)
Apple, raw 1 small (100 g)	3	0.4	58
Applesauce, sweet 1 cup (300 g)	3	0.6	273
Apricots, raw 2–3 med (100 g)	4	0.8	51
Banana 2 tbs (23 g)	4	0.2	16
Cantaloupe 1 cup diced	4	1.6	72
Dates, dried 2 (20 g)	5	0.4	54
Grapefruit, raw 1 medium (200 g)	3	1.0	82
Oranges, raw ½ small (50 g)	6	0.4	25
Orange juice ¼ cup (50 g)	6	0.4	20
Peaches, raw 1 tbs (16 g)	5	0.1	6
Peaches, canned ½ peach and 1 tbs syrup (50 g)	7	0.2	39
Pineapple, canned 3 large slices and syrup (300 g)	7	0.9	222
Strawberries, fresh 30 large (300 g)	3	2.4	111
Tangerine 1 small (50 g)	6	0.4	23
Watermelon 2 cups (400 g)	4	2.0	104

GERBER'S STRAINED AND JUNIOR FRUITS

In 7-tbsp (100-g) amounts

Applesauce	1	0.2	81
Apricots with Tapioca	2	0.5	80
Bananas with Tapioca	6	0.3	88
Peaches	21	0.6	82

Table continues on following page

TABLE 13–20.   SERVING LISTS FOR METHIONINE-RESTRICTED DIET (Continued)

BREADS/CEREALS

Contains per serving an average of 20 mg methionine, 1.5 g protein, and 55 kcal.

	Methionine (mg)	Protein (g)	Energy (kcal)
Bread, Italian (enriched), 1 slice (20 g)	23	1.8	55
Bread, Raisin, 1 slice (23 g)	22	1.5	60
Bread, Roman Meal, 1 slice (23 g)	19	2.4	60
Cornflakes, $\frac{3}{4}$ cup (18 g)	18	1.5	72
Wheat, Shredded, $\frac{3}{4}$ biscuit (15 g)	22	1.6	63
Farina, enriched, cooked, $\frac{1}{3}$ cup	15	1.3	50
Oatmeal, cooked, $\frac{1}{4}$ cup	21	1.4	37
Rice, brown and white, cooked, 6 tbs	19	1.0	51
Macaroni, cooked tender, $\frac{1}{3}$ cup	24	1.6	50
Noodles, cooked tender, $\frac{1}{4}$ cup	28	1.7	50
Baby Cereals			
Barley (1 tbs), dry measure	5	0.3	8
Oatmeal (1 tbs), dry measure	7	0.3	9
Rice (1 tbs), dry measure	4	0.2	5
Mixed (1 tbs), dry measure	5	0.3	9

FATS

Contains per serving an average of 2 mg methionine, 0.1 g protein, and 65 kcal.

	Methionine (mg)	Protein (g)	Energy (kcal)
Butter, 1 tbs (14 g)	2	0.1	102
Coffee-Rich Liquid 1 tbs (14 g)	3	0.1	24
French Dressing 1 tbs (14 g)	2	0.1	57
Margarine 2 tsp (10 g)	2	0.1	72
Mayonnaise 1 tbs (14 g)	3	0.1	101
Thousand Island Dressing 1 tbs (14 g)	2	0.1	70
Whipping Cream, Heavy 1 tsp	2	0.1	17

Table continues on following page

TABLE 13–20.   SERVING LISTS FOR METHIONINE-RESTRICTED DIET (Concluded)

FREE FOODS

These foods contain little or no protein and may be used as desired in the diet as long as appetite is not depressed by their use and the child is not overweight.

	Methionine (mg)	Protein (g)	Energy (kcal)
Candies:			
Gumdrops, 1 large			35
Hard candy, 2 pieces			39
Other sweets: Jelly beans, 10			110
Lollipops, 1 medium (2¼″ diam)			108
Corn Syrup, 1 tbs			58
Danish Dessert, ½ cup			123
Fruit Ices, ½ cup			69
Kool Aid, ½ cup			53
Maple Syrup, 1 tbs			50
Molasses, 1 tbs			46
Popsicle, 1 twin bar			95
Start, liquid, ½ cup			60
Sugar, granulated, 1 tbs			43
Tang, liquid, ½ cup			59

3. Calculate the number of calories supplied by the Methionaid and add MJ Product 80056 to meet the minimum caloric requirement.

4. Calculate a volume of formula to accommodate this combination of Methionaid and 80056 at a concentration of approximately 20 kcal/oz, which generally will also meet the usual fluid requirement of 150 to 200 ml/kg for infants.

5. Add sufficient natural protein (*e.g.*, evaporated milk, whole cow's milk, commercial formula, or solid food) to meet the methionine requirement.

6. By calculating the formula in this way, greater flexibility will be possible when changes are introduced in the amount of methionine prescribed. Only the natural protein source being added to the diet will have to be altered.

TABLE 13–21.   SUMMARY GUIDE FOR DIET PLANNING
METHIONINE-RESTRICTED DIET

Food Group (per serving)	Methionine (mg)	Protein (g)	Energy (kcal)
Vegetables			
Group 1	10	0.7	10
Group 2	10	1.5	35
Fruits	5	0.8	75
Bread/Cereals	20	1.5	55
Fats	2	0.1	65

TABLE 13–22.   SAMPLE DIETARY PRESCRIPTION AND CALCULATION

CASE: A 1-month-old infant weighing 4 kg was just diagnosed as having homocystinuria. Calculate an appropriate diet using Methionaid.

STEP 1: Calculate requirements using Table 13–20.

Methionine 4 kg × 42 mg/kg = 168 mg
Protein   4 kg × 2.0 g/kg = 8 g
Energy   4 kg × 120 kcal/kg = 480 kcal
Fluid   4 kg × 200 ml/kg = 800 ml

STEP 2: Calculate the amount of Methionaid needed based on protein requirement.

$$100 \text{ g Methionaid} = 63 \text{ g protein (see Table 13–18)}$$
$$8 \text{ g protein} \times \frac{100 \text{ g Methionaid}}{63 \text{ g protein}} = 12.7 \text{ g Methionaid}$$

STEP 3: Determine amount of MJ 80056 needed.

$$100 \text{ g Methionaid} = 250 \text{ kcal (Table 13–18)}$$
$$12.7 \text{ g Methionaid} \times \frac{250 \text{ kcal}}{100 \text{ g}} = 32 \text{ kcal}$$
480 kcal required − 32 kcal from Methionaid = 448 kcal to be derived from 80056
$$100 \text{ g } 80056 = 490 \text{ kcal}$$
$$448 \text{ kcal needed} \times \frac{100 \text{ g } 80056}{490 \text{ kcal}} = 91.5 \text{ g } 80056$$

STEP 4: Calculate volume of fluid.

12.7 g of Methionaid and 91.5 g 80056 will provide approximately 480 kcal. Twenty-eight fl oz of water must be added so as to provide a formula concentration of 20 kcal/oz (740 ml)

STEP 5: Calculate amount of natural protein to be added.

$$30 \text{ ml of whole cow's milk} = 26 \text{ mg methionine}$$
$$168 \text{ mg methionine needed} \times \frac{30 \text{ ml whole milk}}{26 \text{ mg methionine}} = 194 \text{ ml whole milk}$$

STEP 6: Compare the final prescription with the calculated nutritional requirements.

	Amount	Methionine (mg)	Protein (g)	Energy (kcal)		Fluid (ml)
Methionaid	12.7 g	0	8	32		
80056	91.5 g	0	0	448		
Water q/s	740 ml	0	0	0	q/s	740
Whole Cow's milk	194 ml	168	7.1	129		194
TOTALS		168	15.1	609		934

The final prescription provides adequate protein, calories, and fluid, and exactly the prescribed amount of methionine.

Type I Glycogen Storage Disease

David L. Valle, M.D., and
Barbara Jean Cavagnaro-Wong, R.D.

INTRODUCTION

Type I glycogen storage disease disrupts both glycogenolysis and gluconeogenesis. Normal biochemical and hormonal homeostatic systems aimed at maintaining blood glucose in a narrow concentration range may aggravate the metabolic abnormalities characteristic of this disorder.

GOAL OF THERAPY

The goal of therapy for patients with this disease is maintenance of near-normal levels of blood glucose in order to provide adequate amounts of glucose for cerebral metabolism and to reduce gluconeogenesis and glycogenolysis (both of which accentuate metabolic acidosis in this disorder).

DIETARY THERAPY

Nature of the Defect

Type I glycogen storage disease, or von Gierke's disease, is an inherited disorder of glucose homeostasis resulting from decreased activity of glucose-6-phosphatase. Infants with this disorder usually are symptomatic within the first few days of life. They are often irritable, have frequent episodes of vomiting, and show poor weight gain. They have massive hepatomegaly, nephromegaly, and a cherubic appearance caused by prominent cheeks. Laboratory abnormalities include chronic hypoglycemia and metabolic acidosis, along with increased plasma concentrations of lactic acid, ketone bodies, cholesterol, triglycerides, and uric acid.

The microsomal enzyme glucose-6-phosphatase is found in the liver and to a lesser extent in the kidneys and gut and catalyzes the cleavage of glucose-6-phosphate to glucose and inorganic phosphate. This reaction is the final common step in both glycogenolysis and gluconeogenesis. Since these two processes are the major mechanisms for glucose production, the disorder has profound effects on glucose homeostasis (Fig. 13–11).

In normal individuals, blood glucose rises after the ingestion of a meal and then gradually decreases as liver and peripheral tissues utilize glucose. Within 2 to 3 hours after a meal, blood glucose returns to preprandial levels. If there is no additional dietary intake, the blood sugar is maintained at near-normal lev-

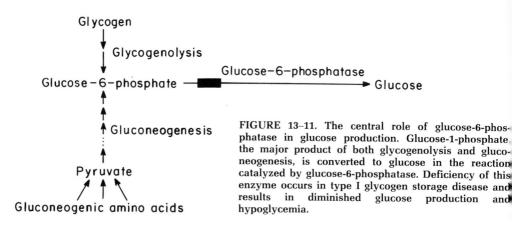

FIGURE 13–11. The central role of glucose-6-phosphatase in glucose production. Glucose-1-phosphate, the major product of both glycogenolysis and gluconeogenesis, is converted to glucose in the reaction catalyzed by glucose-6-phosphatase. Deficiency of this enzyme occurs in type I glycogen storage disease and results in diminished glucose production and hypoglycemia.

els by the release of glucose from the liver. This glucose production, which involves both glycogenolysis and gluconeogenesis, is stimulated by a decline in insulin levels as well as the release of glucagon, cortisol, and epinephrine. Glucose-6-phosphate is a common product of both gluconeogenesis and glycogenolysis.

Since individuals with type I glycogen storage disease cannot convert glucose-6-phosphate to glucose, their blood glucose levels fall rapidly during fasting. Continued stimulation of glycogenolysis and gluconeogenesis causes hepatic glucose-6-phosphate to increase to high levels. Instead of being hydrolyzed, glucose-6-phosphate becomes a substrate for glycolysis, resulting in increased production of lactate and acetyl-CoA. Hexose monophosphate shunt activity may also increase in response to the high levels of glucose-6-phosphate resulting in enhanced production of ribose phosphate and NADPH. The high concentrations of serum uric acid in part result from increased tissue levels of ribose phosphate (a precursor of uric acid) and serum lactate (an inhibitor of renal urate excretion).

These biochemical derangements produce extensive long-term consequences. Early in life, patients with type I glycogen storage disease may have seizures because of severe hypoglycemia. Even if proper metabolic control is not achieved, cerebral metabolism adapts to the utilization of ketones as an energy source and, eventually, hypoglycemia no longer induces neurologic symptoms. Nonetheless, poor linear growth is prominent. Accumulation of fat and glycogen causes massive hepatomegaly. For reasons that are not clear, older patients develop hepatic adenomas that occasionally undergo malignant transformation. Bleeding problems are common in early childhood. Widespread xanthomas may occur. Hyperuricemia may lead to uric acid nephropathy and, later in childhood, to clinical gout.

Type I glycogen storage disease, an autosomal recessive trait with no ethnic predilection, occurs with a frequency of about 1/100,000 live births. As with other rare genetic disorders, there is heterogeneity among the mutant genes causing a reduction in the function of glucose-6-phosphatase. In about 5 to 10 per cent of patients with both clinical and laboratory manifestations of this type of glycogen storage disease, the activity of hepatic glucose-6-phosphatase is normal. This disorder is designated as type Ib glycogen storage disease (the more common form with reduced enzyme activity is type Ia). Glucose-6-phosphatase is apparently bound to the luminal side of the membranes of the smooth endoplasmic reticulum, and a specific transport system is required for cytoplasmic glucose-6-phosphate to traverse the membrane and reach the enzyme. This transport system appears to be defective in the type Ib patients. Since both types Ia and Ib glycogen storage disease demonstrate an inability to hydrolyze glucose-6-phosphate, clinical manifestations are similar.

Rationale for Dietary Therapy

Maintenance of normal blood glucose concentrations by frequent (or even continuous) oral feeding provides substrate for cerebral metabolism and prevents the metabolic derangements that lead to lactic acidosis and hyperlipidemia.

Results of Dietary Therapy

The standard therapy, consisting of frequent feedings rich in glucose content, usually corrects the acidosis and hyperlipidemia partially. Liver size often decreases but does not return to normal. Hepatic adenomas also may decrease in size and number. Linear growth improves but final adult height is less than that predicted by parental heights. The bleeding tendency resolves.

As infants with type I glycogen storage disease become older, it becomes more difficult to maintain the frequent (every 3 hr) feeding schedule. A number of recent reports suggest that good results can be obtained by coupling frequent daytime feedings with continuous nocturnal nasogastric infusion of a mixture of glucose polymers and protein. Approximately one-third of the daily caloric requirements are provided by the infusion. Patients treated in this fashion have exhibited improved linear growth; decreased plasma levels of lactate, uric acid, and triglycerides; and possible reduction in the number of hepatic adenomas. Since the nasogastric infusion prevents nocturnal hypoglycemia, cerebral metabolism once again becomes dependent on glucose rather than ketone bodies. Thus, these patients may be at greater risk for symptomatic hypoglycemia.

PATIENT IDENTIFICATION AND DIAGNOSIS

The clinical picture of hepatomegaly, growth failure, metabolic acidosis, hyperuricemia, and hyperlipidemia strongly suggests type I glycogen storage disease. Lack of significant rise in blood sugar (40 per cent increment over fasting) within 30 minutes of receiving parenteral glucagon helps to confirm this diagnosis. Failure to develop hyperglycemia following infusion of galactose or fructose also suggests the diagnosis, but these tests may accentuate lactic acidosis and add little to the glucagon stimulation test.

Confirmation of the diagnosis requires measurement of glucose-6-phosphatase activity in a liver biopsy specimen. Ideally, this assay should be performed by experienced investigators who can prepare the fresh liver sample in two different ways. In one, the vesicles of endoplasmic reticulum are disrupted (thereby bypassing the need for an intact glucose-6-phosphate transport system); in the other, the vesicles remain intact. Type Ia patients lack activity in both samples, while those with type Ib lack activity only in the sample with intact vesicles.

DIETARY PRINCIPLES

The central principle in the dietary management of type I glycogen storage disease is to maintain adequate levels of blood sugar by providing oral glucose and glucose polymers. Gluconeogenic amino acids or other sugars (galactose, fructose) are not helpful, since glucose-6-phosphatase activity is necessary for their conversion to glucose. Galactose and fructose are avoided, because they may accentuate lactic acidosis.

The need to prevent hypoglycemia and maintain normal uric acid levels and a normal acid-base balance should be kept in mind. The diet should have a normal protein content but should restrict fat moderately, while maintaining a normal caloric intake. Frequent feedings of carbohydrate (glucose) must be given throughout a 24-hour period, especially during infancy, to maintain glucose homeostasis and prevent hypoglycemia. As discussed earlier, nocturnal nasogastric infusions of glucose with frequent intermittent daytime feedings improve growth and correct many of the metabolic abnormalities.

The only allowable carbohydrate sources are glucose or glucose polymers. Fructose and galactose are converted to lactic acid in the liver and will raise the serum lactate level without contributing to the blood sugar. RCF (Ross) is a carbohydrate-free soy protein formula base that may be used during infancy in conjunction with water and Polycose (as a source of glucose) (Table 13–23). RCF allows prescription of the amount and type of carbohydrate that an infant can tolerate with the assurance that other nutrient needs will be met so long as volume intake is adequate. Allowable solid foods may be introduced as the child grows. A suggested galactose-, sucrose-, fructose-free diet is detailed in Table 13–24.

There is some evidence that exchanging medium-chain triglycerides for dietary saturated fats may lower plasma triglycerides and cholesterol, relieve xanthomas, and diminish hepatomegaly. However, the same changes also occur when the blood sugar is controlled properly.

TABLE 13–23. SPECIAL DIETARY PRODUCTS FOR TYPE I GLYCOGEN STORAGE DISEASE*

Nutrient	RCF (Ross carbohydrate-free soy protein formula base) (per 1000 ml)[†]		Polycose (Ross Laboratories)	
	UNDILUTED	DILUTED[‡]	100 G POWDER	100 ML LIQUID
Calories	810	680	380	200
Protein (g)	40	20		
Fat (g)	72	36		
Carbohydrate (g)	0.1	70	94	50
Vitamin A, IU		2500		
Vitamin D, IU		400		
Vitamin E, IU		17		
Vitamin C (mg)		55		
Folic Acid (mcg)		0.10		
Thiamine (mg)		0.40		
Riboflavin (mg)		0.60		
Niacin (mg)		9.0		
Vitamin B$_6$ (mg)		0.40		
Vitamin B$_{12}$ (mcg)		3.0		
Biotin (mcg)		3.0		
Pantothenic Acid (mg)		5.0		
Vitamin K$_1$ (mg)		0.15		
Calcium (mg)	1400	700	60	30
Phosphorus (mg)	1000	500	13	6
Iodine (mcg)	0.20	0.10		
Iron (mg)	3.0	1.5		
Magnesium (mg)	100	50		
Copper (mg)	1.0	0.5		
Chloride (mg)	1060	530	213	107
Potassium (mg)	1420	710	39	20
Sodium (mg)	600	300	115	58
Manganese (mg)	0.40	0.20		

*From Ross Laboratories, Columbus, Ohio 43216, 1981.
†This product (RCF) is deficient in iron; an additional 5.3 mg of iron/l should be supplied from other sources.
‡With equal volume of 14% carbohydrate solution (7 tbs Polycose in 12 oz water).

TABLE 13–24.   GALACTOSE-, SUCROSE-, FRUCTOSE-FREE DIET

Foods Permitted	Foods Omitted
MILK AND MILK PRODUCTS	
Special formula—made of RCF*, Polycose* (or dextrose), and water.	Milk of any kind: skim, dried, evaporated, condensed, malted. Cheeses and cheese spreads. Yogurt, ice cream, and sherbets. Any food containing milk or milk products, lactose, casein, whey, curds, or dry-milk solids.
EGGS, MEAT, FISH, FOWL	
Eggs, beef, chicken, turkey, fish, lamb, veal, pork. Fresh, frozen, or canned. Only permitted foods may be added.	Creamed or breaded meat, fish, or fowl. Meats containing milk or milk products, such as frankfurters. Organ meats such as liver, pancreas, kidney, and brain. Meats in which sugar is used in processing, such as ham, bacon, and luncheon meats.
VEGETABLES	
Asparagus, broccoli, carrots, cauliflower, celery, corn, cucumber, green beans, wax beans, lettuce, and spinach. Only permitted foods may be added.	Sugar beets, peas, lima beans, soybeans, legumes. Creamed, breaded, or buttered vegetables. Any canned or frozen vegetable in which lactose has been used in processing.
FRUIT	
None.	All.
POTATOES, BREAD, CEREAL PRODUCTS	
White potatoes and potato chips.	Any creamed, buttered, breaded, or mashed potatoes. French-fried potatoes and instant potatoes if lactose or milk has been added during processing. Sweet potatoes.
Breads, rolls, and crackers in which only allowed ingredients are used. Macaroni, noodles, spaghetti, and rice. Flour: plain and self-rising. Baking powder and baking soda.	Prepared mixes such as muffins, biscuits, waffles, and pancakes. All breads, rolls, and crackers when omitted ingredients are used in preparation. (Read labels carefully or contact company.)

*Ross Laboratories.

Note: Labels should be read carefully and any products that contain milk, lactose, casein, whey, dry milk solids, curds, sugar, fruit, or other omitted items should not be used. Lactalbumin and calcium compounds do not contain lactose and need not be omitted from the diet.

TABLE 13–24. GALACTOSE-, SUCROSE-, FRUCTOSE-FREE DIET (Concluded)

Foods Permitted	Foods Omitted
All cooked and ready-to-eat cereals, except those omitted.	Instant Cream of Wheat. Sugar-coated cereals. Dry cereals with added skim milk powder or lactose, such as Special K and Total (read labels carefully).
FATS	
Oil shortenings, dressings without sugar or milk and milk products, MCT oil, milk-free margarine.	Regular margarines, butter, cream, cream cheese, mayonnaise, salad dressings made with sugar or containing milk or milk products.
SOUPS	
Clear soups, consommé, clear broths made from allowed vegetables.	Cream soups, chowders, commercially prepared soups that contain lactose, most vegetable soups (check labels).
DESSERTS	
Dietetic jello, any dessert homemade from allowed ingredients.	All desserts containing sugar, such as cake, pie, cookies, candy, puddings, jello, ice cream, sherbet, and others. Any dessert containing honey, fruit, chocolate, or milk.
BEVERAGES	
Special formula made of RCF, Polycose, and water. Vegetable juices except tomato. Ground coffee, tea.	Milk and milk-containing drinks, fruit juices, carbonated and noncarbonated soft drinks, instant coffee, cocoa, malted milk, Ovaltine, tomato juice.
MISCELLANEOUS	
Nuts; peanut butter with no added sugar, honey, molasses, or milk fillers; some pickles; unbuttered popcorn; corn syrup; olives; aspartame; saccharine; pure spices and herbs; prepared mustard; and vinegar, garlic, glucose, maltose, dextrose, and starch.	Gravy, white sauce, chocolate, all candy, monosodium glutamate (Accent), chewing gum, some spice blends, catsup, chili sauces, other sauces containing sugar, tomato sauce, tomato paste, most pickles, maple syrup, jam, jellies, preserves. Fructose, galactose, lactose, sucrose (table sugar), mannitol, sorbitol, and all other carbohydrates not composed of glucose only.

BIBLIOGRAPHY

Introduction

American Academy of Pediatrics, Committee on Nutrition: Special diets for infants with inborn errors of amino acid metabolism. Pediatrics 57:783–792, 1976.

Phenylketonuria

Acosta, P. B., and Elsas, L. J.: Dietary Management of Inherited Metabolic Disease: Phenylketonuria, Galactosemia, Tyrosinemia, Homocystinuria, Maple Syrup Urine Disease. Atlanta, ACELMU Publishers, 1976.

Acosta, P. B., and Wenz, E.: Diet Management of PKU for Infants and Preschool Children. U.S. Department of Health, Education and Welfare, Pub. No. (HSA) 77-5209, 1977. (Superintendent of Documents, U.S. Government Printing Office, Washington, DC 20402.)

Ernest, A. E., McCabe, E. R. B., Neifer, M. R., and O'Flynn, M. E.: Guide to Breast Feeding the Infant with PKU. U.S. Department of Health, Education and Welfare, Pub. No. (HSA) 79-5110, 1979. (Superintendent of Documents, U.S. Government Printing Office, Washington, DC 20402.)

Levy, H. L., Lenke, R. R., and Crocker, A. C.: Maternal PKU: Proceedings of a Conference. U.S. Department of Health, Education and Welfare, Pub. No. (HSA) 81-5299, 1981. (Superintendent of Documents, U.S. Government Printing Office, Washington, DC 20402.)

Levy, H. L., and Waisbren, S.E.: Effects of untreated maternal phenylketonuria and hyperphenylalaninemia on the fetus. N Engl J Med 309:1269–1274, 1983.

Scriver, C. R., and Clow, C. L.: Phenylketonuria: Epitome of human biochemical genetics. N Engl J Med 303:1394–1400, 1980.

Tourian, A., and Sidboury, J. B.: Phenylketonuria and hyperphenylalaninemia. In Stanbury, J. B., Wyngaarden, J. B., Frederickson, D. S., Goldstein, J. L., and Brown, M. S. (Eds.): The Metabolic Basis of Inherited Disease. New York, McGraw-Hill Book Co., 1983, pp. 270–286.

Williamson, M. L., Koch, R., Azen, C., and Charge, C.: Correlates of intelligence test results in treated phenylketonuria children. Pediatrics 68:161–167, 1981.

Galactosemia

Fishler, K., Donnell, G. N. Bergren, W. R., and Koch, R.: Intellectual and personality development in children with galactosemia. Pediatrics 50:412–419, 1972.

Fishler, K., Koch, R., Donnell, G. N., and Wenz, E.: Developmental aspects of galactosemia from infancy to childhood. Clin Pediatr 19:38, 1980.

Komrower, G. M., and Lee, D. H.: Long-term follow-up of galactosemia. Arch Dis Child 45:367–373, 1970.

Pickering, W. R., and Howell, R. R.: Galactokinase deficiency: Clinical and biochemical findings in a new kindred. J Pediatr 81:50–55, 1972.

Segal, S.: Disorders of galactose metabolism. In Stanbury, J. B., Wyngaarden, J. B., Frederickson, D. S., Goldstein, J. L., and Brown, M. S. (Eds.): The Metabolic Basis of Inherited Disease. New York, McGraw-Hill Book Co., 1983, pp. 167–191.

Maple Syrup Urine Disease

Acosta, P. B., and Elsas, L. J.: Dietary Management of Inherited Metabolic Disease: Phenylketonuria, Galactosemia, Tyrosinemia, Homocystinuria, Maple Syrup Urine Disease. Atlanta, ACELMU Publishers, 1976.

American Academy of Pediatrics, Committee on Nutrition: Special diets for infants with inborn errors of amino acid metabolism. Pediatrics 57:783–792, 1976.

Clow, C. L., Reade, T. M., and Scriver, C. R.: Outcome of early and long-term management of classical maple syrup urine disease. Pediatrics 68:856–862, 1981.

Committee for Improvement of Hereditary Disease Management: Management of maple syrup urine disease in Canada. Can Med Assoc J 115:1005–1010, 1976.

Scriver, C. R., and Rosenberg, L. E.: Amino Acid Metabolism and Its Disorders. Philadelphia, W. B. Saunders Co., 1973, pp. 207–233, 256–289.

Tanaka, K., and Rosenberg, L. D.: Disorders of branched-chain amino acid and organic acid metabolism. In Stanburg, J. B., Wyngaarden, J. B., Frederickson, D. S., Goldstein, J. L., and Brown, M. S. (Eds.): The Metabolic Basis of Inherited Disease. New York, McGraw-Hill Book Co., 1983, pp. 440–473.

Congenital Hyperammonemia and Related Disorders

Bachmann, C., Krahenbul, S., Colombo, J. P., Schubiger, G., Jaggi, K. H., and Tonz, O.: N-acetylglutamate synthetase deficiency: a disorder of ammonia detoxication. N Engl J Med 304:543, 1981.

Batshaw, M. L., Brusilow, S., Waber, L., Blom, W., Brubakk, A. M., Burton, B. D., Cann, H. M., Kerr, D., Mamunes, P., Matalon, R., Myerberg, D., and Schafer, I. A.: Treatment of inborn errors of urea synthesis. Activation of alternative pathways of waste nitrogen synthesis and excretion. N Engl J Med 306:1387–1392, 1982.

Brusilow, S. W., Batshaw, M. L., and Waber, L.: Neonatal hyperammonemic coma. Adv Pediatr 29:69–103, 1982.

Brusilow, S. W., Batshaw, M. L., and Walser, M.: Use of ketoacids in inborn errors of urea synthesis. In Winick, M. (Ed.): Nutritional Management of Genetic Disorders. New York, John Wiley and Sons, 1979, pp. 65–75.

Grisolia, S., Baguena, R., and Mayor, F. (Eds.): The Urea Cycle. New York, Wiley Interscience, 1976.

Kraus, B.: The Barbara Kraus Dictionary of Protein. New York, Harpers Magazine Press, 1975.

Lowenthal, A., and Mori, A. (Eds.): Urea Cycle Diseases. New York, Plenum Press, 1982.

Michels, V. V., Potts, E., Walser, M., and Beaudet, A. L.: Ornithine transcarbamylase deficiency: Long-term survival. Clin Genet 22:211, 1982.

Nutritive Value of American Foods in Common Units. Agriculture Handbook #456. U.S. Government Printing Office, 1975.

Pennington, J. A. T., and Church, H. N.: Bowes and Church's Food Values of Portions Commonly Used. Philadelphia, J.B. Lippincott Co., 1980.

Read, E., Wenz, E., Duffy, R. A., Wellman, N. S., Acosta, A., and Acosta, P. B.: The PKU Cookbook. Albuquerque, University of New Mexico Printing Plant, 1976.

Schuett, V. E.: Low Protein Food List. Madison, Wisc., University of Wisconsin Press, 1981.

Walser, M.: Urea cycle disorders and other congenital hyperammonemic syndromes. In Stanbury, J. B., Wyngaarden, J. B., Frederickson, D. S., Goldstein, J. L., and Brown, J. S. (Eds.): The Metabolic Basis of Inherited Disease, New York, McGraw-Hill Book Co., 1983.

Homocystinuria from Cystathioninc-β-Synthase Deficiency

American Academy of Pediatrics, Committee on Nutrition: Special diets for infants with inborn errors of amino acid metabolism. Pediatrics 57:783–792, 1976.

Mudd, S. H., and Levy, H. L.: Disorders of Transulfuration. In Stanbury, J. B., Wyngaarden, J. B., Frederickson, D. S., Goldstein, J. L., and Brown, M. S. (Eds.): The Metabolic Basis of Inherited Disease. New York, McGraw-Hill Book Co., 1983, pp. 522–559.

Scriver, C. R., and Rosenberg, L. E.: Amino Acid Metabolism and Its Disorders. Philadelphia, W. B. Saunders Co., 1973, pp. 207–233, 256–289.

Seashore, M.R., Durant, J. L. and Rosenberg, L.E.,: Studies on the mechanism of pyridoxine-responsive homocystinuria. Pediatr Res 6:187–193, 1972.

Valle, D., Pai, G. S., Thomas, G. H., and Pyeritz, R.: Homocystinuria due to cystathionine β-synthase deficiency: Clinical manifestations and therapy. Johns Hopkins Med J 146:110–117, 1980.

Wilcken, B., and Turner, G.: Homocystinuria in New South Wales. Arch Dis Child 63:242–245, 1978.

Type I Glycogen Storage Disease

Ballas, L. M., and Arion, W. J.: Measurement of glucose-6-phosphate penetration into liver microsomes. Confirmation of substrate transport in glucose-6-phosphate system. J Biol Chem 252:8512–8518, 1977.

Greene, H. L., Slonim, A. E., Burr, I. M., and Moran, J. R.: Type I glycogen storage disease: 5 years of management with nocturnal intragastric feeding. J Pediatr 96:590–595, 1980.

Howell, R. R., and Williams, J. C.: The glycogen storage diseases. In Stanbury, J. B., Wyngaarden, J. B., Frederickson, D. S., Goldstein, J. L., and Brown, M. S. (Eds.): The Metabolic Basis of Inherited Disease. New York, McGraw-Hill Book Co., 1983, pp. 141–166.

Narisawa, K., Igarashi, Y., Otomo, H., and Tada, K.: A new variant of glycogen storage disease type I probably due to a defect in the glucose-6-phosphate transport system. Biochem Biophys Res Comm 83:1360–1364, 1978.

Segal, S.: Disorders of galactose metabolism. In Stanbury, J. B., Wyngaarden, J. B., Frederickson, D. S., Goldstein, J. L., and Brown, M. S. (Eds.): The Metabolic Basis of Inherited Disease. New York, McGraw-Hill Book Co., 1983, pp. 167–191.

14

ALCOHOL

Mackenzie Walser, M.D.

INTRODUCTION

Alcohol is not only a significant nutrient in the diet of the United States and other countries but also a major public health problem. Recent studies have shed new light on the relationship between alcohol consumption and damage to vital organs and have also pointed to a beneficial effect at relatively low intakes.

ALCOHOL CONSUMPTION PATTERNS

Although it is often assumed that protein, fat, and carbohydrate are the only energy sources in normal diets, alcohol comprises at least 5 per cent of the total *calculated* caloric intake of the United States population. This amounts to 25 g (32 ml) of alcohol per adult per day. Much higher average intakes are reported in several European countries.

Alcohol is consumed in significant amounts (one or more drinks a month) by half of the adult United States population. "Heavy drinkers" (defined as those consuming more than 50 g [64 ml] per day of alcohol per 70 kg body weight) comprise about 15 per cent of men and 9 per cent of women in this country. Heavy drinkers are most common between 45 and 49 years of age, while nondrinkers are most commonly found among those aged 50 to 70. These and other aspects of drinking practices in the United States population have been reviewed in detail by Cahalan *et al.*

While it is often supposed that the alcohol-drinking population can be clearly separated into two groups—"social drinkers" and alcoholics—the distinction certainly cannot be made on the basis of a bimodal distribution of alcohol intake. The exact distribution of alcohol intake is not known precisely, but it is clearly not bimodal. Some have speculated that the distribution may be log normal, with a mode at about 32 g of ethanol/day. ("Mode" is defined as the most prevalent value.) However, Cahalan *et al.* found that light drinkers (<25 g/day) were only twice as common as moderate (25 to 50 g/day) or heavy (>50 g/day) drinkers. Maximum possible consumption is about 340 g/day (per 70 kg); the maximal rate of alcohol metabolism is about 14 g/hr (per 70 kg). Higher intakes reported anecdotally must be inaccurate, since the resulting accumulation of alcohol would be fatal.

Since alcohol is consumed in significant amounts by half the United States adult population, and average intake is 25 g per day per adult, it follows that drinkers consume an average of 50 g (64 ml) of alcohol per day. Consumption is greatest on weekends and lowest on Tuesdays.

The ethanol content of common beverages is summarized in Table 14-1. In addition to ethanol, these beverages contain varying amounts of other closely related organic compounds, including methanol, propanol, isobutyl alcohol, isoamyl alcohol, ethyl acetate, ethyl formate, and acetaldehyde. The concentration of these congeners varies enormously among different beverages, being highest in whiskey and brandy (100 to 200 mg/dl) and lowest in gin and vodka (about 3 mg/dl). These substances have been implicated in the genesis of the typical "hangover," although there is no firm evidence on this point; their long-term toxicity is unknown.

ALCOHOL AS A NUTRIENT

Animal studies have repeatedly shown that the energy derived from alcohol is close to the theoretical value of 7 kcal/g. However, in humans this is not the case, at least not with heavy alcohol intakes. Moderate drinkers consume somewhat fewer nonalcoholic calories than do nondrinkers, but heavy drinkers

TABLE 14-1.   ETHANOL CONTENT OF SOME COMMON BEVERAGES

Beverage	Source	% Ethanol, v/v	Serving Size (oz)	Ethanol Content per Serving (g)	Nonintoxicating No. of Servings*		
					50 KG	70 KG	90 KG
Beer	Cereals	4	12	11	3	4	5
Table wine	Grapes	10–14	4	9–13	3	4	5
Whiskey	Cereals	40–45	1½	14–16	2	3	3½
Rum	Molasses	40–45	1½	14–16	2	3	3½
Gin	Grain	40–45	1½	14–16	2	3	3½
Vodka	Grain	40–45	1½	14–16	2	3	3½
Brandy	Wine	40–45	1½	14–16	2	3	3½

*"Nonintoxicating" is defined here as a quantity just *insufficient* to induce a blood alcohol level of 0.1% in a person of average fatness/leanness (body water 60% of body weight), even if ingested over a short time span. Nondrinkers or young persons may become intoxicated at lower blood levels.

often consume nearly the same quantity of nonalcoholic calories as do non-drinkers (contrary to popular impression). This has been shown in surveys of entire communities, such as those in southern California and in France. Furthermore, obesity is less common in alcoholics than nonalcoholics. These findings appear to invalidate the conclusions of a few metabolic studies carried out decades ago in normal volunteers, which are the only rationale for asserting that alcohol yields its full caloric value in man. More recent metabolic studies have confirmed that at high intakes, alcohol fails to yield its full caloric value. Doubtless there is a small percentage of very heavy drinkers who eat little, but these constitute a small minority; their weight loss may well be secondary to inadequate energy intake.

Thus, alcohol consumed in excess of 50 g/day yields substantially less than 7 kcal/g in humans and may in fact yield very little energy. One possible explanation is that malabsorption caused by alcohol impairs the caloric value of other nutrients. Another possibility is that microsomal oxidation of ethanol, which is believed to play a significant role in alcohol metabolism only at relatively high doses, fails to yield any utilizable energy.

BENEFICIAL EFFECTS OF ALCOHOL CONSUMPTION

In addition to its psychologic effects, which presumably account for its widespread consumption, alcohol has some beneficial effects on physical health. Most significant is a reduced incidence of myocardial infarction in moderate drinkers, an observation made repeatedly in both men and women. The mechanism of this effect may be (1) an alcohol-related increase in high-density lipoproteins, a known protective factor against myocardial infarction; (2) a decrease in low-density lipoprotein, which is known to be atherogenic; or (3) an alcohol-induced change in platelet aggregation. Also, the reduction in stress consequent to alcohol ingestion could be a factor. These beneficial effects of alcohol have been reviewed by Turner *et al.*

DELETERIOUS EFFECTS OF ALCOHOL

Intoxication and Addiction

Intoxication is certainly the most prevalent and probably the most damaging adverse effect of alcohol consumption. Alcohol is freely distributed throughout the total body water and is almost completely oxidized at a rate of only 7 to 8 g/hr (in a 70-kg subject). Hence, the ingestion of 50 g of alcohol within an hour or two by a 70-kg subject can produce a blood alcohol level of 0.1 per cent, the legal level of intoxication as defined by most states (see Table 14–1). Consequences of intoxication such as traffic accidents and social disruption are well known, but the prevalence of intoxication is not fully recognized. Since about one-half of the adult population in the United States consumes an average of 50 g/day (often over a short time span) and since this can cause a blood alcohol level of 0.1 per cent in a 70-kg person, it would appear that perhaps 10 per cent of the adult population becomes legally intoxicated each day and an even higher percentage on weekends.

Simple and relatively inexpensive devices that detect intoxication by breath analysis are now available.

Ethanol becomes physically addictive in susceptible individuals at intakes as low as 60 g/day.

Hepatic Toxicity

Cirrhosis of the liver accounts for about 35,000 deaths per year in the United States, and more than 90 per cent of these cases are caused by alcohol ingestion. Cirrhosis is the fourth most common cause of death in white males. Alcoholic hepatitis and fatty infiltration of the liver secondary to alcohol ingestion are even more common than cirrhosis. Although it has often been believed that most heavy drinkers do not develop severe liver disease, this may be a misconception. As shown in Figure 14–1, one-half of those men in whom the product of alcohol intake in g/kg/day times years of consumption equals 25 will develop "severe liver disease." The latter term includes fatty liver with inflammatory changes (about one-third), alcoholic hepatitis (one-third), and cirrhosis (one-third); at least 80 per cent of those in whom this product amounts to 100 will develop these problems.

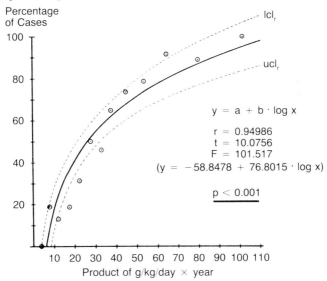

FIGURE 14–1. Correlation between total amount of ethanol per kg of body weight consumed during drinking life and incidence of severe liver damage (n = 108; severe steatofibrosis with inflammatory reactions, chronic alcoholic hepatitis, and cirrhosis of the liver) in 265 male alcoholics (Lelbach, 1972).

ucl$_r$; lcl$_r$ = upper and lower confidence limits of regression.

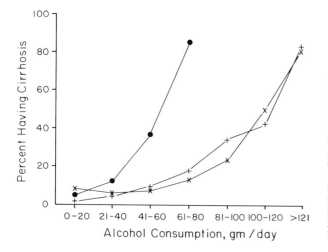

FIGURE 14-2. Incidence of "ascitic cirrhosis" (including all etiologies) in men and women aged 45 or more in two communities in France, as a function of reported alcohol intake in grams per day, according to the reports by Pequignot and associates. Cirrhosis increases significantly in women drinking 21–40 g per day and in men drinking 61–80 g per day. Solid circles, women (Bouches-du-Rhone); crosses, men (Bouches-du-Rhone); plus signs, men (Ille-et-Vilaine).

The study illustrated in Figure 14–1 did not include any moderate drinkers. There is in fact little information on the important question of how much alcohol can be consumed without danger of liver damage. Studies comparing the alcohol consumption of patients with cirrhosis and ascites, irrespective of etiology, with that of healthy individuals identified from voter lists have been reported from two communities in France (Fig. 14–2). There was no increase in the incidence of cirrhosis in men until consumption exceeded at least 40 or perhaps 60 g/day. A majority of men whose alcoholic intake was over 121 g/day had cirrhosis. (Lelbach, in Figure 14–1, found substantially fewer cirrhotic individuals among his heavy drinkers, but this is of no significance because his study population consisted of individuals who had entered an alcohol sanitarium for treatment, rather than of individuals representative of the population at large.)

The results of alcohol intake in women are strikingly different. Consumption of as little as 21 to 40 g/day was associated with a statistically significant increase in the incidence of cirrhosis in women, and the majority of women whose alcohol intake was over 61 g/day had cirrhosis (duration of intake was not considered, but all subjects were over 45 years old). Whether these results are applicable to the United States remains to be established; the difficulty in obtaining reliable estimates of alcohol consumption confounds all such studies.

Nevertheless, as alcohol consumption by women has increased toward that by men, it has been found that women are becoming more susceptible to liver damage from alcohol. There has been a dramatic increase in alcoholic liver disease in women; the male-to-female ratio is now approximately 2:1 for cirrhosis and about 1:1 for alcoholic hepatitis. Furthermore, the number of years of ingestion of over 100 g/day before cirrhosis develops averages 13.5 years in women, compared with 20.0 years in men. It is clear that this difference in susceptibility cannot be attributed solely to the lesser total body weights or lean body weights of women. Differences in immunologic responses directed against host liver cells may play a role.

It is a common misconception that adverse effects of alcohol, especially on the liver, can be prevented by eating a well-balanced diet and, in particular, by ingesting adequate protein. There is no evidence to support this view, although, as noted subsequently, there are some data to suggest that certain types of malnutrition may increase susceptibility to the hepatotoxicity of alcohol. The ingestion of food along with alcohol delays its absorption and, therefore, results in a lower peak blood level than if alcohol were taken alone. However, the relationship between liver disease and alcohol intake appears to be identical both in wine-drinking countries in which intake is spaced throughout most of the day and in countries in which most heavy drinking occurs in the evening. Thiamine deficiency plays a major role in certain forms of alcohol-related brain damage, notably Wernicke's encephalopathy; however, secondary effects of alcohol on thiamine absorption and metabolism are probably at least as important as inadequate dietary thiamine in the induction of this syndrome.

Alcohol may exert its toxic effect on the liver in several ways. Increased synthesis and decreased degradation of fatty acids leads to fatty infiltration. Hepatocellular damage may be secondary to hypoxia in the centrilobular regions or to cellular enlargement. Alcohol stimulates hepatic fibrinogenesis and inhibits hepatocyte regeneration. Enhanced humoral and cellular immune responses to specific liver antigens also occur. Nutritional deficiencies secondary to alcohol intake may also contribute to liver disease. These include inadequate dietary intake of folic acid, thiamine, riboflavin, nicotinic acid, and pyridoxine. Malabsorption of folic acid, thiamine, and vitamin B_{12}, as well as alteration in the metabolism of folic acid, thiamine, and pyridoxine, result from alcohol ingestion. These vitamin abnormalities may play a role in the induction of liver damage.

Various alcoholic beverages do not differ in their hepatotoxicity when compared for ethanol content per gram, despite the fact that they vary greatly in content of nonalcohol calories and that small amounts of vitamins are present in some.

The Nervous System

The effects of alcohol that are toxic to the nervous system—other than acute intoxication and the secondary hazards of trauma—include induction of peripheral neuropathy, delirium tremens, Wernicke's encephalopathy, Korsakoff's psychosis, and a global form of dementia. Some cerebral atrophy or shrinkage is detectable on CT scanning in a high percentage of heavy drinkers. To some degree, cerebral atrophy can be reversed by abstinence. The significance of this shrinkage and the role of fluid shifts or nutritional deficiencies in causing it are not known. Thiamine is useful in combating most forms of chronic neurotoxicity secondary to alcohol ingestion.

Esophageal and Other Types of Cancer

Alcohol intake in excess of 80 g/day is associated with an 18-fold increase in the incidence of esophageal cancer and intakes from 41 to 80 g/day with a two- to fourfold increase. The incidence of some other types of cancer, such as carcinoma of the oral cavity, is also increased in association with alcohol intake.

Deleterious Effects of Alcohol During Pregnancy

Consumption of as little as 24 g/day of ethanol during pregnancy is associated with reduced birth weight of the fetus. Ingestion of as little as 7 g/day leads to an increase in the rate of spontaneous abortion. High intakes often result in a pattern of birth defects including mental retardation known as the fetal alcohol syndrome.

Gastrointestinal Disease

Malabsorption of disaccharides, thiamine, vitamin B_{12}, folic acid, and fat occurs frequently in chronic alcoholics. When liver disease develops, further deficiencies of the B vitamins may occur as the result of impaired metabolism. Gastritis and acute pancreatitis are also common in alcoholics. Hypertriglyceridemia is common in heavy drinkers and may be a factor in the development of acute pancreatitis.

Malnutrition

Alcoholics who have adequate sources of income do not usually exhibit malnutrition. However, derelict alcoholics admitted to municipal hospitals often show signs of protein and vitamin deficiency. Deficiencies of folate (which may lead to anemia), pyridoxine, thiamine, niacin, and vitamin A can occur. Alcohol increases the requirements for folic acid and vitamin B_{12}. Zinc deficiency may impair taste, smell, and dark adaptation vision.

Whether malnutrition contributes to the development of liver disease in alcoholics is uncertain. In particular, there is no evidence that a dietary lack of lipotropic factors (such as choline) plays any role in the development of alcoholic liver disease in humans, even though it definitely can do so in rats. On the other hand, pyridoxine deficiency, which may occur in alcoholics, probably does enhance alcoholic hepatotoxicity.

Hematopoietic Effects

Both directly and secondary to vitamin insufficiency, alcohol consumption can result in anemia and other hematopoietic abnormalities.

Conclusions

The findings summarized here make it clear that alcohol consumption in the United States is far more prevalent and more deleterious than is commonly believed. In part, this may be related to certain widespread misconceptions. These include the beliefs that (1) only alcoholics are at risk from alcohol, (2) liver damage is rare even among alcoholics, (3) alcohol, even in large quantities, is a useful source of energy, (4) a good diet prevents alcoholic liver damage, and (5) an intake of 50 g/day is not only safe but beneficial in both sexes. In fact, it is difficult, if not impossible, to define a safe level of alcohol intake. Clearly, no level of alcohol intake is without risk in pregnancy. In nonpregnant women of average size, the ingestion of 20 g/day is probably safe, but 60 g/day evidently is not. In average-sized men, 40 g/day is probably safe, but 80 g/day apparently is not.

BIBLIOGRAPHY

Alcoholic brain damage. Lancet 1:477–478, 1981.

Argeriou, M.: Daily alcohol consumption patterns in Boston; some findings and a partial test of the Tuesday hypothesis. J Stud Alcohol 36:1578–1583 , 1975.

Cahalan, D., Cisin, I.H., and Crossley, H. M.: American Drinking Practices: A National Survey of Behavior and Attitudes Related to Alcoholic Beverages. Report No. 3. Washington, DC, Social Research Group, George Washington University, 1967.

Castelli, W. P., Doyle, J. T., Gordon, T., et al.: Alcohol and blood lipids: The cooperative lipoprotein phenotyping study. Lancet 2:153–155, 1977.

Ernst, N., Fisher, M., Smith, W., et al.: The association of plasma high-density lipoprotein cholesterol with dietary intake and alcohol consumption: The lipid research clinics program prevalence study. Circulation 62 (Suppl IV):41–52, 1980.

Gavaler, J. S.: Sex-related differences in ethanol induced liver disease: Artifactual or real? Alcoholism 6:186–196, 1982.

Haut, M. J., and Cowan, D. H.: The effect of ethanol on hemostatic properties of human blood platelets. Am J Med 56:22–33, 1974.

Jones, B. R., Barrett-Connor, E., Criqui, M. H., et al.: A community study of calorie and nutrient intake in drinkers and nondrinkers of alcohol. Am J Clin Nutr 35:135–139, 1982.

Lelbach, W. K.: Dosis-Wirkungs-Beziehung bei Alkohol-Leberschaden. Deut Med Wschr 97:1435–1436, 1972.

Lieber, C. S.: Medical Disorders of Alcoholism: Pathogenesis and Treatment. Philadelphia, W. B. Saunders Co., 1982.

MacSween, R. N. M.: Alcohol and cancer. Br Med Bull 38:31–33, 1982.

Mezey, E.: Alcoholic liver disease. Prog Liv Dis 7:555–572, 1982.

Miller, D. R., and Hayes, K. C.: Vitamin excess and toxicity. In Hathcock, J. N. (Ed.): Nutritional Toxicology, Vol. 1. New York, Academic Press, 1982, pp. 81–133.

Morgan, M. Y.: Alcohol and nutrition. Br Med Bull 38:21–29, 1982.

Pequignot, G., Chabert, C., Eydoux, H., et al.: Augmentation du risque de cirrhose en fonction de la ration d'alcool. Rev Alcool 20:191–202, 1974.

Pequignot, G., and Tuyns, A. J.: Comparative toxicity of ethanol on various organs. In Stock, C., Bode, J. C., and Sarles, H. (Eds.): Alcool et Tractus Digestif, Les Editions de l'Institute National de la Santé et de la Récherche Medicale, Strasbourg, 1980, pp. 17–32.

Pequignot, G., Tuyns, A. J., and Berta, J. L.: Ascitic cirrhosis in relation to alcohol consumption. Int J Epidemiol 7:113–120, 1978.

Pirola, R. C., and Lieber, C. S.: Hypothesis: Energy wastage in alcoholism and drug abuse: Possible role of hepatic microsomal enzymes. Am J Clin Nutr 29:90–93, 1976.

Roggin, G. M., Iber, F. L., Kater, R. M. H., *et al.*: Malabsorption in the chronic alcoholic. Johns Hop kins Med J 125:321–330, 1969.

Rosenberg, L., Slone, D., Shapiro, S., *et al.*: Alcoholic beverages and myocardial infarction in young women. Am J Pub Health 71:82–85, 1981.

Saunders, J. B., Davis, M., and Williams, R.: Do women develop alcoholic liver disease more readily than men? Br Med J 282:1140–1143, 1981.

Sherlock, S.: Alcohol-related liver disease: Clinical aspects and management. Br Med Bull 38:67–70 1982.

Smith, R.: Alcohol and alcoholism: The relation between consumption and damage. Br Med 283:895–898, 1981.

Surgeon General's advisory on alcohol and pregnancy. FDA Drug Bull 11:9–10, 1981.

Turner, T. B., Bennett, V. L., and Hernandez, H.: The beneficial side of moderate alcohol use. Johns Hopkins Med J 148:53–63, 1981.

Wilkinson, P., Santamaria, J. N., and Rankin, J. G.: Epidemiology of alcoholic cirrhosis. Aust Anr Med 18:222–226, 1969.

APPENDICES

TABLE A–1.   FOOD AND NUTRITION BOARD, NATIONAL ACADEMY OF SCIENCES—NATIONAL RESEARCH COUNCIL RECOMMENDED DAILY DIETARY ALLOWANCES,[a] REVISED 1980

Designed for the maintenance of good nutrition of practically all healthy people in the U.S.A.

		Weight		Height			Fat-Soluble Vitamins		
	Age (years)	(kg)	(lb)	(cm)	(in)	Protein (g)	VITAMIN A (μG RE)[b]	VITAMIN D (μG)[c]	VITAMIN E (MG α-TE)[d]
Infants	0.0–0.5	6	13	60	24	kg $\times$ 2.2	420	10	3
	0.5–1.0	9	20	71	28	kg $\times$ 2.0	400	10	4
Children	1–3	13	29	90	35	23	400	10	5
	4–6	20	44	112	44	30	500	10	6
	7–10	28	62	132	52	34	700	10	7
Males	11–14	45	99	157	62	45	1000	10	8
	15–18	66	145	176	69	56	1000	10	10
	19–22	70	154	177	70	56	1000	7.5	10
	23–50	70	154	178	70	56	1000	5	10
	51+	70	151	178	70	56	1000	5	10
Females	11–14	46	101	157	62	46	800	10	8
	15–18	55	120	163	64	46	800	10	8
	19–22	55	120	163	64	44	800	7.5	8
	23–50	55	120	163	64	44	800	5	8
	51+	55	120	163	64	44	800	5	8
Pregnant						+30	+200	+5	+2
Lactating						+20	+400	+5	+3

[a]The allowances are intended to provide for individual variations among most normal persons as they live in the United States under usual environmental stresses. Diets should be based on a variety of common foods in order to provide other nutrients for which human requirements have been less well defined.

[b]Retinol equivalents. 1 retinol equivalent = 1 μg retinol or 6 μg β carotene.

[c]As cholecalciferol. 10 μg cholecalciferol = 400 IU of vitamin D.

[d]α-tocopherol equivalents. 1 mg d-α tocopherol = 1 α-TE.

[e]1 NE (niacin equivalent) is equal to 1 mg of niacin or 60 mg of dietary tryptophan.

[f]The folacin allowances refer to dietary sources as determined by *Lactobacillus casei* assay after treatment with enzymes (conjugases) to make polyglutamyl forms of the vitamin available to the test organism.

[g]The recommended dietary allowance for vitamin B_{12} in infants is based on average concentration of the vitamin in human milk. The allowances after weaning are based on energy intake (as recommended by the American Academy of Pediatrics) and consideration of other factors, such as intestinal absorption.

[h]The increased requirement during pregnancy cannot be met by the iron content of habitual American diets nor by the existing iron stores of many women; therefore, the use of 30–60 mg of supplemental iron is recommended. Iron needs during lactation are not substantially different from those of nonpregnant women, but continued supplementation of the mother for 2–3 months after parturition is advisable in order to replenish stores depleted by pregnancy.

(From Recommended Daily Allowances, 9th Rev. Ed. National Academy of Sciences, Washington, DC, 1980.)

Water-Soluble Vitamins

VITAMIN C (MG)	THIAMINE (MG)	RIBOFLAVIN (MG)	NIACIN (MG NE)[e]	VITAMIN B$_6$ (MG)	FOLACIN[f] (μG)	VITAMIN B$_{12}$ (μG)
35	0.3	0.4	6	0.3	30	0.5[g]
35	0.5	0.6	8	0.6	45	1.5
45	0.7	0.8	9	0.9	100	2.0
45	0.9	1.0	11	1.3	200	2.5
45	1.2	1.4	16	1.6	300	3.0
50	1.4	1.6	18	1.8	400	3.0
60	1.4	1.7	18	2.0	400	3.0
60	1.5	1.7	19	2.2	400	3.0
60	1.4	1.6	18	2.2	400	3.0
60	1.2	1.4	16	2.2	400	3.0
50	1.1	1.3	15	1.8	400	3.0
60	1.1	1.3	14	2.0	400	3.0
60	1.1	1.3	14	2.0	400	3.0
60	1.0	1.2	13	2.0	400	3.0
60	1.0	1.2	13	2.0	400	3.0
+20	+0.4	+0.3	+2	+0.6	+400	+1.0
+40	+0.5	+0.5	+5	+0.5	+100	+1.0

Minerals

CALCIUM (MG)	PHOSPHORUS (MG)	MAGNESIUM (MG)	IRON (MG)	ZINC (MG)	IODINE (μG)
360	240	50	10	3	40
540	360	70	15	5	50
800	800	150	15	10	70
800	800	200	10	10	90
800	800	250	10	10	120
1200	1200	350	18	15	150
1200	1200	400	18	15	150
800	800	350	10	15	150
800	800	350	10	15	150
800	800	350	10	15	150
1200	1200	300	18	15	150
1200	1200	300	18	15	150
800	800	300	18	15	150
800	800	300	18	15	150
800	800	300	10	15	150
+400	+400	+150	[h]	+5	+25
+400	+400	+150	[h]	+10	+50

TABLE A–2.   MEAN HEIGHTS AND WEIGHTS AND RECOMMENDED ENERGY INTAKE[a]

Category	Age (Years)	Weight (kg)	Weight (lb)	Height (cm)	Height (in)	Energy Needs (With Range) (kcal)		(MJ)
Infants	0.0–0.5	6	13	60	24	kg × 115	(95–145)	kg × 0.48
	0.5–1.0	9	20	71	28	kg × 105	(80–135)	kg × 0.44
Children	1–3	13	29	90	35	1300	(900–1800)	5.5
	4–6	20	44	112	44	1700	(1300–2300)	7.1
	7–10	28	62	132	52	2400	(1650–3300)	10.1
Males	11–14	45	99	157	62	2700	(2000–3700)	11.3
	15–18	66	145	176	69	2800	(2100–3900)	11.8
	19–22	70	154	177	70	2900	(2500–3300)	12.2
	23–50	70	154	178	70	2700	(2300–3100)	11.3
	51–75	70	154	178	70	2400	(2000–2800)	10.1
	76+	70	154	178	70	2050	(1650–2450)	8.6
Females	11–14	46	101	157	62	2200	(1500–3000)	9.2
	15–18	55	120	163	64	2100	(1200–3000)	8.8
	19–22	55	120	163	64	2100	(1700–2500)	8.8
	23–50	55	120	163	64	2000	(1600–2400)	8.4
	51–75	55	120	163	64	1800	(1400–2200)	7.6
	76+	55	120	163	64	1600	(1200–2000)	6.7
Pregnancy						+300		
Lactation						+500		

[a]The data in this table have been assembled from the observed median heights and weights of children, together with desirable weights for adults for the mean heights of men (70 in) and women (64 in) between the ages of 18 and 34 years as surveyed in the U.S. population (HEW/NCHS data).

The energy allowances for the young adults are for men and women doing light work. The allowances for the two older age groups represent mean energy needs over these age spans, allowing for a 2 per cent decrease in basal (resting) metabolic rate per decade and a reduction in activity of 200 kcal/day for men and women between 51 and 75 years, 500 kcal for men over 75 years, and 400 kcal for women over 75 years. The customary range of daily energy output is shown in parentheses for adults and is based on a variation in energy needs of ±400 kcal at any one age, emphasizing the wide range of energy intakes appropriate for any group of people.

Energy allowances for children through age 18 are based on median energy intakes of children of these ages followed in longitudinal growth studies. The values in parentheses are 10th and 90th percentiles of energy intake, to indicate the range of energy consumption among children of these ages.

(From Recommended Daily Allowances, 9th Rev. Ed. National Academy of Sciences, Washington, DC, 1980.)

TABLE A–3. EXAMPLES OF DAILY ENERGY EXPENDITURES OF MATURE WOMEN AND MEN IN LIGHT OCCUPATIONS

Activity Category[a]	Time (hr)	Man, 70 kg		Woman, 58 kg	
		Rate (kcal/min)	Total [kcal (kj)]	Rate (kcal/min)	Total [kcal (kj)]
Sleeping, reclining	8	1.0–1.2	540(2270)	0.9–1.1	440(1850)
Very light	12	up to 2.5	1300(5460)	up to 2.0	900(3780)
Seated and standing activities, painting trades, auto and truck driving, laboratory work, typing, playing musical instruments, sewing, ironing					
Light	3	2.5–4.9	600(2520)	2.0–3.9	450(1890)
Walking on level, 2.5–3 mph, tailoring, pressing, garage work, electrical trades, carpentry, restaurant trades, cannery workers, washing clothes, shopping with light load, golf, sailing, table tennis, volleyball					
Moderate	1	5.0–7.4	300(1260)	4.0–5.9	240(1010)
Walking 3.5–4 mph, plastering, weeding and hoeing, loading and stacking bales, scrubbing floors, shopping with heavy load, cycling, skiing, tennis, dancing					
Heavy	0	7.5–12.0		6.0–10.0	
Walking with load uphill, tree felling, work with pick and shovel, basketball, swimming, climbing, football					
Total	24		2740(11,500)		2030(8530)

[a]Data from Durnin and Passmore, 1967. (From Recommended Daily Allowances, 9th Rev. Ed. National Academy of Sciences, Washington, DC, 1980.)

TABLE A–4.   ESTIMATED SAFE AND ADEQUATE DAILY DIETARY INTAKES OF SELECTED VITAMINS AND MINERALS[a]

	Age (Years)	Vitamins		
		VITAMIN K (µG)	BIOTIN (µG)	PANTO-THENIC ACID (MG)
Infants	0–0.5	12	35	2
	0.5–1	10–20	50	3
Children	1–3	15–30	65	3
and	4–6	20–40	85	3–4
Adolescents	7–10	30–60	120	4–5
	11 +	50–100	100–200	4–7
Adults		70–140	100–200	4–7

	Age (Years)	Trace Elements[b]					
		COPPER (MG)	MAN-GANESE (MG)	FLUORIDE (MG)	CHROMIUM (MG)	SELENIUM (MG)	MOLYB-DENUM (MG)
Infants	0–0.5	0.5–0.7	0.5–0.7	0.1–0.5	0.01–0.04	0.01–0.04	0.03–0.06
	0.5–1	0.7–1.0	0.7–1.0	0.2–1.0	0.02–0.06	0.02–0.06	0.04–0.08
Children	1–3	1.0–1.5	1.0–1.5	0.5–1.5	0.02–0.08	0.02–0.08	0.05–0.1
and	4–6	1.5–2.0	1.5–2.0	1.0–2.5	0.03–0.12	0.03–0.12	0.06–0.15
Adolescents	7–10	2.0–2.5	2.0–3.0	1.5–2.5	0.05–0.2	0.05–0.2	0.10–0.3
	11 +	2.0–3.0	2.5–5.0	1.5–2.5	0.05–0.2	0.05–0.2	0.15–0.5
Adults		2.0–3.0	2.5–5.0	1.5–4.0	0.05–0.2	0.05–0.2	0.15–0.5

	Age (Years)	Electrolytes		
		SODIUM (MG)	POTASSIUM (MG)	CHLORIDE (MG)
Infants	0–0.5	115–350	350–925	275–700
	0.5–1	250–750	425–1275	400–1200
Children	1–3	325–975	550–1650	500–1500
and	4–6	450–1350	775–2325	700–2100
Adolescents	7–10	600–1800	1000–3000	925–2775
	11 +	900–2700	1525–4575	1400–4200
Adults		1100–3300	1875–5625	1700–5100

[a] Because there is less information on which to base allowances, these figures are not given in the main table of RDA and are provided here in the form of ranges of recommended intakes.
[b] Since the toxic levels for many trace elements may be only several times usual intakes, the upper levels for the trace elements given in this table should not be habitually exceeded. (From Recommended Daily Allowances, 9th Rev. Ed., National Academy of Sciences, Washington, DC, 1980.)

TABLE A–5. ESTIMATED AMINO ACID REQUIREMENTS*

Amino Acid	Requirement/kg of Body Wt (mg/Day)			Amino Acid Pattern for High-Quality Protein (mg/g of Protein)[†]
	INFANT (4–6 MO)	CHILD (10–12 YR)	ADULT	
Histidine	33	?	?	17
Isoleucine	83	28	12	42
Leucine	135	42	16	70
Lysine	99	44	12	51
Total S-containing amino acids	49	22	10	26
Total aromatic amino acids	141	22	16	73
Threonine	68	28	8	35
Tryptophan	21	4	3	11
Valine	92	25	14	48

*From Recommended Daily Allowances, 9th Rev. Ed. National Academy of Sciences, Washington, DC, 1980.
[†]Two grams/kg of body weight/day of protein of the quality listed in column 4 would meet the amino acid needs of the infant.

TABLE A–6.   VITAMINS*

Vitamin	RDA for Healthy Adult Male (Milligrams)[†]	Dietary Sources	Major Body Functions	Deficiency	Excess
WATER-SOLUBLE					
VITAMIN B$_1$ (THIAMINE)	1.4	Pork, organ meats, whole grains, legumes	Coenzyme (thiamine pyrophosphate) in reactions involving the removal of carbon dioxide	Beriberi (peripheral nerve changes, edema, heart failure)	None reported
VITAMIN B$_2$ (RIBOFLAVIN)	1.6	Widely distributed in foods	Constituent of two flavin nucleotide coenzymes involved in energy metabolism (FAD and FMN)	Reddened lips, cracks at corner of mouth (cheilosis), lesions of eye	None reported
NIACIN	18	Liver, lean meats, grains, legumes (can be formed from tryptophan)	Constituent of two coenzymes involved in oxidation-reduction reactions (NAD and NADP)	Pellagra (skin and gastrointestinal lesions, nervous, mental disorders)	Flushing, burning, and tingling around neck, face, and hands
VITAMIN B$_6$ (PYRIDOXINE)	2.2	Meats, vegetables, whole-grain cereals	Coenzyme (pyridoxal phosphate) involved in amino acid metabolism	Irritability, convulsions, muscular twitching, dermatitis near eyes, kidney stones	None reported
PANTOTHENIC ACID	4–7	Widely distributed in foods	Constituent of coenzyme A, which plays a central role in energy metabolism	Fatigue, sleep disturbances, impaired coordination, nausea (rare in man)	None reported
FOLACIN	0.4	Legumes, green vegetables, whole-wheat products	Coenzyme (reduced form) involved in transfer of single-carbon units in nucleic acid and amino acid metabolism	Anemia, gastrointestinal disturbances, diarrhea, red tongue	None reported
VITAMIN B$_{12}$	0.003	Muscle meats, eggs, dairy products (not present in plant foods)	Coenzyme involved in transfer of single-carbon units in nucleic acid metabolism	Pernicious anemia, neurologic disorders	None reported

*VITAMINS are organic molecules needed in very small amounts in the diet of higher animals. Most of the water-soluble (B complex) vitamins act as coenzymes, or organic catalysts; the four fat-soluble vitamins (A, D, E, and K) have more diverse functions. Although low vitamin intake can result in deficiency disease, the misguided use of high-potency vitamin pills can also have undesirable effects.
[†]RDAs are adjusted to the 1980 levels.
From Scrimshaw, N.S., and Young, V.R.: The Requirements of Human Nutrition. Sci Am 235:50–64, 1976.

TABLE A–6.   VITAMINS* (Continued)

Vitamin	RDA for Healthy Adult Male (Milligrams)[†]	Dietary Sources	Major Body Functions	Deficiency	Excess
BIOTIN	0.2–0.5	Legumes, vegetables, meats	Coenzyme required for fat synthesis, amino acid metabolism, and glycogen (animal-starch) formation	Fatigue, depression, nausea, dermatitis, muscular pains	None reported
CHOLINE	Not established. Usual diet provides 500–900	All foods containing phospholipids (egg yolk, liver, grains, legumes)	Constituent of phospholipids. Precursor of putative neurotransmitter acetylcholine	Not reported in humans	None reported
VITAMIN C (ASCORBIC ACID)	60	Citrus fruits, tomatoes, green peppers, salad greens	Maintains intercellular matrix of cartilage, bone, and dentine. Important in collagen synthesis	Scurvy (degeneration of skin, teeth, blood vessels, epithelial hemorrhages)	Relatively nontoxic. Possibility of kidney stones
FAT-SOLUBLE					
VITAMIN A (RETINOL)	1 (1000 μg RE)	Provitamin A (betacarotene) widely distributed in green vegetables. Retinol present in milk, butter, cheese, fortified margarine	Constituent of rhodopsin (visual pigment). Maintenance of epithelial tissues. Role in mucopolysaccharide synthesis	Xerophthalmia (keratinization of ocular tissue), night blindness, permanent blindness	Headache, vomiting, peeling of skin, anorexia, swelling of long bones
VITAMIN D	0.01 (5 μg)	Cod-liver oil, eggs, dairy products, fortified milk, and margarine	Promotes growth and mineralization of bones. Increases absorption of calcium.	Rickets (bone deformities) in children. Osteomalacia in adults	Vomiting, diarrhea, loss of weight, kidney damage
VITAMIN E (TOCOPHEROL)	10	Seeds, green leafy vegetables, margarines, shortenings	Functions as an antioxidant to prevent cell-membrane damage	Possibly anemia	Relatively nontoxic
VITAMIN K (PHYLLOQUINONE)	0.03 0.07–0.14	Green leafy vegetables. Small amount in cereals, fruits, and meats	Important in blood clotting (involved in formation of active prothrombin)	Conditioned deficiencies associated with severe bleeding, internal hemorrhages	Relatively nontoxic. Synthetic forms at high doses may cause jaundice

TABLE A–7. ESSENTIAL MINERALS*

Mineral	Amount in Adult Body (Grams)	RDA†for Healthy Adult Male (Milligrams)	Dietary Sources	Major Body Functions	Deficiency	Excess
CALCIUM	1,500	800	Milk, cheese, dark-green vegetables, dried legumes	Bone and tooth formation Blood clotting Nerve transmission	Stunted growth Rickets, osteoporosis Convulsions	Not reported in man
PHOSPHORUS	860	800	Milk, cheese, meat, poultry, grains	Bone and tooth formation Acid-base balance	Weakness, demineralization of bone Loss of calcium	Erosion of jaw (fossy jaw)
SULFUR	300	(Provided by sulfur amino acids)	Sulfur amino acids (methionine and cystine) in dietary proteins	Constituent of active tissue compounds, cartilage, and tendon	Related to intake and deficiency of sulfur amino acids	Excess sulfur amino acid intake leads to poor growth
POTASSIUM	180	2,500 1875–5625	Meats, milk, many fruits	Acid-base balance Body water balance Nerve function	Muscular weakness Paralysis	Muscular weakness Death
CHLORINE	74	2,000 1700–5100	Common salt	Formation of gastric juice Acid-base balance	Muscle cramps Mental apathy Reduced appetite	Vomiting
SODIUM	64	2,500 1100–3300	Common salt	Acid base balance Body water balance Nerve function	Muscle cramps Mental apathy Reduced appetite	High blood pressure
MAGNESIUM	25	350	Whole grains, green leafy vegetables	Activates enzymes Involved in protein synthesis	Growth failure Behavioral disturbances Weakness, spasms	Diarrhea
IRON	4.5	10	Eggs, lean meats, legumes, whole grains, green leafy vegetables	Constituent of hemoglobin and enzymes involved in energy metabolism	Iron-deficiency anemia (weakness, reduced resistance to infection)	Siderosis Cirrhosis of liver
FLUORINE	2.6	1.5–4	Drinking water, tea, seafood	May be important in maintenance of bone structure	Higher frequency of tooth decay	Mottling of teeth Increased bone density Neurological disturbances

*ESSENTIAL MINERAL ELEMENTS are involved in the electrochemical functions of nerve and muscle, the formation of bones and teeth, the activation of enzymes, and, in the case of iron, the transport of oxygen. The trace minerals nickel, tin, vanadium, and silicon, previously considered to be health hazards, are now known to be essential for animals. Although they are so widely distributed in nature that primary dietary deficiencies are unlikely, changes in the balance among them may have important consequences for health.

(From Scrimshaw, N.S., and Young, V.R.: The Requirements of Human Nutrition. Sci Am 235:50–64, 1976.)

TABLE A–7.   ESSENTIAL MINERALS* (Continued)

Mineral	Amount in Adult Body (Grams)	RDA for Healthy Adult Male (Milligrams)	Dietary Sources	Major Body Functions	Deficiency	Excess
ZINC	2	15	Widely distributed in foods	Constituent of enzymes involved in digestion	Growth failure Small sex glands	Fever, nausea, vomiting, diarrhea
COPPER	0.1	2 2–3	Meats, drinking water	Constituent of enzymes associated with iron metabolism	Anemia, bone changes (rare in man)	Rare metabolic condition (Wilson's disease)
SILICON VANADIUM TIN NICKEL	0.024 0.018 0.017 0.010	Not established	Widely distributed in foods	Function unknown (essential for animals)	Not reported in humans	Industrial exposures: Silicon — silicosis Vanadium — lung irritation Tin — vomiting Nickel — acute pneumonitis
SELENIUM	0.013	0.05–0.2	Seafood, meat, grains	Functions in close association with vitamin E	Anemia (rare)	Gastrointestinal disorders, lung irritation
MANGANESE	0.012	2.5–5	Widely distributed in foods	Constituent of enzymes involved in fat synthesis	In animals: poor growth, disturbances of nervous system, reproductive abnormalities	Poisoning in manganese mines: generalized disease of nervous system
IODINE	0.011	0.15	Marine fish and shellfish, dairy products, many vegetables	Constituent of thyroid hormones	Goiter (enlarged thyroid)	Very high intakes depress thyroid activity
MOLYBDENUM	0.009	0.15–0.5	Legumes, cereals, organ meats	Constituent of some enzymes	Not reported in humans	Inhibition of enzymes
CHROMIUM	0.006	0.05–0.2	Fats, vegetable oils, meats	Involved in glucose and energy metabolism	Impaired ability to metabolize glucose	Occupational exposures: skin and kidney damage
COBALT	0.0015	(Required as vitamin B_{12})	Organ and muscle meats, milk	Constituent of vitamin B_{12}	Not reported in humans	Industrial exposure: dermatitis and diseases of red blood cells
WATER	40,000 (60 % of body weight)	1.5 liters per day	Solid foods, liquids, drinking water	Transport of nutrients Temperature regulation Participates in metabolic reactions	Thirst, dehydration	Headaches, nausea Edema High blood pressure

TABLE A–8.   U.S. RECOMMENDED DAILY ALLOWANCES (U.S. RDAs) FOR ESSENTIAL NUTRIENTS*

Nutrients That MUST Be Declared on the Label:[†]	Infants Birth to 12 mo (tentative)	Children Under 4 Years of Age	Adults and Children 4 or More Years of Age	Pregnant or Lactating Women
Protein (g), PER $\geq$ casein	20	45	45	45
Protein (g), PER $<$ casein	28	65	65	65
Vitamin A (IU)	1,500	2,500	5,000	8,000
Vitamin C (ascorbic acid) (mg)	35	45	60	60
Thiamine (vitamin B_1) (mg)	0.5	0.7	1.5	1.7
Riboflavin (vitamin B_2) (mg)	0.6	0.8	1.7	2.0
Niacin (mg)	8	9	20	20
Calcium (g)	0.6	0.8	1.0	1.3
Iron (mg)	15	10	18	18
Nutrients That MAY Be Declared on the Label:				
Vitamin D (IU)	400	400	400	400
Vitamin E (IU)	5	10	30	30
Vitamin B_6 (mg)	0.4	0.7	2.0	2.5
Folic acid (folacin) (mg)	0.1	0.2	0.4	0.8
Vitamin B_{12} (μg)	2	3	6	8
Phosphorus (g)	0.5	0.8	1.0	1.3
Iodine (μg)	45	70	150	150
Magnesium (mg)	70	200	400	450
Zinc (mg)	5	8	15	15
Copper (mg)	0.6	1	2	2
Biotin (mg)	0.05	0.15	0.3	0.3
Pantothenic acid (mg)	3	5	10	10

*Adapted from Food Technology 28:5, 1974.
[†]Whenever nutrition labeling is required.

TABLE A–9. PERCENTILES FOR WEIGHT AND HEIGHT OF MALES AND FEMALES, 0–18 YEARS[a]

	Males						Females					
	Weight (kg)			Height (cm)			Weight (kg)			Height (cm)		
Age	5	50	95	5	50	95	5	50	95	5	50	95
(Months)												
1	3.16	4.29	5.38	50.4	54.6	58.6	2.97	3.98	4.92	49.2	53.5	56.9
3	4.43	5.98	7.37	56.7	61.1	65.4	4.18	5.40	6.74	55.4	59.5	63.4
6	6.20	7.85	9.46	63.4	67.8	72.3	5.79	7.21	8.73	61.8	65.9	70.2
9	7.52	9.18	10.93	68.0	72.3	77.1	7.00	8.56	10.17	66.1	70.4	75.0
12	8.43	10.15	11.99	71.7	76.1	81.2	7.84	9.53	11.24	69.8	74.3	79.1
18	9.59	11.47	13.44	77.5	82.4	88.1	8.92	10.82	12.76	76.0	80.9	86.1
(Years)												
2	10.49	12.34	15.50	82.5	86.8	94.4	9.95	11.80	14.15	81.6	86.8	93.6
3	12.05	14.62	17.77	89.0	94.9	102.0	11.61	14.10	17.22	88.3	94.1	100.6
4	13.64	16.69	20.27	95.8	102.9	109.9	13.11	15.96	19.91	95.0	101.6	108.3
5	15.27	18.67	23.09	102.0	109.9	117.0	14.55	17.66	22.62	101.1	108.4	115.6
6	16.93	20.69	26.34	107.7	116.1	123.5	16.05	19.52	25.75	106.6	114.6	122.7
7	18.64	22.85	30.12	113.0	121.7	129.7	17.71	21.84	29.68	111.8	120.6	129.5
8	20.40	25.30	34.51	118.1	127.0	135.7	19.62	24.84	34.71	116.9	126.4	136.2
9	22.25	28.13	39.58	122.9	132.2	141.8	21.82	28.46	40.64	122.1	132.2	142.9
10	24.33	31.44	45.27	127.7	137.5	148.1	24.36	32.55	47.17	127.5	138.3	149.5
11	26.80	35.30	51.47	132.6	143.3	154.9	27.24	36.95	54.00	133.5	144.8	156.2
12	29.85	39.78	58.09	137.6	149.7	162.3	30.52	41.53	60.81	139.8	151.5	162.7
13	33.64	44.95	65.02	142.9	156.5	169.8	34.14	46.10	67.30	145.2	157.1	168.1
14	38.22	50.77	72.13	148.8	163.1	176.7	37.76	50.28	73.08	148.7	160.4	171.3
15	43.11	56.71	79.12	155.2	169.0	181.9	40.99	53.68	77.78	150.5	161.8	172.8
16	47.74	62.10	85.62	161.1	173.5	185.4	43.41	55.89	80.99	151.6	162.4	173.3
17	51.50	66.31	91.31	164.9	176.2	187.3	44.74	56.69	82.46	152.7	163.1	173.5
18	53.97	68.88	95.76	165.7	176.8	187.6	45.26	56.62	82.47	153.6	163.7	173.6

[a]Data in this table have been used to derive weight and height reference points in the present report: It is not intended that they necessarily be considered standards of normal growth and development. Data pertaining to infants 2–18 months of age are taken from longitudinal growth studies at Fels Research Institute. Ages are exact, and infants were measured in the recumbent position. The measurements were based on some 867 children followed longitudinally at the institute between 1929 and 1975. Data pertaining to children between 2 and 18 years of age were collected between 1962 and 1974 by the National Center for Health Statistics and involve some 20,000 individuals comprising nationally representative samples in three studies conducted between 1960 and 1974. In these studies, children were measured in the standing position with no upward pressure exerted on the mastoid processes. In the previous edition of this report, data for children up to six years of age were taken from longitudinal growth studies in Iowa and Boston, where children were measured in the recumbent position. This explains the systematically smaller heights for 2–5-year-old children in this current table compared with those represented in previous editions. In this table, actual age is represented. (From Recommended Daily Allowances, 9th Rev. Ed., National Academy of Sciences, Washington, DC, 1980.)

TABLE A–10.   MEN'S AND WOMEN'S WEIGHTS ACCORDING TO FRAME SIZE

Height Ft	In	Small Frame	Medium Frame	Large Frame
Men				
5	2	128–134	131–141	138–150
5	3	130–136	133–143	140–153
5	4	132–138	135–145	142–156
5	5	134–140	137–148	144–160
5	6	136–142	139–151	146–164
5	7	138–145	142–154	149–168
5	8	140–148	145–157	152–172
5	9	142–151	148–160	155–176
5	10	144–154	151–163	158–180
5	11	146–157	154–166	161–184
6	0	149–160	157–170	164–188
6	1	152–164	160–174	168–192
6	2	155–168	164–178	172–197
6	3	158–172	167–182	176–202
6	4	162–176	171–187	181–207
Women				
4	10	102–111	109–121	118–131
4	11	103–113	111–123	120–134
5	0	104–115	113–126	122–137
5	1	106–118	115–129	125–140
5	2	108–121	118–132	128–143
5	3	111–124	121–135	131–147
5	4	114–127	124–138	134–151
5	5	117–130	127–141	137–155
5	6	120–133	130–144	140–158
5	7	123–136	133–147	143–163
5	8	126–139	138–150	146–167
5	9	129–142	139–153	149–170
5	10	132–145	142–156	152–173
5	11	135–148	145–159	156–176
6	0	138–151	148–162	158–179

Note: Weights at ages 25–59 based on lowest mortality. Weight in pounds according to frame (in indoor clothing weighing 5 lb for men and 3 lb for women; shoes with 1" heels).

Note also that these weight tables record systematically heavier weights than the 1959 tables. There is controversy as to whether these new desirable weights are too high. (Garrison, R.J., Feinleib, M., Castelli, W.P., and McNamara, P.: Cigarette smoking as a confounder of the relationship between relative weight and long-term mortality. JAMA 249:2199–2203, 1983.)

Source of basic data: 1979 Build Study, Society of Actuaries and Association of Life Insurance Medical Directors of America, 1980. From Metropolitan Life Insurance Co., 1983.

TABLE A–10A. BODY FRAME TYPE $\dfrac{\text{Height (cm)}}{\text{Wrist (cm)}}$

Frame	Male	Female
Small	10.4	11.1
Medium	9.6–10.4	10.1–11.0
Large	9.6	10.1

Note: Wrist measurement should be taken on the right wrist. Use body frame size in conjunction with 1983 Metropolitan Height Weight Tables to determine desirable weight range. (From Grant, J.P.: Handbook of Total Parenteral Nutrition. Philadelphia, W.B. Saunders Co., 1980, p. 15.)

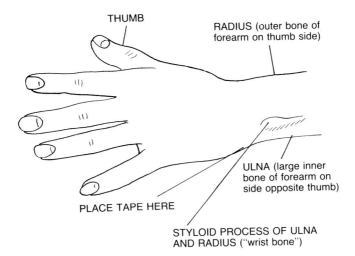

FIGURE A–1. To measure wrist circumference, place soft measuring tape around smallest part of wrist distal (toward the fingers) to styloid process of radius and ulna ("wrist bone"). Convert to centimeters if necessary. (From Anne Grant, MS., R.D.: Nutritional Assessment Guidelines. Berkeley, CA, Cutter Laboratories, Inc. Diagram from Lindner, P., and Lindner, D.: How to Assess Degrees of Fatness. Cambridge Scientific Industries, 101 Virginia Avenue, Cambridge, MD 21613.)

TABLE A–11. CALORIC REQUIREMENTS IN CHILDREN AND ADOLESCENTS*

Age	Range of Energy Needs (kcal)	
1–3 yr	900–1800	
4–6 yr	1300–2300	
7–10 yr	1650–3300	
	Male	Female
11–14 yr	2000–3700	1500–3000
15–18 yr	2100–3900	1600–3000
19–22 yr	2500–3300	1700–2500

Protein: 15–20% of total calories
Fat: 30–35% of total calories

*From Recommended Daily Allowances, 9th Rev. Ed., National Academy of Sciences, Washington, DC, 1980.

TABLE A–12. GUIDE FOR ADJUSTING CALORIC REQUIREMENTS IN ADULTS ACCORDING TO ACTIVITY (KCAL/KG/DAY, BASED ON IDEAL WEIGHT)

	Sedentary*	Moderate Activity	Strenuous Activity
Overweight	20	25	30
Normal weight	25	30	35
Underweight	30	35	40

*The value ordinarily used for an elderly sedentary patient is 15 kcal/kg.

TABLE A–13.   EXCHANGE LISTS FOR MEAL PLANNING

The use of "exchanges" in planning meals allows for variety in the diet and enables the user to follow the guidelines of the prescribed diet under varying circumstances. An exchange has four essential characteristics: it allows choice, it specifies portion size, and it is both a caloric trade-off and a nutritional equivalent.

Procedure for Using Exchange Lists

1. Each item on an exchange list is interchangeable with any other item in the amount specified, *i.e.*, under "bread exchanges" 1 slice of white bread is an exchange for ½ cup cooked cereal.

2. Foods on different lists or from different groups are not interchangeable, *i.e.*, 1 slice of bread is not an exchange for 1 oz of meat.

3. If 1 exchange on a food list or group is allowed on the meal plan, it means that any item on that list or in that group may be used in the amount specified. If 2 exchanges are allowed it means that a double portion of any food may be used or 2 different items in the amount specified, *i.e.*, 2 slices of bread, or 1 slice of bread and ½ cup cooked cereal.

4. Sample Menu: 2 Meat Exchanges   2 oz roast beef
           1 Vegetable Exchange   ½ cup carrot sticks
           2 Fat Exchanges   2 tsp mayonnaise
           2 Bread Exchanges   1 small corn on cob + 1 slice bread

5. Special instructions for the individual exchange lists are given with the appropriate list.

List 1: Milk Exchanges (Includes Nonfat, Low-Fat, and Whole Milk)

One exchange of nonfat milk contains 12 g of carbohydrate, 8 g of protein, a trace of fat, and 80 calories.

This list shows the kinds and amounts of milk or milk products to use for 1 milk exchange. Low-fat and whole milk contain saturated fat.

NONFAT FORTIFIED MILK

Skim or Nonfat Milk	**1 cup**
Powdered (Nonfat Dry, Before Adding Liquid)	⅓ cup
Canned, Evaporated—Skim Milk	½ cup
Buttermilk Made from Skim Milk	**1 cup**
Yogurt Made from Skim Milk (Plain, Unflavored)	**1 cup**

LOW-FAT FORTIFIED MILK

1% fat fortified milk (omit ½ fat exchange)	1 cup
2% fat fortified milk (omit 1 fat exchange)	1 cup
Yogurt made from 2% fortified milk (plain, unflavored) (omit 1 fat exchange)	1 cup

WHOLE MILK (OMIT 2 FAT EXCHANGES)

Whole milk	1 cup
Canned, evaporated whole milk	½ cup
Buttermilk made from whole milk	1 cup
Yogurt made from whole milk (plain, unflavored)	1 cup

Table continues on following page

TABLE A–13. EXCHANGE LISTS FOR MEAL PLANNING (Continued)

List 2: Vegetable Exchanges

One exchange of vegetables contains about 5 g of carbohydrate, 2 g of protein, and 25 calories. This list shows the kinds of vegetables to use for 1 vegetable exchange. One exchange is ½ cup.

Asparagus	Mustard
Bean sprouts	Spinach
Beets	Turnip
Broccoli	Mushrooms
Brussels sprouts	Okra
Cabbage	Onions
Carrots	Rhubarb
Cauliflower	Rutabaga
Celery	Sauerkraut
Eggplant	String beans, green or yellow
Green pepper	Summer squash
Greens:	Tomatoes
Beet	Tomato juice
Chards	Turnips
Collards	Vegetable juice cocktail
Dandelion	Zucchini
Kale	

The following raw vegetables may be used as desired:

Chicory	Lettuce
Chinese cabbage	Parsley
Cucumbers	Pickles, dill
Endive	Radishes
Escarole	Watercress

Starchy vegetables are found in the Bread Exchange List.

List 3: Fruit Exchanges

One exchange of fruit contains 10 g of carbohydrate and 40 calories.
This list shows the kind and amounts of fruits to use for 1 fruit exchange:

Apple	1 small	Grapes	12
Apple juice	⅓ cup	Grape juice	¼ cup
Applesauce	½ cup	Mango	½ small
(unsweetened)		Melon	¼ small
Apricots, fresh	2 medium	Cantaloupe	¼ small
Apricots, dried	4 halves	Honeydew	⅛ medium
Banana	½ small	Watermelon	1 cup
Berries		Nectarine	1 small
Blackberries	½ cup	Orange	1 small
Blueberries	½ cup	Orange juice	½ cup
Raspberries	½ cup	Papaya	¾ cup
Strawberries	¾ cup	Peach	1 medium
Cherries	10 large	Pear	1 small
Cider	⅓ cup	Persimmon, native	1 medium
Cranberries (as desired		Pineapple	½ cup
if no sugar is added)		Pineapple juice	⅓ cup
Dates	2	Plums	2 medium
Figs, fresh	1	Prunes	2 medium
Figs, dried	1	Prune juice	¼ cup
Grapefruit	½	Raisins	2 tbs
Grapefruit juice	½ cup	Tangerine	1 medium

Table continues on following page

List 4: Bread Exchanges (Includes Bread, Cereal, and Starchy Vegetables)

One exchange of bread contains 15 g of carbohydrate, 2 g of protein, and 70 calories.

This list shows the kinds and amounts of bread, cereals, starchy vegetables, and prepared foods to use for 1 bread exchange.

BREAD

White (including French and Italian)	1 slice
Whole wheat	1 slice
Rye or pumpernickel	1 slice
Raisin	1 slice
Bagel, small	$\frac{1}{2}$
English muffin, small	$\frac{1}{2}$
Plain roll, bread	1
Frankfurter roll	$\frac{1}{2}$
Hamburger roll	$\frac{1}{2}$
Dried bread crumbs	3 tbs
Tortilla, 6"	1

CEREAL

Bran flakes	$\frac{1}{2}$ cup
Other ready-to-eat unsweetened cereal	$\frac{3}{4}$ cup
Puffed cereal (unfrosted)	1 cup
Cereal (cooked)	$\frac{1}{2}$ cup
Grits (cooked)	$\frac{1}{2}$ cup
Rice or barley (cooked)	$\frac{1}{2}$ cup
Pasta (cooked), spaghetti, noodles, macaroni	$\frac{1}{2}$ cup
Popcorn (popped, no fat added, large kernel)	3 cups
Cornmeal (dry)	2 tbs
Flour	$2\frac{1}{2}$ tbs
Wheat germ	$\frac{1}{4}$ cup

CRACKERS

Arrowroot	3
Graham, $2\frac{1}{2}$" sq	2
Matzoh, 4" × 6"	$\frac{1}{2}$
Oyster	20
Pretzels, $3\frac{1}{8}$" long × $\frac{1}{8}$" diameter	25
Rye wafers, 2" × $3\frac{1}{2}$"	3
Saltines	6
Soda, $2\frac{1}{2}$" sq	4

DRIED BEANS, PEAS, AND LENTILS

Beans, peas, lentils (dried and cooked)	$\frac{1}{2}$ cup
Baked beans, no pork (canned)	$\frac{1}{4}$ cup

STARCHY VEGETABLES

Corn	$\frac{1}{3}$ cup
Corn on cob	1 small
Lima beans	$\frac{1}{2}$ cup
Parsnips	$\frac{2}{3}$ cup
Peas, green (canned or frozen)	$\frac{1}{2}$ cup
Potato, white	1 small
Potato (mashed)	$\frac{1}{2}$ cup
Pumpkin	$\frac{3}{4}$ cup
Winter squash, acorn, or butternut	$\frac{1}{2}$ cup
Yam or sweet potato	$\frac{1}{4}$ cup

PREPARED FOODS

Biscuit, 2" diameter (omit 1 fat exchange)	1
Corn Bread, 2" × 2" × 1" (omit 1 fat exchange)	1

Table continues on following page

TABLE A–13. EXCHANGE LISTS FOR MEAL PLANNING (Continued)

PREPARED FOODS (CONTINUED)

Corn muffin, 2″ diameter (omit 1 fat exchange)	1
Crackers, round butter type (omit 1 fat exchange)	5
Muffin, plain small (omit 1 fat exchange)	1
Potatoes, French-fried, length 2″ to 3½″ (omit 1 fat exchange)	8
Potato or corn chips (omit 2 fat exchanges)	15
Pancake, 5″ × ½″ (omit 1 fat exchange)	1
Waffle, 5″ × ½″ (omit 1 fat exchange)	1

List 5: Meat Exchanges, Lean Meat

One exchange of lean meat (1 oz) contains 7 g of protein, 3 g of fat, and 55 calories.
This list shows the kinds and amounts of lean meat and other protein-rich foods to use for 1 low-fat meat exchange. *Trim off all visible fat.*

BEEF	Baby beef (very lean), chipped beef, chuck, flank steak, tenderloin, plate skirt steak, round (bottom, top), all cuts rump, spare ribs, tripe.	1 oz
LAMB	Leg, rib, sirloin, loin (roast and chops), shank, shoulder.	1 oz
PORK	Leg (whole rump, center shank), ham, smoked (center slices).	1 oz
VEAL	Leg, loin, rib, shank, shoulder, cutlets.	1 oz
POULTRY	Meat *without skin* of chicken, turkey, Cornish hen, guinea hen, pheasant.	1 oz
FISH	Any fresh or frozen.	1 oz
	Canned salmon, tuna, mackerel, crab, and lobster.	¼ cup
	Clams, oysters, scallops, shrimp.	5 or 1 oz
	Sardines, drained.	3
CHEESES (containing less than 5% butterfat)		1 oz
COTTAGE CHEESE (dry and 2% butterfat)		¼ cup
DRIED BEANS AND PEAS (omit 1 bread exchange)		½ cup

Meat Exchanges, Medium-Fat Meat

One exchange of medium-fat meat (1 oz) contains 7 g of protein, 5 g of fat, and 75 calories.
This list shows the kinds and amounts of medium-fat meat and other protein-rich foods to use for 1 medium-fat meat exchange. *Trim off all visible fat.*

BEEF	Ground (15% fat), corned beef (canned), rib eye, round (ground commercial)	1 oz
PORK	Loin (all cuts tenderloin), shoulder arm (picnic), shoulder blade, Boston butt, Canadian bacon, boiled ham	1 oz
LIVER, HEART, KIDNEY, AND SWEETBREADS (these are high in cholesterol)		1 oz
COTTAGE CHEESE, creamed		¼ cup
CHEESE	Mozzarella, ricotta, farmer's cheese, Neuchâtel	1 oz
	Parmesan	3 tbs
EGG	High in cholesterol	1
Peanut butter (omit 2 additional fat exchanges)		2 tbs

TABLE A–13.   EXCHANGE LISTS FOR MEAL PLANNING (Concluded)

Meat Exchanges, High-Fat Meat

One exchange of high-fat meat (1 oz) contains 7 g of protein, 8 g of fat, and 100 calories.

This list shows the kinds and amounts of high-fat meat and other protein-rich food to use for 1 high-fat meat exchange. *Trim off all visible fat.*

BEEF	Brisket, corned beef (brisket), ground beef (more than 20% fat), hamburger (commercial), chuck (ground commercial), roasts (rib), steaks (club and rib)	1 oz
LAMB	Breast	1 oz
PORK	Spare ribs, loin (back ribs), pork (ground), country-style ham, deviled ham	1 oz
VEAL	Breast	1 oz
POULTRY	Capon, duck (domestic), goose	1 oz
CHEESE	Cheddar types	1 oz
COLD CUTS		$4\frac{1}{2}'' \times \frac{1}{8}''$ slice
FRANKFURTER		1 small

List 6: Fat Exchanges

Contains 5 g fat, 45 calories. One fat exchange is the amount listed.

POLYUNSATURATED FATS (PREDOMINATE)

*Margarine	1 tsp	‡Italian dressing	1 tbs
‡Mayonnaise	1 tsp	Oil (safflower, sunflower, corn, cottonseed, soy)	1 tsp
‡Salad dressing, mayonnaise type	2 tsp		
‡French dressing	1 tbs	Walnuts	6 small

MONOUNSATURATED FATS (PREDOMINATE)

†Avocado (4″ diam)	$\frac{1}{8}$	†Pecans	2 lge whole
†Oil, olive	1 tsp	†Peanuts:	
†Oil, peanut	1 tsp	Spanish	20 whole
†Olives	5 small	Virginia	10 whole
†Almonds	10 whole	†Nuts, other	6 small

SATURATED FATS

Margarine, regular stick	1 tsp	Cream, light	2 tbs
Butter	1 tsp	Cream, sour	2 tbs
Bacon fat	1 tsp	Cream, heavy	1 tbs
Bacon, crisp	1 strip	Cream cheese	1 tbs
Lard	1 tsp	Salt pork	$\frac{3}{4}''$ cube

*Made with corn, cottonseed, safflower, soy, or sunflower oil only.

†Fat content is primarily monounsaturated.

‡If made with corn, cottonseed, safflower, soy, or sunflower oil, can be used on fat-modified diet.

Adapted from Exchange Lists for Meal Planning. American Diabetes Association, Inc., and The American Dietetic Association, 1976.)

INDEX

Page numbers in *italics* indicate illustrations. Page
numbers followed by (t) indicate tables.

Body frame type, according to wrist
    circumference, 385t
Bolus feeding, for enteral alimentation, 82
Branched-chain ketoacidemia, 321–331, *322,*
    324t–331t. See also *Maple syrup urine
    disease.*
Breads, sodium content of, 217t–218t
Breast, cancer of, fat intake and, 3
Breast feeding, 38–39, 40t–41t, 42
    initiation of, 39, 42
    on demand, 42
    phenylalanine-restricted diet and, 313
Burns, parenteral nutrition in, 87

Calcific nephrolithiasis, calcium restriction for,
    225, 226t
Calcium, in vegan diet, 33
    restriction of, 225–226, 226t
Calcium carbonate, in chronic renal failure, 182
Calcium requirement, during pregnancy, 52
Calcium salts, in chronic renal failure, 182
Calcium supplementation, and prevention of
    osteoporosis, 5
    for chronic renal failure, 181
Caloric distribution, in insulin-dependent
    diabetes, 136
    in non-insulin-dependent diabetes, 135
Caloric intake, for weight loss in obesity, 125,
    129
Caloric requirements, for children and
    adolescents, 386t
    in adults, 386t
Calories, in ketogenic diet, 277
Cancer, alcohol and, 368
    diet and, 3
    of breast, fat intake and, 3
Candy, sodium content of, 221t
Carbamoyl phosphate synthetase deficiency,
    332, 334
    diagnosis of, 337–338
    results of dietary therapy for, 336
Carbohydrate(s), amount of, in ketogenic diet,
    277–278
    in normal diet, 2
Carbohydrate disorders, 133–146, 137–143t
Carbohydrate intake, in diabetes mellitus, 135–
    138, 137t
Casec, for dietary supplementation, 118t
Catheter sepsis, during total parenteral
    nutrition, 102
Celiac disease, fat restriction for, 148
    gluten-free diet for, 251–254, 252t–255t
    milk restriction for, 248
Central venous catheters, technical
    complications of, 100–101
Central venous thrombosis, during total
    parenteral nutrition, 101
Cereals, sodium content of, 217t–218t
Cheeses, sodium content of, 215t

Children, caloric requirements for, 386t
    on vegetarian diet, 34
Cholecystitis, fat-restricted diet for, 147–148
Cholelithiasis, fat-restricted diet for, 147–148
Cholesterol, content of, in foods, 161t–168t
    dietary measures for reduction of, 159–160,
        160–161, 162t–170t, 171–173, 172t–173t
    dietary modification of levels of, 153–176,
        153t–174t
    HDL, determination of level of, 159
    high-fiber intake and, 160
    LDL, determination of level of, 159
    reduction of, 158–161, 161t–170t, 171–173, 172t–
        173t
Chromium, in diet, 105
    trivalent, in total parenteral nutrition, 105
Cigarette smoking, during pregnancy, 54
Cimetidine, for gastroesophageal reflux, 257
    for peptic ulcer disease, 261
Cirrhosis, ascites, incidence of, *366*
    of liver, alcohol and, 365–367, *365–366*
Citrulline, for hyperammonemia, 340t
Citrullinemia, *333,* 334
Clear liquid diet, 62, 63t, 65
Colon, cancer of, fat intake and, 3
    diverticular disease of, high-fiber diet and,
        238
Colonic obstruction, dietary management of,
    260
Congenital hyperammonemia, and related
    disorders, 331–342, *332–337,* 340t–342t
Congestive heart failure, sodium restriction for,
    212–213
Constant infusion, for enteral feedings, 82
Constipation, high-fiber diet for, 238
Controlyte, for dietary supplementation, 118t
Copper, in vegan diet, 33
Copper deficiency, resulting from total
    parenteral nutrition, 105
Coronary artery disease, high-fat diet and, 2
    hypercholesterolemia and, 156
Cotazem, for pancreatic enzyme
    supplementation, 266
Cotazym S, for pancreatic enzyme
    supplementation, 266
Cow's milk, composition of, 326t
CPS deficiency. See *Carbamoyl phosphate
    synthetase deficiency.*
Creatinine excretion, and lean body mass, 21–23
    expected, in men of ideal weight, 24t
        in women of ideal weight, 24t
    linear regression of, according to various
        authors, 22t
    24-hour, of normal children, in relation to
        height, 23t
Creatinine-height index, in nutritional
    assessment, 21–23, 22t–24t, 25
    vs. nitrogen retention, 25
Cyproheptadine, to increase appetite, 117
Cystathionine-β-synthase deficiency, and
    homocystinuria, 342–352, *343,* 346t–353t